Practical Cardio-Oncology

T0298537

Edited by

Susan F. Dent, MD, FRCPC
Duke Cancer Institute
Durham, North Carolina, USA

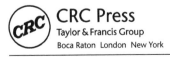

CRC Press
Taylor & Francis Group
Boca Raton London New York

CRC Press is an imprint of the
Taylor & Francis Group, an **informa** business

CRC Press
Taylor & Francis Group
6000 Broken Sound Parkway NW, Suite 300
Boca Raton, FL 33487-2742

First issued in paperback 2021

ISBN 13: 978-1-03-208931-7 (pbk)
ISBN 13: 978-1-138-29696-1 (hbk)

This book contains information obtained from authentic and highly regarded sources. While all reasonable efforts have been made to publish reliable data and information, neither the author[s] nor the publisher can accept any legal responsibility or liability for any errors or omissions that may be made. The publishers wish to make clear that any views or opinions expressed in this book by individual editors, authors or contributors are personal to them and do not necessarily reflect the views/opinions of the publishers. The information or guidance contained in this book is intended for use by medical, scientific or health-care professionals and is provided strictly as a supplement to the medical or other professional's own judgement, their knowledge of the patient's medical history, relevant manufacturer's instructions and the appropriate best practice guidelines. Because of the rapid advances in medical science, any information or advice on dosages, procedures or diagnoses should be independently verified. The reader is strongly urged to consult the relevant national drug formulary and the drug companies' and device or material manufacturers' printed instructions, and their websites, before administering or utilizing any of the drugs, devices or materials mentioned in this book. This book does not indicate whether a particular treatment is appropriate or suitable for a particular individual. Ultimately it is the sole responsibility of the medical professional to make his or her own professional judgements, so as to advise and treat patients appropriately. The authors and publishers have also attempted to trace the copyright holders of all material reproduced in this publication and apologize to copyright holders if permission to publish in this form has not been obtained. If any copyright material has not been acknowledged please write and let us know so we may rectify in any future reprint.

Library of Congress Cataloging-in-Publication Data

Names: Dent, Susan (Susan Faye), editor.
Title: Practical cardio-oncology / [edited by] Susan Dent.
Description: Boca Raton : Taylor & Francis, 2020. | Includes bibliographical references and index.
Identifiers: LCCN 2019017173| ISBN 9781138296961 (hardback : alk. paper) | ISBN 9781315099590 (ebook)
Subjects: | MESH: Cardiovascular Diseases--prevention & control | Antineoplastic Agents--adverse effects | Neoplasms--complications | Medical Oncology
Classification: LCC RC280.H45 | NLM WG 120 | DDC 616.99/412--dc23
LC record available at https://lccn.loc.gov/2019017173

Visit the Taylor & Francis Web site at
http://www.taylorandfrancis.com

and the CRC Press Web site at
http://www.crcpress.com

Publisher's Note
The publisher has gone to great lengths to ensure the quality of this reprint but points out that some imperfections in the original copies may be apparent.

Contents

Contributors

Michael Jacob Adams MD MPH FACPM
Department of Public Health Practice
University of Rochester
Rochester, New York

Shahnawaz Amdani MD FACC
Department of Pediatric Cardiology
Cleveland Clinic Children's Hospital
Cleveland, Ohio

Shetal Amin MD
Department of Cardiology
University of South Florida
Tampa, Florida

Neha Bansal MD
Division of Pediatric Cardiology
Children's Hospital at Montefiore
Bronx, New York

Cristina Salvadori Bittar MD
Cardio-Oncology Department
University of São Paulo
São Paulo, Brazil

Joyce Botros BSc MB BCh BAO
Ottawa Hospital Research Institute
Department of Medicine
Ottawa, Canada

Christine Brezden-Masley MD PhD FRCPC
Division of Hematology/Oncology
University of Toronto
Toronto, Canada

Kristina Cahill PA
Division of Cardiology
Department of Medicine
University of South Florida/Memorial
    Hospital of Tampa
and
Morsani School of Medicine
Tampa, Florida

Joe Carver MD
Abramson Cancer Center
University of Pennsylvania
Philadelphia, Pennsylvania

Michael Chetrit MD
Division of Cardiology
McGill University Health Center
Montreal, Canada

Carlo Cipolla MD
Cardiology Division
European Institute of Oncology
Milan, Italy

Palmer H. Cole MD
Division of Cardiology
Department of Medicine
University of South Florida/Memorial
    Hospital of Tampa
and
Morsani School of Medicine
Tampa, Florida

Patrick Collier MD PhD FASE FESC
Cleveland Clinic Lerner College of Medicine of
    Case Western Reserve University
Cardio-Oncology Center
Department of Cardiovascular Imaging
Robert and Suzanne Tomsich Department of
    Cardiovascular Medicine
Sydell and Arnold Miller Family Heart and
    Vascular Institute
The Cleveland Clinic Foundation
Cleveland, Ohio

Susan F. Dent MD FRCPC
Duke Cancer Institute
and
Department of Medicine
Duke University
Durham, North Carolina

Girish Dwivedi MD PhD FASE FESC FRACP
Department of Advanced Clinical and
    Translational Cardiovascular Imaging
Harry Perkins Institute of Medical
    Research
and
Fiona Stanley Hospital
The University of Western Australia
Perth, Australia

Anecita Fadol PhD FNP-BC FAANP
Department of Nursing
University of Texas
Houston, Texas

Sabin Filimon MD
Department of Medicine
McGill University Health Center
Montreal, Canada

Christopher Fleming MD
Department of Hematology and Medical
    Oncology
Taussig Cancer Center
Cleveland, Ohio

Michael G. Fradley MD
Division of Cardiovascular Medicine
University of South Florida
Morsani College of Medicine
and
H. Lee Moffitt Cancer Center and
    Research Institute
Tampa, Florida

Nestor Gahungu MD MBBS FRACP
Department of Cardiology
Royal Perth Hospital
Perth, Australia

Sarju Ganatra MD
Division of Cardiovascular Medicine
Lahey Hospital and Medical Center
Burlington, Massachusetts

and

Dana-Farber Cancer Institute
Boston, Massachusetts

Habibat Garuba MD FRCPC
Department of Medicine
University of Ottawa
Ottawa, Canada

Nina Ghosh MD FRCPC
Department of Medicine
University of Ottawa
Heart Institute
and
Merivale Cardiovascular Consultants
Queensway Carleton Hospital
Ottawa, Canada

Melkon Hacobian MD
Department of Medicine
University of California Los Angeles
Los Angeles, California

Ludhmila Abrahão Hajjar MD
Department of Cardio-Oncology
Instituto do Cancer
University of São Paulo
São Paulo, Brazil

Gregory R. Hartlage MD
Department of Cardiology
University of South Florida
Tampa, Florida

Joerg Herrmann MD
Department of Cardiovascular Diseases
and
Cardio-Oncology Clinic
Mayo Clinic College of Medicine and Science
Rochester, Minnesota

Josee Ivars BSc MSc
Faculty of Health Sciences
McMaster University
Hamilton, Canada

Christopher B. Johnson MD FRCPC
Department of Medicine
The Ottawa Hospital General Campus
and
University of Ottawa
Ottawa, Canada

Gretchen Kimmick MD MS
Duke Cancer Institute
Department of Medicine
Duke University
Durham, North Carolina

Girish Kunapareddy MD
Department of Hematology and Medical
    Oncology
Taussig Cancer Center
Cleveland Clinic
Cleveland, Ohio

Angeline Law MD FRCPC
Department of Medicine
University of Ottawa
Ottawa, Canada

Felicity Lee MBBS FRACP
Department of Advanced Clinical and
    Translational Cardiovascular Imaging
Harry Perkins Institute of Medical Research
and
Fiona Stanley Hospital
The University of Western Australia
Perth, Australia

Daniel J. Lenihan MD FACC
Cardiovascular Division
Washington University in St. Louis
St. Louis, Missouri

Emma Rachel Lipshultz BA
University of Miami Miller School
    of Medicine
Miami, Florida

and

Department of Pediatric Oncology
Dana-Farber Cancer Institute
Boston, Massachusetts

Steven E. Lipshultz MD FAAP FAHA
University at Buffalo Jacobs School of
    Medicine and Biomedical Sciences
Pediatric Chief-of-Service
Kaleida Health
and
Medical Director of Pediatric Services Business
    Development
John R. Oishei Children's Hospital
and
University of Buffalo Medical Director of
    Pediatrics
Buffalo, New York

Heather Lounder BSc candidate (class 2021)
Biology Department
Queen's University
Kingston, Canada

Alexander R. Lyon MD
Department of Cardiology
Royal Brompton Hospital
and
National Heart and Lung Institute
Imperial College
London, United Kingdom

Cesar Alberto Morales-Pabon MD
Department of Cardiology
University of South Florida
Tampa, Florida

Negar Mousavi MD
Division of Cardiology
McGill University Health Center
Montreal, Canada

Aarti A. Patel MD
Department of Cardiology
University of South Florida
Tampa, Florida

Marilia Harumi Higuchi dos Santos Rehder MD PhD
Cardio-Oncology Department
University of São Paulo
São Paulo, Brazil

Moira Rushton-Marovac MD FRCPC
Department of Medicine
University of Ottawa
Ottawa, Canada

Chirag Shah MD
Department of Radiation Oncology
Taussig Cancer Center
Cleveland Clinic
Cleveland, Ohio

Adarsh Sidda MD
Department of Internal Medicine
Summa Health
Akron, Ohio

**Carolina Maria Pinto Domingues Carvalho
Silva** MD PhD
Cardio-Oncology Department
University of São Paulo
São Paulo, Brazil

Millee Singh MD
Department of Cardiology
University of South Florida
Tampa, Florida

Gary Small MB PhD MRCP
Department of Medicine
University of Ottawa
Ottawa, Canada

Sebastian Szmit MD
Department of Pulmonary Circulation
Thromboembolic Diseases and Cardiology
Centre of Postgraduate Medical Education
European Health Centre
Otwock, Poland

Li-Ling Tan MD
Department of Cardiology
Royal Brompton Hospital
London, United Kingdom

and

Department of Cardiology
National University Heart Centre Singapore
Singapore

Grace Tang MSc
Division of Hematology/Oncology
St. Michael's Hospital
Toronto, Canada

Hassan Tariq MD
Department of Cardiology
University of South Florida
Tampa, Florida

Mirela Tuzovic MD
Department of Medicine
University of California Los Angeles
Los Angeles, California

Eric H. Yang MD
Department of Medicine
University of California Los Angeles
Los Angeles, California

Sean Zheng MD
Department of Cardiology
Royal Brompton Hospital
London, United Kingdom

PART I

Introduction

Cardio-oncology: How a new discipline arrived

SUSAN F. DENT, NESTOR GAHUNGU, MOIRA RUSHTON-MAROVAC, JOSEE IVARS, CARLO CIPOLLA, AND DANIEL J. LENIHAN

INTRODUCTION

Mortality rates due to cancer have decreased over the last 30 years owing to improvements in early detection strategies, improved surgical approaches, and advances in cancer treatments (1–3). By 2026, it is expected there will be over 20 million cancer survivors in the USA alone (1). Cancer survivors are at risk, not only of cancer recurrence, but of the long-term consequences of their treatment, including cardiotoxicity. Cardiovascular disease is now the second leading cause of morbidity and mortality in cancer survivors (2). Conventional chemotherapy and targeted therapies are associated with cardiac damage, including left ventricular (LV) dysfunction and heart failure, treatment-induced hypertension, thromboembolic events, coronary vasospasm, and arrhythmias. Early and late effects of radiation therapy can lead to coronary artery disease, pericardial disease, valvular heart disease, and arrhythmias. Cardio-oncology has emerged as an essential discipline in medicine, in response to the combined decision-making necessary to optimize the care of cancer patients receiving cardiotoxic cancer therapy. This chapter will focus on the history of cardio-oncology, the present landscape, and briefly discuss future challenges and directions.

CANCER AND HEART DISEASE

Cancer and cardiovascular disease account for over 45% of deaths in the USA (3). Mortality rates due to cancer alone have decreased over the last 30 years owing to improvements in early detection strategies, improved surgical approaches, and advances in cancer treatments (1,3). Modern treatments have led to an improvement in the chances of surviving a diagnosis of cancer: 5-year survival rate for early breast cancer increased from 70% in 1990 to 88% in 2012 (4,5). Similar improvements have been seen in other solid and hematological malignancies (3). By 2026, it is expected that there will be over 20 million cancer survivors in the USA alone (1). Established and novel treatments such as anthracyclines, HER-2-targeted agents, and immunotherapy, typically used in the treatment of a wide range of cancers, are associated with an increased risk of cardiovascular injury, including cardiomyopathy and heart failure (6).

The incidence of cancer treatment related cardiovascular injury varies widely depending on the specific cancer therapy prescribed, duration of therapy, and underlying patient comorbidities. The population is aging—by 2050 over 20% of the U.S. population will be over 65 years of age (7); a risk factor for the development of both cancer and heart disease. Other common shared risk factors include obesity, tobacco use, and lack of exercise. Given the overlap of risk factors for both cancer and heart disease, patients may have established cardiovascular disease prior to the detection of their cancer (8), placing them at a greater risk of cardiovascular complications. This presents a great challenge to healthcare professionals, especially oncologists, who are tasked with prescribing cancer therapies which may have a detrimental impact on cardiovascular health. Consequently, although current cancer treatments can achieve desirable clinical outcomes, patients with existing cardiovascular (CV) comorbidities and those at significant risk of cancer-related CV complications, may be denied life-preserving cancer therapies due to the overwhelming risk of cardiotoxicity and the unknown extent of its deleterious effects.

The interplay of cancer and heart disease and the respective metabolic pathways is complex. Our knowledge of the CV effects of chemotherapeutic drugs continues to stem from clinical trials in cancer patients that shed light on these shared functional pathways (9).

It is speculated that cardiac dysfunction, in some patients, may result from cancer agents that cause transient myocardial dysfunction like the phenomenon known as myocardial stunning. In 2005, a classification first proposed in an editorial published in the *Journal of Clinical Oncology* (10) classified cardiac dysfunction into two distinct types, namely Type 1 and Type 2. Type 1 was thought to be due to anthracycline-induced myocardial damage and more likely to be permanent and irreversible, whereas Type 2 was secondary to trastuzumab-induced myocardial dysfunction and had a higher likelihood of recovery. However, based on our current knowledge of the mechanisms of cancer therapy related cardiac dysfunction with different cancer agents, this classification should be considered overly simplistic and irrelevant in clinical practice today. There are now over nine classes of cancer drugs that may, through different mechanisms of action, cause CV dysfunction (e.g., rhythm disturbances, severe hypertension, valvular heart disease, cardiac ischemia) in cancer

patients (11). These CV complications depend on the prescribed cancer regimen, duration, and the patient's preexisting comorbidities.

This advancing level of complexity sparked a need for research in this field and set the stage for the development of the new discipline of cardio-oncology, which aims to improve the overall clinical outcomes of patients with cancers. Oncologists and cardiologists are called together in a partnership to provide collaborative care for cancer patients receiving cardiotoxic therapy. This has resulted in the development of several clinical guidelines with recommendations on screening techniques, the use of biomarkers and cardiac imaging for detecting cardiac injury, as well as risk assessment and stratification of cancer patients. These guidelines have been largely based on data from the adult breast cancer literature, as it pertains to the CV toxicity of anthracyclines and HER-2-targeted agents. Further research is needed to develop evidence-based recommendations in other solid and hematological malignancies.

Cancer treatment and cardiotoxicity: The basis for cardio-oncology

Daunorubicin was the first anthracycline-based cancer therapy to be identified from the soil bacterium *Streptomyces peucetius* in the 1950s (12). Since this discovery, several other anthracycline drugs have been discovered and found to be effective as chemotherapeutic agents (13,14).

Cardiotoxicity as a concept became recognized in the 1960s when anthracyclines were found to be strongly associated with an increased risk of cardiomyopathy and heart failure in a dose-dependent manner (15,16). In 1979, a retrospective analysis of 4018 patient records found that clinically overt congestive heart failure (CHF) occurred in 2.2% of patients who had received anthracycline-based therapies (16). The cumulative incidence of CHF increased from 3% in patients receiving doxorubicin at a moderate dose (400 mg/m²) to 18% in those being treated with high doses (700 mg/m²) (16). Subsequent studies demonstrated that subclinical LV dysfunction, not measured in earlier studies, was highly prevalent among patients receiving anthracycline chemotherapy (17). As shown by Swain et al. in a large retrospective analysis of data from three phase III prospective trials of breast and lung cancer treatment with doxorubicin, the prevalence of subclinical LV dysfunction or overt clinical CHF can be as high as 54% in patients receiving a cumulative dose of doxorubicin at 500 mg/m², while up to 48% of patients receiving high doses (cumulative doses of 700 mg/m²) of doxorubicin would be expected to develop clinically overt CHF (18).

Since the first documented complete cure of a human solid tumor by chemotherapy in 1953, significant milestones have been made in cancer treatments, offering cancer patients a better chance of survival. Some recent advances include the discovery of monoclonal antibodies, such as trastuzumab, and tyrosine kinase inhibitors, such as imatinib.

Trastuzumab is a monoclonal antibody, initially approved by the U.S. Food and Drug Administration (FDA) in 1998, for treatment of women with human epidermal growth factor receptor-2 (HER-2)-positive metastatic breast cancer. The addition of trastuzumab to standard anthracycline based chemotherapy (given concurrently) was associated with improved clinical outcomes, including a longer time to disease progression, a higher rate of objective response, and a 20% reduction in the risk of death at one year, when compared to patients receiving chemotherapy alone (19). However, trastuzumab significantly increased the risk of cardiotoxicity; overall, 28% of patients receiving anthracycline, cyclophosphamide, and trastuzumab experienced cardiotoxicity compared to 8% treated with chemotherapy alone. Furthermore, the risk of developing New York Heart Association (NYHA) cardiac dysfunction class III or IV was highest among patients who had received trastuzumab compared to the non-trastuzumab group (16% vs. 3%) (19). Trastuzumab (for one year) was approved by the FDA in 2006 for women with early stage HER-2-positive breast cancer, with a recommendation for close cardiac monitoring (every 3 months while on treatment) and avoidance of concurrent administration with anthracycline chemotherapy.

Between 2001 and 2017, at least 76 targeted anticancer therapies were approved by the U.S. FDA (20). Targeted therapies were expected to reduce cancer therapy-related toxicity to nontarget tissues while offering a higher chance of cure. However, advanced immunotherapies, small molecule kinase inhibitors, proteasome and histone deacetylases targeting inhibitors, and monoclonal antibodies, have all been associated with deleterious cardiotoxic effects, including hypertension and LV dysfunction (20). Therefore, cardiotoxicity remains a threat to the potential curative rates that can be achieved with current and evolving novel cancer treatments.

Radiotherapy, a well-recognized and established adjuvant therapy used in over 50% of cancers, is also associated with potential CV toxicity (21). High-energy particles and other forms of radiation interfere with cell proliferation and viability, which is the basis for its use in oncology (22). The first reported use of radiation therapy for treatment of cancer dates as far back as 1903 when S.W. Goldberg and Efim London used it to successfully cure two patients with basal cell carcinoma of the skin (23). Since then, radiation therapy has become an integral part of treatment used to improve clinical outcomes in cancer patients. In breast cancer, radiotherapy reduces the risk of local cancer recurrence and mortality by 50% and 17%, respectively, after breast conservation surgery (24). In patients with Hodgkin's lymphoma, combination therapy with chemotherapy and radiotherapy increases the chances of survival by over 70% (25).

While the addition of radiotherapy to chemotherapy improves cure rates and reduces recurrence, exposure of ionizing radiation to other tissues, such as the myocardium and CV system, can lead to deleterious tissue damage, particularly if the dose exceeds more than 30 Gy (26).

Similar to chemotherapy, radiotherapy-induced cardiac complications were first reported in the 1960s and included pericardial diseases, cardiomyopathy, coronary artery disease, valvular disease, and conduction abnormalities (27). While traditional radiation modalities involved large radiation doses over a large field, current approaches are more targeted and use low radiation doses to minimize unwanted exposures. Consequently, the challenge for treating clinicians is the difficulty in predicting the dose of radiation that would be safe and yet effective in cancer treatment, particularly as CV complications occur much later after completion of therapy. Darby et al. recently demonstrated that the rates of major coronary events increased linearly with the mean dose to the heart by 7.4% per gray in women with breast cancer who received radiotherapy. This incremental increase in major coronary artery events started within 5 years of exposure to ionizing radiation, but continued to increase up to 20 years after exposure (28).

CARDIO-ONCOLOGY: AN EMERGING MULTIDISCIPLINARY FIELD

Cardiotoxicity resulting from cancer treatments remains a challenging issue given the escalation of newer targeted therapies being introduced into clinical practice. Favorable benefits of current and emerging cancer therapies may be offset by the CV morbidity and mortality related to cancer treatments, which in turn impact clinical outcomes irrespective of oncologic prognosis. CV complications can develop early or many years following completion of cancer therapy. In the Childhood Cancer Survivor Study, a retrospective analysis of 14,358 individuals who had survived childhood malignancies, Mulrooney et al. found that the risk of developing congestive heart failure 5 years or more after the diagnosis of cancer was 2.4-fold higher after exposure to anthracycline treatment at doses $\geq$250 mg/m² compared to those who were not exposed to anthracyclines (29). The Childhood Cancer Survivor Study also demonstrated an 8.2-fold higher rate of cardiac death compared with the age-matched and sex-matched national average 15 to 25 years after diagnosis and treatment of childhood cancer. In the study by Darby et al., major CV events were shown to occur 20 years after radiotherapy in women with breast cancer (28).

Adult cancer survivors are not only exposed to the risks of chemotherapeutic agents, but also the aging effects on CV health. Chemotherapy and radiotherapy can have synergistic or additive effects on the risk of cardiac complications, which are more severe with advancing age and preexisting CV risk factors. The extent of cardiotoxicity associated with a proposed cancer therapy may be difficult to predict because the extent to which each risk factor contributes to the overall cardiovascular risk is largely unknown (30). Early diagnosis and routine management of CV risk factors during and after completion of cancer therapy are necessary to improve CV and overall clinical outcomes while optimizing cancer survival rates.

Cardio-oncology as a discipline has developed from recognition of the complexities involved in treating patients with cancer who are at risk of or develop cancer therapy related cardiac dysfunction. In a nationwide online survey of 444 adult and pediatric cardiology division chiefs and CV fellowship training directors, 39% of participants did not feel confident dealing with the specific CV needs of cancer patients (31). This alarming statistic alone speaks to the need for coordinated care, communication and education between oncologists and cardiologists.

The concept of cardio-oncology has its origins in the 1960s, when early observations demonstrating that anthracyclines caused dose-dependent cardiomyopathy and heart failure led to modifications of anthracycline-based treatment regimens with limitations on cumulative doses (16). These early studies also spurred an interest in research toward a better understanding of the mechanisms, as well as methods of early detection, prevention, and treatment of cancer-related cardiotoxicity. Since the publication of the first observational studies, there has been a considerable increase in research into mechanisms of cardiotoxicity (32,33), new cancer therapeutics (32), serum cardiac biomarkers (34), and imaging techniques (35) for risk stratification, as well as clinical trials investigating cardioprotective strategies (36).

While cardio-oncology remains a developing specialty, collaboration between oncologists and cardiologists is not a new concept. For years, collaboration has existed between these disciplines, but placed an emphasis on oncologists being able to recognize cardiotoxicity and referring patients to cardiologists on an "ad hoc" basis. This approach resulted in significant vulnerability, in part owing to the lack of understanding by cardiologists of the mechanism of action and importance of cancer therapies, thus resulting in poor CV and overall clinical outcomes. In a study evaluating treatment practices for cancer therapy-related asymptomatic decreases in LV ejection fraction, only 42% of patients who exhibited echocardiographic evidence of LV dysfunction were seen by cardiologists (37). Furthermore, knowledge of cancer treatment-related cardiotoxicity among cardiologists was variable due to their limited exposure to patients with cancer, which contributed to poor CV health (38). Cardio-oncology as a specialty has evolved in the twenty-first century to provide a formalized approach to addressing the complex CV needs of patients with cancer, with the goal of optimizing patient care in a multidisciplinary approach. The growing need for a partnership between oncologists and cardiologists with expertise in cardio-oncology has subsequently led to the development of cardio-oncology clinics and rapidly expanding cardio-oncology programs across the world.

Cardio-oncology clinics

As a highly specialized field of medicine, cardio-oncology seeks to enhance the overall safety and effectiveness of cancer treatment while simultaneously screening for and managing CV risk. The joint expertise between cardiologists and oncologists has the potential to improve clinical decision making and optimize screening and treatment of CV complications related to ageing and cancer treatment. This approach also offers an appropriate setting for optimization of CV health for patients with cancers who present with concomitant CV diseases, thereby affording these patients opportunities to undergo life-preserving cancer therapies with overall positive net benefits.

The establishment of cardio-oncology clinics allows for coordinated care in a multidisciplinary team, involving radiation and medical oncologists, hematologists, cardiologists, dedicated cardio-oncology nurses and nurse specialists, and other healthcare personnel involved in caring for patients with cancers (39). Such a multidisciplinary approach to the care of patients with complex and potentially life-threatening conditions is supported by strong evidence in favor of improving clinical outcomes. In a meta-analysis of 29 trials comprising 5039 patients with heart failure, it was shown that patients who were treated within the context of a multidisciplinary team had a significantly reduced risk of mortality and rehospitalizations (40). These benefits have also been observed among patients with cancer who are managed by a multidisciplinary team (41). In an observational study performed at the University of Ottawa's Cardio-Oncology Clinic, up to 80% of patients referred to the clinic were able to complete prescribed cancer therapy (42). In major cardio-oncology centers, up to 30% of cardio-oncology referrals are for patients with cancer therapy-related cardiac dysfunction. The remainder of the practice focuses on patients referred for pre-treatment risk stratification and management, and monitoring and treatment of cardiotoxicity during and after cancer treatments (31).

Assessment of the risk of cardiotoxicity prior to initiating cancer treatment is an essential component of the clinic and is a high priority (22,39). This is achieved by establishing baseline CV risk through a comprehensive history and physical examination, focusing on important factors known to increase the risk of cardiotoxicity, such as age (<15 years or >65 years), existing CV disease (cardiomyopathy or heart failure, coronary artery disease, hypertension, diabetes, dyslipidemia), or a history of prior or concurrent exposure to chemotherapeutic agents and/or radiotherapy (22). A detailed medication history that includes any history of prior use of cardioprotective therapies such as beta-blocking agents and angiotensin-receptor blockers (ARBs) or angiotensin-converting enzyme inhibitors (ACE inhibitors), as well as the cardiotoxicity potential and the cumulative doses of proposed treatment regimens are considered in any risk assessment (43). While there are no universally accepted recommendations as to the minimum baseline investigations required, it is preferable that patients, particularly those predicted to be at high risk, have a chest x-ray, 12-lead electrocardiogram (ECG), biomarkers such as troponin levels and/or brain natriuretic peptide (BNP), and echocardiography with strain imaging, depending on risk of cardiotoxicity (39). This comprehensive assessment serves as an important baseline for monitoring cancer therapy-related cardiac complications and may identify high-risk patients who require cardiac optimization therapies prior to commencing cancer treatment (22).

A cardio-oncology clinic also facilitates effective strategies for monitoring of cardiac complications during and after cancer treatments. A proposed protocol for monitoring of cardiotoxicity related to cancer therapies was first developed in the 1970s and 1980s, and was primarily based on a decline in left ventricular ejection fraction (LVEF) observed in patients receiving anthracycline-based therapy (44). Current guidelines emphasize the importance of a careful history and physical examination, and in some instances recommend routine surveillance imaging (e.g., trastuzumab), preferably with a transthoracic echocardiography in high-risk patients, even in absence of symptoms (45). These recommendations are based on low to intermediate quality of evidence, and do not specify the frequency and type of surveillance strategies required during and after treatment with cardiotoxic chemotherapy. The frequency of screening for cardiac complications is therefore at the discretion of the treating oncologist. Similarly, the treating oncologist and cardiologist must decide on whether or not a patient who exhibits evidence of cardiac dysfunction continues cancer treatments, as there are no recommendations offered in current guidelines (45). In the absence of evidence-based guideline recommendations, collaboration between cardiologists and oncologist in a cardio-oncology clinic facilitates early detection of cancer treatment related cardiotoxicity, and allows for the completion of life-preserving cancer treatments while optimizing CV functioning and improving survival and quality of life. Guideline recommendations for screening and monitoring of cardiotoxicity before, during, and after cancer therapies are discussed further in Chapter 6.

A cardio-oncology clinic can take many forms; it can either occupy a physical space within a cardiology practice with open communication between cardiologists and oncologists, or vice versa. Alternatively, cardiologists and oncologists can be staffed simultaneously in the same space (46). Irrespective of the model chosen, there are advantages and disadvantages to each; centers should consider logistical requirements to determine the style of clinic most easily facilitated by the local institutional needs. Ultimately, the success of a cardio-oncology clinic rests on the ability of the clinical and support staff to coordinate clinical activities, advocate for and educate patients, enhance clinical flow, and ensure timely scheduling. The hospital and greater community have a role in promoting the success and encouraging further development and growth of the program. It is recommended that cardio-oncology clinics establish a database for future research purposes and facilitate opportunities for ongoing professional education of all staff (46).

Cardio-oncology programs

Cardio-oncology programs are usually found in tertiary and quaternary hospitals where both comprehensive cancer centers and heart failure programs coexist. Cardio-oncology programs should provide the infrastructure necessary for timely provision of clinical care for cancer patients, including early identification of risk factors for cardiotoxicity, and early detection and treatment of cardiac dysfunction during and after cancer treatment.

Once established, cardio-oncology programs should improve the CV outcomes of patients with cancers, although there are little published data on outcome measures. At MD Anderson Cancer Center,

one of the first comprehensive cancer centers to establish a dedicated cardio-oncology program, the program grew from four general cardiologists into a comprehensive cardio-oncology center, consisting of interventional cardiologists, electrophysiologists, and an advanced heart failure programs (31). The number of new consults and inpatient follow-up visits grew by 48% and 95%, respectively, while the program also witnessed a significant growth in cardiac imaging as well as increasing number of cardiac catheterization and electrophysiology procedures (31). Other success stories have been reported by many large centers, including the Memorial Sloan Kettering Cancer Center, Vanderbilt-Ingram Cancer Center, University of Pennsylvania Abramson Cancer Center, Dana-Farber Cancer Institute, and the Mayo Clinic (31,39).

A dedicated cardio-oncology program should provide education in cardio-oncology for healthcare providers, patients, and their families. Institutions should support continuing medical education events via lectures, web-based tools, and printed material. Current best practices in cardio-oncology are heavily based on expert opinion and low to moderate quality evidence. Research should be an integral component of any cardio-oncology program to generate the knowledge needed to provide high quality evidence-based care.

Where are we now?

EDUCATION AND RESEARCH

Cardio-oncology, as a subspecialty, is undeniably growing at a rapid pace and is now recognized by major cardiology and oncology societies. The past few decades have seen an exponential increase in new publications in the field of cardio-oncology, the emergence of a *Cardio-Oncology Journal*, and the creation of an international-based data registry (47). The birth and growth of the International Cardio-Oncology Society (ICOS) has facilitated significant collaboration among international experts and led to improved educational opportunities, including a rapidly growing number of international conferences specific to the field of cardio-oncology (47,48).

As a developing specialty, cardio-oncology provides clinicians and researchers with a multitude of opportunities in education and research. Basic scientific research on the mechanisms of cardiotoxicity associated with evolving novel cancer therapies, as well as investigation into less cardiotoxic and yet effective cancer treatments, remain areas of greatest need. There is also an urgent need to clarify the methods of detection and monitoring for cardiac dysfunction (47). The role of novel noninvasive cardiac imaging modalities, as well as the use of serum cardiac biomarkers in the early detection of cardiotoxicity in cancer patients, are areas for future research (35).

To optimize the clinical outcomes of patients undergoing treatment with cardiotoxic cancer therapies, a specialist's knowledge and understanding of the challenges in both cardiology and oncology are necessary. While conferences, monthly webinars, and web-based lecture series exist to serve the educational needs of those interested in cardio-oncology, there are only a few centers that offer recognized fellowship programs. Current training programs also suffer from a lack of standardized training requirements (49). In a recent consensus statement of ICOS and the Canadian Cardiac Oncology Network, the need for focused and structured educational fellowship programs was emphasized in order to improve the increasingly complex needs of cancer patients (47). More educational opportunities and formal fellowship programs are therefore required. Over the next few decades, we will likely witness a growing number of dedicated fellowship programs across the world, offering clinical and research opportunities in both cardiology and oncology. Now is an opportune time for trainees interested in cardio-oncology to immerse themselves in this exciting and growing field.

CARDIO-ONCOLOGY SOCIETIES AND GUIDELINES

Several clinical practice guidelines in cardio-oncology offer recommendations on the identification, risk stratification, monitoring, and management of cardiac dysfunction related to cancer treatments. These guidelines are produced by national and international oncology and major CV societies, including the European Society of Cardiology (ESC) (43), the Canadian Cardiovascular Society (50), the American Society of Echocardiography and the European Association of Cardiovascular Imaging (ASE/EACVI) (51), the European Society for Medical Oncology (ESMO) (6), and the American Society of Clinical Oncology (ASCO) (45). Over the last decade, the American College of Cardiology has also shown a growing interest in

the field of cardio-oncology, leading to the recent creation of a Cardio-Oncology Council (31,47).

Furthermore, a growing number of cardio-oncology societies are being developed across the world, including the British Cardio-Oncology Society (http://bc-os.org), the Canadian Cardiac Oncology Network (http://cardiaconcology.ca), and the ICOS (www.ic-os.org). These societies aim to promote education and research, develop best clinical practice guidelines, and promote a better understanding of the effects of cancer treatments on CV health. Collaborations are rapidly developing between local, national, and international communities with the sole goal of improving the care and clinical outcomes of patients with cancer.

As cardio-oncology is still a developing specialty, many aspects of clinical practice remain to be clarified. Current guideline recommendations are based on of low to intermediate quality evidence, and many clinicians are left without guidance on the management of patients with high CV burden undergoing cancer therapies. Evidence is lacking on the optimal surveillance strategies during and following treatment with cardiotoxic cancer therapies. The role of biomarkers in monitoring and early detection of cardiotoxicity remains to be clarified due to conflicting results in the literature.

Furthermore, although many large centers are rapidly developing comprehensive cardio-oncology programs and clinics, there are still many challenging obstacles to overcome. Strong data demonstrating the effectiveness of cardio-oncology programs are still lacking; program pioneers may have trouble acquiring institutional support (52). It is expected that the rapid growth of this novel specialty, as well as the growing national and international collaborations, will help close these knowledge gaps in the next few years. Existing cardio-oncology programs will be expected to grow, while new societies will develop in countries such as Australia, where such societies have not yet formed. Stronger evidence-based clinical recommendations, informed by large international multicenter clinical trials, will continue to be developed, and will be expected to improve clinical practice in cardio-oncology.

OUTLINE OF BOOK CHAPTERS

The aim of this book is to provide healthcare professionals with a practical guide outlining the application of our current knowledge in cardio-oncology.

Changes in cancer treatments and associated CV toxicity, as well as strategies for minimizing this risk, are reviewed. Primary and secondary preventative strategies are discussed in the context of evidence-based medical practice. Cardiac imaging modalities for assessment of cardiotoxicity and the role of serum biomarkers are explored. The long-term CV consequences of cancer therapy are discussed in chapters on adult and childhood cancer survivorship. Physicians will gain a better understanding of risk assessment, an overview of the current guidelines, treatment, prevention and detection strategies, and management in the context of survivorship.

A practical approach to setting up a cardio-oncology clinic as well as easy-to-implement guidelines are provided for readers. Nursing roles in cardio-oncology, including a practical approach to assessment, monitoring, and treating cancer therapy-related cardiac complications are discussed. Clinical factors are brought together in a presentation of case studies to emphasize key learning points. In the final chapters, the current state in cardio-oncology training, clinical care, education, and future research are presented.

REFERENCES

1. Miller KD et al. Cancer treatment and survivorship statistics, 2016. *CA Cancer J Clin.* 2016;66(4):271–9.
2. Reulen RC et al. Long-term cause-specific mortality among survivors of childhood cancer. *JAMA.* 2010;304(2):172–9.
3. DeSantis CE et al. Cancer treatment and survivorship statistics, 2014. *CA Cancer J Clin.* 2014;64(4):252–71.
4. Siegel R et al. Cancer treatment and survivorship statistics, 2012. *CA Cancer J Clin.* 2012;62(4):220–41.
5. DeSantis C et al. Breast cancer statistics, 2013. *CA Cancer J Clin.* 2014;64(1):52–62.
6. Curigliano G et al. Cardiovascular toxicity induced by chemotherapy, targeted agents and radiotherapy: ESMO Clinical Practice Guidelines. *Ann Oncol.* 2012;23(Suppl 7):vii155–166.
7. Colby SL, Ortman JM. *Projections of the size and composition of the US population: 2014 to 2060: Population estimates and projections.* 2017.
8. Cubbon RM, Lyon AR. Cardio-oncology: Concepts and practice. *Indian Heart J.* 2016;68(Suppl 1):S77–85.
9. Bellinger AM et al. Cardio-oncology: How new targeted cancer therapies and precision medicine can inform cardiovascular discovery. *Circulation* 2015;132(23):2248–58.
10. Ewer MS, Lippman SM. Type II chemotherapy-related cardiac dysfunction: Time to recognize a new entity. *J Clin Oncol.* 2005; 23(13):2900–2.
11. Curigliano G et al. Cardiotoxicity of anticancer treatments: Epidemiology, detection, and management. *CA Cancer J Clin.* 2016;66(4):309–25.
12. Di Marco A, Cassinelli G, Arcamone F. The discovery of daunorubicin. *Cancer Treat Rep.* 1981;65(Suppl 4):3–8.
13. Arcamone F et al. Adriamycin, 14-hydroxy-daunomycin, a new antitumor antibiotic from *S. peucetius* var. caesius. *Biotechnol Bioeng.* 1969;11(6):1101–10.
14. Di Marco A, Gaetani M, Scarpinato B. Adriamycin (NSC-123,127): A new antibiotic with antitumor activity. *Cancer Chemother Rep.* 1969;53(1):33–7.
15. Lefrak EA et al. A clinicopathologic analysis of adriamycin cardiotoxicity. *Cancer* 1973;32(2):302–14.
16. Von Hoff DD et al. Risk factors for doxorubicin-induced congestive heart failure. *Ann Intern Med.* 1979;91(5):710–7.
17. Alexander J et al. Serial assessment of doxorubicin cardiotoxicity with quantitative radionuclide angiocardiography. *N Engl J Med.* 1979;300(6):278–83.
18. Swain SM, Whaley FS, Ewer MS. Congestive heart failure in patients treated with doxorubicin: A retrospective analysis of three trials. *Cancer* 2003;97(11):2869–79.
19. Slamon DJ et al. Use of chemotherapy plus a monoclonal antibody against HER2 for metastatic breast cancer that overexpresses HER2. *N Engl J Med.* 2001;344(11):783–92.
20. Zheng PP, Li J, Kros JM. Breakthroughs in modern cancer therapy and elusive cardiotoxicity: Critical research-practice gaps, challenges, and insights. *Med Res Rev.* 2018;38(1):325–76.

21. Darby SC et al. Radiation-related heart disease: Current knowledge and future prospects. *Int J Radiat Oncol Biol Phys.* 2010;76(3):656–65.

22. Herrmann J et al. Evaluation and management of patients with heart disease and cancer: Cardio-oncology. *Mayo Clin Proc.* 2014;89(9):1287–306.

23. Goldberg S, London E. XXIV. Zur Frage der Beziehungen zwischen Bequerelstrahlen und Hautaffectionen. *Dermatology* 1903; 10(5):457–62.

24. Darby S et al. Effect of radiotherapy after breast-conserving surgery on 10-year recurrence and 15-year breast cancer death: Meta-analysis of individual patient data for 10,801 women in 17 randomised trials. *Lancet* 2011;378(9804):1707–16.

25. André MPE. Combination chemoradiotherapy in early Hodgkin Lmphoma. *Hematol/ Oncol Clinics.* 2014;28(1):33–47.

26. Groarke JD et al. Cardiovascular complications of radiation therapy for thoracic malignancies: The role for non-invasive imaging for detection of cardiovascular disease. *Eur Heart J.* 2014;35(10):612–23.

27. Cohn KE et al. Heart disease following radiation. *Med (Baltim).* 1967;46(3):281–98.

28. Darby SC et al. Risk of ischemic heart disease in women after radiotherapy for breast cancer. *N Engl J Med.* 2013;368(11):987–98.

29. Mulrooney DA et al. Cardiac outcomes in a cohort of adult survivors of childhood and adolescent cancer: Retrospective analysis of the Childhood Cancer Survivor Study cohort. *BMJ.* 2009;339:b4606.

30. Tilemann LM et al. Cardio-oncology: Conflicting priorities of anticancer treatment and cardiovascular outcome. *Clin Res Cardiol.* 2018;107(4):271–80.

31. Barac A et al. Cardiovascular health of patients with cancer and cancer survivors: A roadmap to the next level. *J Am Coll Cardiol.* 2015;65(25):2739–46.

32. Duran JM et al. Sorafenib cardiotoxicity increases mortality after myocardial infarction. *Circ Res.* 2014;114(11):1700–12.

33. Zhang S et al. Identification of the molecular basis of doxorubicin-induced cardiotoxicity. *Nat Med.* 2012;18(11):1639–42.

34. Cardinale D et al. Prognostic value of troponin I in cardiac risk stratification of cancer patients undergoing high-dose chemotherapy. *Circulation* 2004;109(22):2749–54.

35. Jiji RS, Kramer CM, Salerno M. Non-invasive imaging and monitoring cardiotoxicity of cancer therapeutic drugs. *J Nucl Cardiol.* 2012;19(2):377–88.

36. Bosch X et al. Enalapril and carvedilol for preventing chemotherapy-induced left ventricular systolic dysfunction in patients with malignant hemopathies: The overcome trial (prevention of left ventricular dysfunction with enalapril and carvedilol in patients submitted to intensive chemotherapy for the treatment of malignant hemopathies). *J Am Coll Cardiol.* 2013;61(23):2355–62.

37. Yoon GJ et al. Left ventricular dysfunction in patients receiving cardiotoxic cancer therapies are clinicians responding optimally? *J Am Coll Cardiol.* 2010;56(20):1644–50.

38. Chen CL, Steingart R. Cardiac disease and heart failure in cancer patients: Is our training adequate to provide optimal care? *Heart Fail Clin.* 2011;7(3):357–62.

39. Barros-Gomes S et al. Rationale for setting up a cardio-oncology unit: Our experience at Mayo Clinic. *Cardio-Oncol.* 2016;2(1):5.

40. McAlister FA et al. Multidisciplinary strategies for the management of heart failure patients at high risk for admission: A systematic review of randomized trials. *J Am Coll Cardiol.* 2004;44(4):810–9.

41. Parent S, Pituskin E, Paterson DI. The cardio-oncology program: A multidisciplinary approach to the care of cancer patients with cardiovascular disease. *Can J Cardiol.* 2016;32(7):847–51.

42. Sulpher J et al. Clinical experience of patients referred to a multidisciplinary cardiac oncology clinic: An observational study. *J Oncol.* 2015;2015:671232.

43. Zamorano JL et al. 2016 ESC position paper on cancer treatments and cardiovascular toxicity developed under the auspices of the ESC committee for practice guidelines: The task force for cancer treatments and cardiovascular toxicity of the European Society of Cardiology (ESC). *Eur Heart J.* 2016;37(36):2768–801.

44. Schwartz RG et al. Congestive heart failure and left ventricular dysfunction complicating doxorubicin therapy. Seven-year experience using serial radionuclide angiocardiography. *Am J Med*. 1987;82(6):1109–18.

45. Armenian SH et al. Prevention and monitoring of cardiac dysfunction in survivors of adult cancers: American Society of Clinical Oncology clinical practice guideline. *J Clin Oncol*. 2017;35(8):893–911.

46. Snipelisky D et al. How to develop a cardio-oncology clinic. *Heart Fail Clin*. 2017;13(2):347–59.

47. Lenihan DJ et al. Cardio-oncology training: A proposal from the International Cardioncology Society and Canadian Cardiac Oncology Network for a new multidisciplinary specialty. *J Card Fail*. 2016;22(6): 465–71.

48. Lenihan DJ, Cardinale D, Cipolla CM. The compelling need for a cardiology and oncology partnership and the birth of the International Cardi-Oncology Society. *Prog Cardiovasc Dis*. 2010;53(2):88–93.

49. Halperin JL et al. ACC 2015 core cardiovascular training statement (COCATS 4) (revision of COCATS 3). *A Report of the ACC Competency Management Committee* 2015;65(17):1721–3.

50. Virani SA et al. Canadian Cardiovascular Society guidelines for evaluation and management of cardiovascular complications of cancer therapy. *Can J Cardiol*. 2016; 32(7):831–41.

51. Plana JC et al. Expert consensus for multimodality imaging evaluation of adult patients during and after cancer therapy: A report from the American Society of Echocardiography and the European Association of Cardiovascular Imaging. *J Am Soc Echocardiogr*. 2014;27(9):911–39.

52. Okwuosa TM, Yeh ETH, Barac A. Burgeoning cardio-oncology programs. *Chall Oppor Early Career Cardiologists/Fac Dir*. 2015; 66(10):1193–7.

PART II

Clinical aspects of cardio-oncology

2

Current imaging strategies in cardio-oncology

MIRELA TUZOVIC, MELKON HACOBIAN, AND ERIC H. YANG

INTRODUCTION

The increasing number of cancer survivors is a reflection of the advancements that have been made in early detection, and treatment with chemotherapy, targeted therapies, immunotherapy and radiation (1). Cancer therapies can cause a range of cardiovascular adverse effects, including congestive heart failure, angina symptoms, acute coronary syndrome, stroke, arrhythmias, accelerated atherosclerosis, and peripheral arterial disease (2). Structural and functional changes of the cardiovascular endothelium owing to chemotherapeutic agents can lead to both short- and long-term sequelae that may impact long-term mortality and quality of life, even if the patient's malignancy is successfully treated. The presence of traditional cardiovascular risk factors is associated with increased risk of developing cardiovascular complications from cancer treatments. Cardiovascular imaging plays a crucial role in detecting both subclinical changes and symptomatic disease (3,4).

Although the frequency of screening for cardiotoxicity in patients undergoing active treatments and cancer survivors remains a topic of debate and ongoing research, screening and early diagnosis of cardiovascular complications of cancer treatments can potentially attenuate or prevent significant morbidity and mortality in cancer patients. Many different imaging modalities have been used for detection and monitoring of chemotherapeutic-related cardiotoxicity. Here, we highlight the important advantages and disadvantages, as well as the specific applications of transthoracic echocardiography (TTE), cardiac magnetic resonance imaging (CMR), multigated cardiac blood pool imaging (MUGA), nuclear perfusion scans, positron emission tomography (PET), computed tomography (CT), and vascular ultrasound in cancer patients receiving chemotherapy and/or radiotherapy with potential short- and long-term cardiovascular toxicity. We also review the cardiotoxicity surveillance recommendations from the Children's Oncology Group, International Late Effects of Childhood Cancer Guidelines, as well as five different society-endorsed statements.

IMAGING CLASSIFICATION OF CARDIOTOXICITY

The American Society of Echocardiography (ASE) and the European Association of Cardiovascular Imaging (EACI) define cancer therapeutic-related cardiac dysfunction (CTRCD) as a reduction in left ventricular ejection fraction (LVEF) of >10% to a value of <53% which should be confirmed on a follow-up study in 2–3 weeks (5). Table 2.1 lists the classifications of severity of left ventricular (LV) dysfunction, as well as the American College of Cardiology (ACC) and American Heart Association (AHA) stages of heart failure, which can also be applied to patients who develop cancer therapy-related cardiomyopathy.

While most of the guidelines on imaging for the detection of cardiotoxicity focus on LVEF assessment, other chemotherapeutic-related cardiac effects, including radiation-induced cardiac disease, coronary artery thrombosis, and vasospasm, will be mentioned here when appropriate. The cardio-oncologist now has access to a variety of multimodality imaging options to assess for cardiotoxicity, and it is critical to understand the strengths and weakness of each modality as well as the evidence to date regarding their indications (Table 2.2).

Transthoracic echocardiography

TTE is the most commonly used method for evaluation of cardiac dysfunction from various causes. Echocardiography enables a comprehensive assessment of cardiac function, structure, valvular disease, and the pericardium. LVEF and right ventricular (RV) function are important parameters to assess when CTRCD is suspected, while pericardial and valve thickening are more common manifestations of radiation-induced cardiac disease. While chemotherapy-induced cardiotoxicity can affect the RV as well as the LV, changes in RV function is not known to be associated with worse outcomes. TTE also enables assessment of diastolic dysfunction; however, these changes have not been reliably predictive of cardiotoxicity (6).

TTE has tremendous advantages when compared to other imaging modalities because it is widely available, inexpensive, portable, and is not associated with radiation exposure. The main limitations include limited accuracy and reproducible measurements. LVEF measurement using 2D TTE biplane method (Figure 2.1) has a temporal variability/coefficient of variation of 7.4% (7), which is important to highlight because the measurement variability is close to the definition of cardiotoxicity (defined as a drop in LVEF of 10% or more (5)). Measurement variability is the result of a number of factors including poor acoustic windows and body habitus which can affect the quality of the

images as well as the geometric assumptions used to estimate 3D volumes from 2D images. Some of these limitations are minimized with 3D echocardiography measurements (Figure 2.2), which are not reliant on geometric assumptions. For example, LVEF assessment with 3D echocardiography has a temporal variability/coefficient of variation of 4.0% (7). Recognizing this, the ASE encourages use of 3D echocardiography whenever possible (5).

Echocardiography-based deformation imaging (also known as strain imaging), has become an essential tool for cardiotoxicity surveillance. While reduction in LVEF correlates with clinical cardiotoxicity, changes in strain are more sensitive, appear prior to LVEF reduction, and are suggestive of subclinical cardiotoxicity. Global longitudinal strain (GLS) is a measure of the average change in length of the left ventricular in the longitudinal direction in the apical four-, three-, and two-chamber views. GLS has been found to be the best predictor of cardiotoxicity due to anthracycline use (Figure 2.3). A fall in GLS between 10% and 15% is associated with development of both symptomatic and asymptomatic cardiotoxicity (8,9). A reduction of 15% from baseline is considered abnormal and suggestive of cardiac injury (10). A longitudinal strain <19% at the completion of anthracycline therapy has been associated with late development of cardiotoxicity (11). Although LV radial and circumferential strain are often measured, global radial and circumferential strain have not been correlated with cardiotoxicity. The European Society of Cardiology (ESC) and ASE recommend performing GLS measurements at the time of LVEF assessment (5,10). It is important to highlight that there are significant variations in normal strain values between vendors and tracking algorithms, therefore using the same software and vendor for follow-up studies is important (5).

Multigated cardiac blood pool imaging

MUGA is a nuclear-based imaging modality that uses a radiotracer to tag red blood cells which are counted as they flow through the heart allowing for an highly accurate assessment of cardiac function. MUGA was the first imaging study used for LVEF assessment as a way to define and track cardiotoxicity (Figure 2.4). The initial recommendations for anthracycline-induced cardiotoxicity monitoring were based on

Table 2.1 Different classification schemes for cardiac toxicity and heart failure

Classification system	Low	Severity Intermediate	High
Oncology derived			
LV systolic dysfunction (CTCAE, version 4.03)	–	Symptomatic as a result of a drop in EF; responsive to intervention	Refractory or poorly controlled HF owing to EF drop; intervention such as LVAD, vasopressor support, or heart transplantation indicated	Death
Heart failure (CTCAE, version 4.03)	Asymptomatic with abnormal biomarkers or imaging	Symptoms with mild to moderate activity or exertion	Severe with symptoms at rest or with minimal activity or exertion; intervention indicated	Life-threatening consequences; urgent intervention indicated (e.g., continuous IV therapy or mechanical hemodynamic support)	Death
Decreased ejection fraction (CTCAE, version 4.03)	–	Resting EF 40–50%; 10–19% drop from baseline	Resting EF 20–39%; >20% drop from baseline	Resting EF <20%	–
Cardiac Review and Evaluation Committee	Any of 4 criteria confirms cardiac dysfunction: cardiomyopathy, reduced LVEF (global or more severe in the septum); symptoms of HF; signs associated with HF (S3 gallop and/or tachycardia); and decrease in LVEF from baseline ≥5% to <55% with accompanying signs or symptoms of HF or decline in LVEF ≥10% to <55% without accompanying signs of symptoms of HF		–
Cardiology derived			
Heart failure stage (ACC/AHA)	Stage A, at risk (e.g., patients receiving cardiotoxic medications but without structural heart disease or symptoms)	Stage B, structural heart disease (hypertrophy, low EF, valve disease)	Stage C, structural heart disease with prior or current symptoms	Stage D, refractory HF requiring specialized interventions	–
NYHA symptom classification	Grade I, no limitations of activity	Grade II, mild limitation of activity; grade III, marked limitation of activity	Grade IV, confined to bed or chair	–

Source: Adapted from Khouri MG et al. *Circulation.* 2012;126:2749–63.
Abbreviations: CTCAE, Common Terminology Criteria for Adverse Events; EF, ejection fraction; HF, heart failure; IV, intravenous; LVAD, left ventricular assist device; LVEF, left ventricular ejection fraction.

Table 2.2 Imaging modalities currently used to evaluate cardiotoxicity

Modality	Pros	Cons
MUGA	Reproducibility	Involves radiation
	Accuracy	Not able to evaluate other cardiac structures
CMR	Accuracy	Not easily available at all centers
	Can evaluate other cardiac structures	Higher costs
	Can evaluate myocardial perfusion, viability and fibrosis	
TTE (2D/3D)	Easy accessibility	Not as accurate in evaluating LVEF when compared to MUGA and CMR and can miss small changes in LV contractility (use of contrast is recommended in 2D images if two contiguous segments are not well visualized in apical views)
	Portability	
	No radiation	
	Can evaluate other cardiac structures and pulmonary hypertension	
	Can use speckle tracking to evaluate for subclinical markers like myocardial deformation	

Abbreviations: MUGA, multigated blood pool acquisition; CMR, cardiac magnetic resonance imaging; TTE, transthoracic echocardiogram; 2D, 2-dimensional imaging; 3D, 3-dimensional imaging; LVEF, left ventricular ejection fraction.

LVEF assessment by MUGA (12). Compared to echocardiography, MUGA-derived cardiac functional assessment is more accurate with less measurement variability (13); however, it does not assess valvular or pericardial disease, and it provides limited information about RV function. In addition, it is both more costly than echocardiography and exposes the patient to radiation which can become significant if multiple follow-up studies are needed. In light of these limitations and concerns, MUGA is less commonly used as the first-line study than echocardiography. It remains a good option for highly accurate LVEF assessment when echocardiography is suboptimal or the LVEF measurement is uncertain.

Cardiac magnetic resonance imaging

CMR is a newer and powerful imaging modality that manipulates magnetic fields to generate high resolution cardiac images. CMR is recognized by the ACC as a potential method for cardiotoxicity screening, and it is considered a gold standard study for assessment of LV function (14). CMR can assess both systolic and diastolic myocardial function, myocardial structure, and provide assessment of valve function. Using various sequencing methods, CMR can be adapted to provide virtually any information including pericardial thickness, myocardial fibrosis/scar, and evidence of infiltrative disease. It provides tissue characterization for cardiac masses

as well. It does not expose the patient to any radiation. Compared to echocardiography, images are higher resolution and more reproducible; therefore, when discontinuation of chemotherapy is being considered due to cardiotoxicity, CMR should be used to verify the LVEF (5).

While CMR is considered a very safe test, deposits of gadolinium, which is the main contrast used in CMR, have recently been noted in the brains of patients undergoing multiple CMR studies. This has raised some concern and has prompted an Food and Drug Administration (FDA). Drug Safety warning (15). The potential effects of gadolinium retention are currently being monitored and the FDA has expressed that based on current knowledge, the benefits of magnetic resonance imaging (MRI) continue to outweigh any potential harm. In patients with kidney dysfunction and a glomerular filtration rate (GFR) of less than 30 mL/min/1.73 m^2, gadolinium is contraindicated due to risk of a progressive condition called nephrogenic systemic fibrosis. Despite its breadth and accuracy, CMR use is limited for multiple reasons. It is expensive and not available in many centers. It requires long exam times with significant patient cooperation and long periods of breath-holding. In patients with pacemaker/defibrillator or breast implants, image quality can be limited by artifact.

CMR is well-recognized as a reliable study for evaluation of cardiotoxicity, and many types of

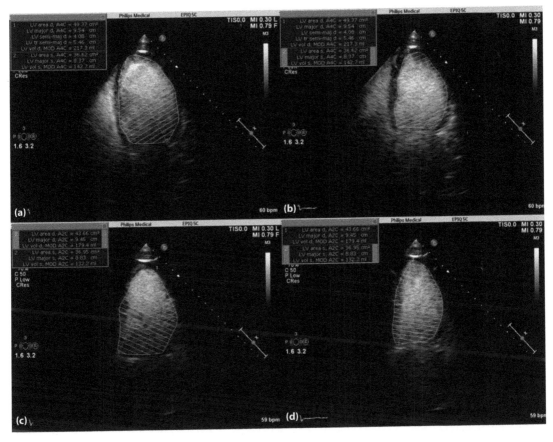

Figure 2.1 Example of contrast echocardiography in a 72-year-old male with a history of metastatic fibrosarcoma who underwent a total cumulative dosing of 446 mg/m² of doxorubicin, olaratumab, and stereotactic body radiation therapy to the right middle lung lobe for a total dose of 50 Gy, with anthracycline and radiation associated cardiomyopathy. The LV endocardium is opacified with injection of perfluten lipid microspheres (Definity, Lantheus, Billerica, MA) allowing for more accurate assessment of LV function and to evaluate for thrombus. Biplanar quantification of LVEF, using modified Simpson's rule, was estimated at 30%. Panel (a): Apical four-chamber view in end-diastole. Panel (b): Apical four-chamber view in end-systole. Panel (c): Apical two-chamber view in end-diastole. Panel (d): Apical two-chamber view in end-systole. (MOD: method of disks.)

changes following anthracycline and trastuzumab treatment have been reported. Change in CMR-derived LV mass has been shown to predict cardiovascular events in patients with anthracycline cardiomyopathy (16). CMR can detect myocardial edema owing to acute inflammation after anthracycline administration as well as an increase in extracellular volume which may correlate with myocardial fibrosis (17,18). Patients with breast cancer and trastuzumab-induced cardiomyopathy have been shown to have mid-myocardial hyperenhancement (19) (Figure 2.5). In contrast, late gadolinium enhancement (LGE), which is associated with fibrosis/scar, is rare in anthracycline

cardiotoxicity (16) and is largely helpful in excluding other etiologies of cardiomyopathy including prior myocardial infarction or amyloidosis.

Nuclear perfusion imaging

Nuclear perfusion imaging is used to assess for coronary artery flow obstruction in patients with symptoms or signs of ischemia. It does also provide an assessment of LV function; however, this is not the test of choice for LVEF assessment due to low reliability compared to echocardiography. Therefore, in patients with suspected cardiotoxicity—as defined by a change in LVEF—this test is not routinely

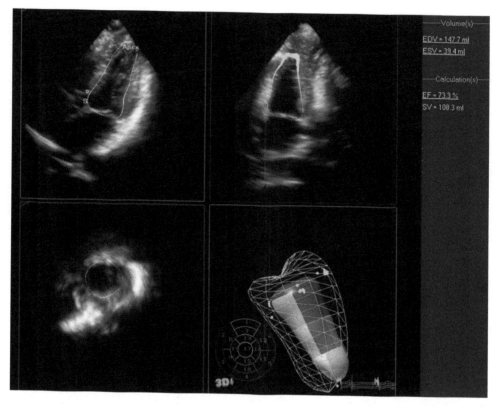

Figure 2.2 Example of 3D volumetric transthoracic echocardiographic assessment of left ventricular ejection fraction. (EDV: end-diastolic volume; ESV: end systolic volume; EF: ejection fraction; SV: stroke volume.)

performed. With chemotherapeutic agents associated with vascular thrombosis and vasospasm such as 5-flourouracil, tyrosine kinase inhibitors (TKI), and vascular endothelial growth factor (VEGF) inhibitors TKIs, perfusion imaging can be helpful to evaluate for cardiac ischemia in patients with cardiac symptoms. Screening with nuclear perfusion imaging in the asymptomatic patient prior to or during chemotherapy has not been well studied and is not generally recommended. One key exception is screening for coronary artery disease (CAD) in patients who have received prior chest or breast radiation. Patients with chest and/or breast radiation are at particularly high risk of CAD and have an estimated incidence of radiation-induced heart disease 5–10 years after treatment of 10%–30% (20). Based on one study, the prevalence of CAD based on coronary CT angiography in Hodgkin's lymphoma survivors was up to 39% with a significant percentage of high risk lesions (left main or proximal left anterior descending artery) (21). The EACI and ASE recommend screening with a stress test all high-risk patients (including those who received anterior or left-sided chest radiation) 5–10 years postradiation treatment (22).

Positron emission tomography

PET is a nuclear-based imaging technique that uses a biologically active molecule to detect metabolic activity in various tissues. One important application of PET within cardiology is for assessment of myocardial viability. The use of PET imaging for the detection of cardiotoxicity is not well studied. One small study of six female cancer patients undergoing doxorubicin treatment received a PET scan with carbon-11 acetate before and during chemotherapy. In this study, there was no change in the metabolism or blood flow associated with treatment (23). PET using fludeoxyglucose (a glucose analog) may show changes in glucose utilization preceding cardiotoxicity in patients receiving anthracyclines; however, further studies are needed to evaluate the significance of these changes (24).

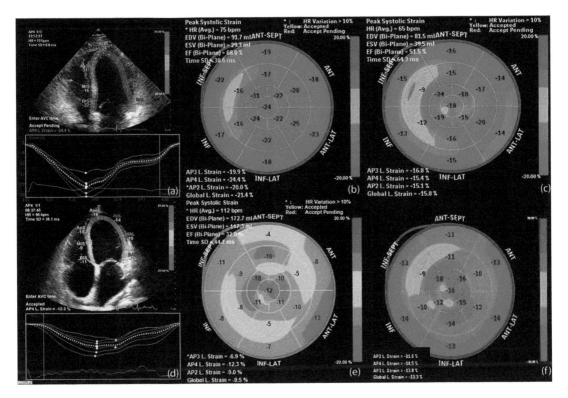

Figure 2.3 Serial transthoracic echocardiographic imaging with speckle tracking of the patient from Figure 2.1: 72-year-old male with a history of metastatic fibrosarcoma who underwent a total cumulative dosing of 446 mg/m^2 of doxorubicin, olaratumab, and stereotactic body radiation therapy to the right middle lung lobe for a total dose of 50 Gy. Panel (a): Speckle tracking in the apical four-chamber view 3 months into treatment, demonstrating normal LVEF quantification of 68% and normal LV strain values in all wall segments. Longitudinal strain curves are noted below imaging. Panel (b): Representative polar map of study done in Panel (a), displaying peak longitudinal strain values using the two-chamber, three-chamber, and four-chamber TTE views with a normal global longitudinal strain (GLS) value of −21.4%. Panel (c): Polar map of LV strain analysis performed 3 months later, showing a decrease in LV function to 52% and a decrease in GLS value to −15.8%. Panel (d): Speckle tracking of four-chamber view of TTE performed 8 months after completion of doxorubicin treatment demonstrates a significant worsening from baseline of strain curves with an LVEF of 21%. Panel (e): Polar map of LV strain value of study done in Panel (d), with a GLS value of −9.5%. Panel (f): Polar map of LV strain performed on TTE study done 5 months later on medical therapy shows a mild improvement in LVEF to 30% and mild improvement in GLS value of −13.3%. (Aps: apical septum; MIS: midseptum; BIS: basal septum; ApL: apical lateral; MAL: mid-anterolateral; BAL: basal anterolateral.)

Cardiac computed tomography

CT scanners obtain high-spatial resolution images providing accurate assessment of LVEF, valve structure, and the pericardium. CT scans are also able to identify the risk and presence of CAD by quantifying coronary calcification and visualizing the coronary artery lumen. Although the accuracy of CT is comparable to echocardiography, CT is not used as first line imaging for assessing cardiac function and structure for cardiotoxicity detection. Coronary CT angiography may have a role

in patients who develop symptoms on particular chemotherapeutic agents that are linked to coronary ischemia/thrombosis, such as 5-fluorouracil, capecitabine, paclitaxel, cisplatin, or VEGF inhibitors (2–3), as cancer patients may be too high risk to undergo invasive coronary angiography.

An important limitation of CT that makes it less appealing for routine use is that it requires high radiation doses (22). Other limitations include the need for iodinated contrast, breath-holding, and poor image quality with elevated heart rates. Coronary artery and valvar disease assessment can

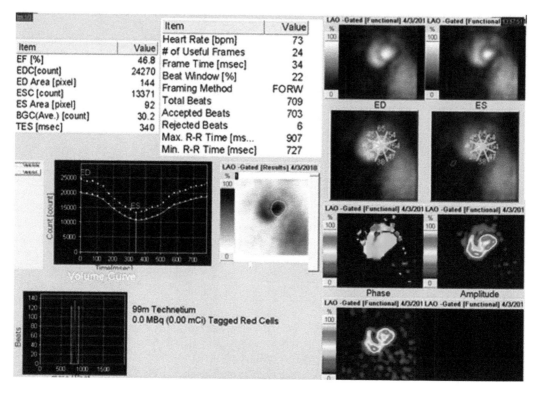

Figure 2.4 Example of multigated acquisition (MUGA) scan in a 32-year-old male with a history of presumed methamphetamine induced cardiomyopathy, diabetes, and obesity with newly diagnosed acute lymphoblastic leukemia undergoing anthracycline treatments. A pretreatment echocardiogram demonstrated suboptimal imaging, even with contrast administration, with an estimated LVEF of 36%. MUGA demonstrated an LVEF of 46.8%. (EF: ejection fraction; EDC: end diastolic count; ESC: end systolic count; TES: time to end of systole; LAO: left anterior oblique.)

also be limited by the presence of calcium blooming, which can overestimate the severity of coronary vessel stenosis (28).

One possible application of CT scanning is risk stratification in cancer patients undergoing chemotherapy with potential cardiotoxicity. PET-CT scans, which are routinely performed for cancer staging, can also potentially provide quantitative coronary artery calcium burden for patients. In contrast to LVEF and valve assessment, CT calcium scores can be obtained without using high radiation exposure and without contrast use. Calcium scores assessed on CT imaging have been shown to predict CAD in patients without clinical cardiovascular disease. The association of high coronary artery calcium scores has been reported in small studies of Hodgkin's lymphoma and breast cancer survivors treated with chemoradiation (25–27). Patients with elevated calcium scores undergoing cardiotoxic chemotherapy should undergo aggressive primary prevention with initiation of statin therapy if tolerated, as they may be at risk of downstream cardiac events (29). In cancer survivors who have undergone mediastinal radiation, cardiac CT can also provide an all-encompassing visualization of cardiac and vascular sequelae, including evaluating for radiation induced aortic, pericardial, valvular, myocardial, and CAD (Figure 2.6).

Carotid ultrasound

Carotid duplex is a noninvasive, relatively inexpensive, and readily available modality to assess extracranial circulation that is not reliant on ionizing radiation. Despite advances in magnetic resonance angiogram and CT angiography, due to other limiting factors (i.e., availability, cost, radiation, iodinated contrast exposure, claustrophobia), these studies may be difficult to perform

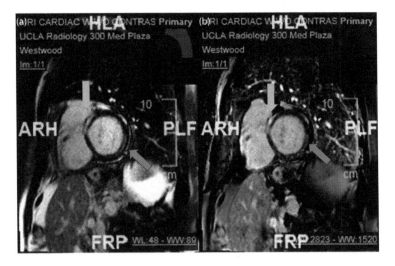

Figure 2.5 Example of cardiac magnetic resonance of patient from Figure 2.1, with anthracycline and radiation associated cardiomyopathy. The view shown is a short axis view of the left ventricle across the mitral valve, with myocardial abnormal delayed enhancement of the basal to mid-interventricular septum (blue arrows) and basal inferolateral wall (red arrows), consistent with a nonischemic pattern. Invasive coronary angiography did not reveal any macrovascular disease. Left ventricular systolic function was severely depressed at 23%. Panel (a): Magnitude only inversion recovery (MAG) images. Panel (b): Phase sensitive inversion recovery (PSIR) images.

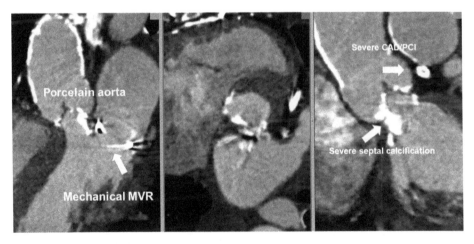

Figure 2.6 Example of cardiac computed tomography angiography (CCTA) in visualizing extent of chemoradiation induced cardiovascular sequelae. Multiplanar reconstructions from a pretranscatheter aortic valve replacement CCTA for a 57-year-old female, who had Hodgkin's lymphoma at the age of 16 who underwent chemotherapy and mediastinal radiation. She presented with severe aortic stenosis, having already had a mechanical mitral valve replacement 3 years prior. A heavily calcified (porcelain) aorta is seen, along with evidence of prior coronary stent placement from radiation induced CAD, along with severe septal calcification. (MVR: mechanical valve replacement; CAD: coronary artery disease; PCI: percutaneous coronary intervention.)

serially (30). For asymptomatic patients with elevated risk for carotid artery disease based on the type of cancer treatment (such as those receiving mediastinal and/or neck radiation), it may be reasonable to obtain serial carotid ultrasounds for monitoring. However, in patients with signs and symptoms of cardiovascular disease, especially treated with high-risk agents such as nilotinib or ponatinib, carotid ultrasound and MR/CT angiography may be considered for further identification of baseline, and accelerated development of atherosclerotic disease with treatments (2).

Measurement of carotid intima-media thickness (CIMT), with B-mode ultrasound is a noninvasive, sensitive, and reproducible technique for identifying and qualifying atherosclerotic burden and cardiovascular risk. CIMT measurements should be limited to the far wall of the common carotid artery, and should be supplemented by a thorough scan of the extracranial carotid arteries for the presence of carotid plaque, which increases the sensitivity for identifying subclinical vascular disease. Carotid plaque is defined as the presence of focal wall thickening that is at least 50% greater than that of the surrounding vessel wall, or as a focal region with CIMT greater than 1.5 mm that protrudes into the lumen, that is distinct from the adjacent boundary. The presence of carotid plaque and CIMT greater than, or equal to 75th percentile for the patient's age, sex, and race, are indicative of increased cardiovascular risk (31). CIMT measurement has been used to identify patients receiving head and neck radiation who are at high cardiovascular risk (32) and may ultimately lead to more effective prevention and improvement in cardiovascular outcomes.

Ankle-brachial index

Ankle-brachial index (ABI) is a simple test, which provides an accurate and rapid way for detecting the presence and severity of lower extremity arterial disease. The ABI is defined as the ratio of the systolic blood pressure in the upper arm compared to the ankle. Brachial and dorsalis pedis arterial systolic pressures are measured by applying an appropriately sized blood pressure cuff and using a continuous wave Doppler probe to record the arterial signal. Values below 0.9 are indicative of peripheral arterial disease (30). ABI can be performed at baseline and annually in asymptomatic patients at risk for peripheral artery disease such as patients receiving abdominal and/or pelvic radiation. In symptomatic patients, especially treated with high-risk agents such as nilotinib or ponatinib, direct visualization with arterial ultrasonography or CT/MR angiography may be indicated (2).

Venous duplex ultrasound

Deep vein thrombosis is a common problem in cancer patients. Compression venous ultrasound is considered the imaging modality of choice for the diagnosis of deep vein thrombosis. Using a high resolution linear array transducer, the deep venous system is usually examined from the level of the inguinal ligament at the common femoral vein to the tibioperoneal trunk. The large veins should be examined in the transverse plane with and without compression every 2–3 cm. Lack of coaptation of the vein wall is consistent with presence of venous thrombosis (30). Venous duplex should be considered in symptomatic cancer patients for detection of thromboembolic disease (2).

IMAGING CARDIOTOXICITY SURVEILLANCE GUIDELINES

A number of society-driven consensus statements (Table 2.3) have been published to outline cardiotoxicity surveillance strategies based on the known time course of LV dysfunction with particular cancer treatments. Data on optimal surveillance continues to be limited due to the relative lack of long-term, wide scale studies examining the effects of potentially cardiotoxic treatments; also confounding this are the ongoing dynamic treatment strategies of malignancies, and development of new chemotherapeutic agents with unknown long-term complications. Nonetheless, these statements can act as a guide for short- and long-term cardiotoxicity surveillance and treatment of cancer patients and survivors.

Children's Oncology Group

The online Children's Oncology Group (COG) Long-Term Follow-Up (LTFU) Guidelines, which were last modified in 2018 (at the time of this writing), provides guidance to healthcare professionals regarding surveillance for organ toxicities related to chemoradiation treatments in the pediatric/young adult population (33). The authors deemed patients at high risk for cardiotoxicity if they received a total cumulative dosing of doxorubicin equivalent of ≥ 250 mg/m^2 in patients. Chest radiation ≥ 35 Gy, in the absence of anthracycline therapy, was also considered a major risk factor for cardiotoxicity. The LTFU guidelines recommend echocardiography as an imaging modality of choice with assessment of ventricular function at baseline, at entry into long-term follow-up, then periodically based on radiation dose, and

Table 2.3 Recommendations for surveillance for cardiac dysfunction according to major societies

Society	Modality of choice	Frequency of LVEF assessment
American Society of Clinical Oncology (ASCO)	1. Echocardiography; MUGA or MRI if echocardiography is not available, with MRI preferred over MUGA	Frequency of surveillance should be determined by the provider based on patient's clinical characteristics
	2. Strain imaging and biomarkers (BNP, troponin) could be considered in conjunction with routine echocardiography	Repeat assessment at 6–12 months after therapy in patients considered at high risk
American Society of Echocardiography (ASE) and European Association of Cardiovascular Imaging (EACVI)	1. Echocardiography, ideally incorporating 3-dimensional imaging and global longitudinal strain	Baseline, end of, and 6 months after therapy associated with type I cardiotoxicity (i.e., anthracyclines)
	2. Consider measuring high-sensitivity troponin in conjunction with imaging	Baseline, every 3 months during therapy associated with type II cardiotoxicity (ie trastuzumab)
European Society for Medical Oncology (ESMO)	1. Echocardiography or MUGA	Baseline, every 3, 6, 9, 12, and 18 months after initiation of treatment
		For patients with metastatic disease, obtain baseline measurement and only repeat if patient develops symptoms of HF
	2. May consider MRI as an alternative	Assessment 4 and 10 years after anthracycline therapy if treated <15 years of age, or >15 years with cumulative dose of >240 mg/m² doxorubicin
European Society of Cardiology (ESC)	1. Echocardiography including 3-dimensional assessment of LVEF and global longitudinal strain	Baseline, every 3 months during therapy (i.e., anthracyclines or trastuzumab) and once after completion
	2. MUGA and MRI may be considered as alterantives	Repeat assessment in 2–3 weeks for any suspected cancer treatment related cardiac dysfunction
Canadian Cardiovascular Society (CCS)	1. Echocardiography including 3-dimensional imaging and strain, MUGA and MRI as alternatives	No specific recommendation
	2. Consider concomitant measurement of biomarkers (BNP, troponin)	
Trastuzumab Labeling	1. Echocardiography or MUGA	Baseline (immediately preceding initiation of trastuzumab), every 3 months during or upon completion of therapy, and at every 6 months for at least 2 years following completion of therapy

Source: Adapted from Florido R et al. J Am Heart Assoc. 2017;6:e006915.
Abbreviations: MUGA, multigated acquisition; MRI, magnetic resonance imaging; BNP, brain natriuretic peptide; LVEF, left ventricular ejection fraction.

cumulative anthracycline dose. In addition, for patients who have received ≥40 Gy of neck radiation, carotid ultrasound is recommended 10 years after treatment to screen for carotid artery disease.

International Late Effects of Childhood Cancer Guidelines

In 2015, the International Late Effects of Childhood Cancer Guideline Harmonization Group attempted to unify different societal consensus statements (North American Children's Oncology Group, Dutch Childhood Oncology Group, UK Children's Cancer and Leukaemia Group, Scottish Intercollegiate Guidelines Network) owing to discordant statements ranging from cutoff doses of anthracyclines deemed to be high risk for developing cardiotoxicity, surveillance imaging modality of choice, as well as frequency of screening in the pediatric/young adult population (34). The total anthracycline cumulative dose considered high risk for developing cardiomyopathy was ≥250 mg/m^2 or a radiation dose of ≥35 Gy chest radiation, or a combination of both treatments with a moderate to high dose of anthracycline (≥100 mg/m^2) and moderate to high dose chest radiation (≥15 Gy). Echocardiography was considered to be the surveillance modality of choice for LV systolic function, but radionuclide angiography and CMR was also reasonable in patients where echocardiography was not technically feasible or optimal. For patients deemed low to high risk, cardiomyopathy surveillance was recommended to begin no later than 2 years after the completion of cardiotoxic therapy, with repeat imaging at 5 years after diagnosis and continued every 5 years afterwards. However, the authors felt that more frequent and life-long cardiomyopathy surveillance was also reasonable for survivors with anthracycline exposure.

European Society of Medical Oncology

Published in 2012, the European Society for Medical Oncology (ESMO) Clinical Practice Guidelines were the product of a multidisciplinary working group that provide guidance on cardiotoxicity surveillance, and a review of known cardiotoxic chemotherapeutics (35). LVEF assessment with echocardiography was regarded as mandatory for baseline cardiac function prior to treatment with potentially cardiotoxic chemotherapy. They also advocated for MUGA and CMR as alternative imaging modalities summarizing their advantages and disadvantages. For echocardiographic protocol, they advised image acquisition by 2D or 3D if available, and assessment of diastolic function and LV volume. At the time this document was written, a "high risk" cumulative dose cutoff of doxorubicin was >500 mg/m^2, which was subsequently lowered in later consensus statements/guidelines from other societies.

For patients receiving anthracycline and/or trastuzumab therapy, it was advised that cardiac function be assessed at baseline, 3, 6, and 9 months during treatments, and then at 12 months and 18 months after the initiation of treatment. The working group acknowledged that limited data were available for elderly patients and "increased vigilance" was recommended for patients ≥60 years old. For patients with metastatic disease, LVEF should be monitored at baseline and then "infrequently" in the absence of symptoms. For long-term cardiotoxicity surveillance, assessment of cardiac function was recommended 4 and 10 years after anthracycline therapy in patients who were treated at <15 years of age, or at age >15 years with a cumulative dose of doxorubicin of >240 mg/m^2 or epirubicin >360 mg/m^2.

During cardiac monitoring, if an LVEF reduction of ≥15% from baseline with normal function (LVEF ≥50%) was noted, anthracyclines and/or trastuzumab could be continued. If LVEF declined to <50% during such treatments, the LVEF should be reassessed after 3 weeks. If the LVEF reduction was confirmed, it was advised to hold chemotherapy and initiate cardioprotective agents with frequent clinical and echocardiographic evaluation. If the LVEF decreased to <40%, it was advised that chemotherapy stop and alternatives be considered, along with initiation of treatment for LV dysfunction.

American Society of Clinical Oncology

In 2016, the American Society of Clinical Oncology (ASCO) published their Clinical Practice Guideline in the Prevention and Monitoring of Cardiac Dysfunction in Survivors of Adult Cancers. An expert panel conducted a systematic review of 104 studies, which comprised of meta-analyses, randomized clinical trials, observational studies, and clinical experience from 1996 to 2016 (36). This ASCO document is notable because the threshold considered high risk for cardiotoxicity was lowered to a doxorubicin cumulative dose of $\geq$250 mg/m^2 or an epirubicin cumulative dose of $\geq$600 mg/m^2. In addition, high-dose radiotherapy (RT) with a total dose of $\geq$30 Gy where the heart is in the treatment field, or a combination of anthracycline and chest RT at any dose was considered high risk for cardiotoxicity as well.

Echocardiography is the preferred diagnostic imaging modality for workup of cardiac dysfunction. CMR and MUGA can be considered if echocardiography is not available or technically feasible, with preference given to CMR. Although there are no specific recommendations of frequency of cardiovascular imaging during treatments, it was recommended that an echocardiogram be performed between 6 and 12 months after completion of cancer-directed therapy in asymptomatic patients considered to be at increased risk of cardiotoxicity.

Canadian Cardiovascular Society

In their 2016 society guidelines, the Canadian Cardiovascular Society (CCS) recommended that patients who received potentially cardiotoxic cancer therapy undergo LVEF assessment before initiation of treatments (37). The same imaging modality should be used to determine LVEF before, during, and after completion of therapy. For those undergoing echocardiographic imaging, myocardial strain imaging be considered as a tool to assist in detecting subclinical cardiotoxicity. They determined that a relative percentage reduction in GLS of <8% was likely not clinically significant, whereas a relative reduction of >15% was likely to be abnormal. The CCS also preferred the use of 3D echocardiography whenever feasible and technically satisfactory (37). The intervals of imaging were not specified in this document.

European Society of Cardiology

The ESC published an ESC Position Paper on cancer treatments and cardiovascular toxicity in 2016. The ESC Task Force determined echocardiography to be the method of choice in the detection of myocardial dysfunction before, during, and after cancer therapy (10). They advocated for 3D echocardiography if endocardial definition was optimal, and for performing 2D biplane Simpson

method if 3D imaging was not available or was suboptimal.

The task force determined that any significant decrease in LVEF (>10%) to a value that does not drop below the lower limit of normal (defined as an LVEF of 50%), should undergo repeated LVEF assessment shortly after and over the duration of cancer treatment. If LVEF decreases >10% to a value below the lower limit of normal, medical treatment should be initiated. The ESC also recommended considering an LVEF assessment at baseline, every 3 months during treatment, and at the end of treatment with either anthracyclines or trastuzumab. While they supported long-term surveillance after cancer treatment, no specific frequency was recommended.

American Society of Echocardiography/European Association of Cardiovascular Imaging

The ASE and European Association of Cardiovascular Imaging (EACVI) released a joint expert consensus statement in 2014, providing a proposed cardio-oncology echocardiography protocol (Table 2.4), and cardiotoxicity surveillance intervals based on the types of chemotherapeutic agents being used (5). The classifications of CTRCD were divided into "Type I" (associated with anthracycline use and permanent/irreversible myocardial damage if not treated) and "Type II" CTRCD (associated with trastuzumab and tyrosine kinase inhibitors, which is more reversible with discontinuation of therapy and/or initiation of treatment). Although this classification system is oversimplified and may not be applicable to a variety of other novel cancer treatments (i.e., targeted therapies, immunotherapy), the document focuses on more commonly used treatments with known cardiotoxic profiles. Further research efforts are needed to document short- and long-term cardiovascular outcomes for current and future cancer therapy agents in order to provide a more nuanced, accurate classification system for physicians to provide adequate imaging surveillance for cancer patients during and after their treatments.

For patients undergoing treatments associated with potential irreversible (Type I) cardiotoxicity, it is advised to obtain an LVEF assessment at baseline, at the end of treatment, and 6 months later for doxorubicin equivalent doses of <240 mg/m^2, along with serial biomarker assessments. For doses

Table 2.4 ASE/EACVI recommended cardio-oncology echocardiogram protocol

- Standard transthoracic echocardiography
  - In accordance with ASE/EAE guidelines and IAC-Echo
- 2D strain imaging acquisition
  - Apical three-, four-, and two-chamber views
- Acquire ≥3 cardiac cycles
  - Images obtained simultaneously maintaining the same 2D frame rate and imaging depth
    - Frame rate between 40 and 90 frames/sec or ≥40% of HR
  - Aortic VTI (aortic ejection time)
- 2D strain imaging analysis
  - Quantify segmental and global strain (GLS)
  - Display the segmental strain curves from apical views in a quad format
  - Display the global strain in a bull's-eye plot
- 2D strain imaging pitfalls
  - Ectopy
  - Breathing translation
- 3D imaging acquisition
  - Apical four-chamber full volume to assess LV volumes and LVEF calculation
  - Single and multiple beats optimizing spatial and temporal resolution
- Reporting
  - Timing of echocardiography with respect to the IV infusion (number of days before or after)
- Vital signs (BP, HR)
- 3D LVEF/2D biplane Simpson's method
- GLS (echocardiography machine, software, and version used)
- In the absence of GLS, measurement of medial and lateral s' and MAPSE
- RV: TAPSE, s', FAC

Source: Adapted from Plana JC et al. *J Am Soc Echocardiogr.* 2014;27:911–39.
Abbreviations: ASE/EACVI, American Society of Echocardiography/European Association of Cardiovascular Imaging; BP, blood pressure; FAC, fractional area change; HR, heart rate; IAC-Echo, Intersocietal Accreditation Commission Echocardiography; MAPSE, mitral annular plane systolic excursion; TAPSE, tricuspid annular plane systolic excursion; RV, right ventricle; VTI, velocity-time integral.

that exceed 240 mg/m², LVEF assessment is advised prior to each additional 50 mg/m². In addition, the ASE/EACVI consensus statement prefers that 3D echocardiography be used for LVEF assessment; however, if this is not feasible, contrast echocardiography with GLS and troponin-I assessment can be considered. Cardiology consultation is advised for a reduction in LVEF to <53%, abnormal GLS value, and/or elevation in troponin levels. If abnormal LVEF values are seen during surveillance, CMR was advised for confirmation of LV dysfunction.

For patients who are receiving cancer treatments with potentially reversible (Type II) cardiotoxicity, such as trastuzumab, or following treatment associated with potentially irreversible cardiotoxicity, LVEF/GLS/troponin-I assessment is advised at baseline and every 3 months until treatment is finished. Long-term surveillance is not advised. As

with the CCS guidelines, a GLS relative percentage decrease of <8% was unlikely to be clinically significant, where as a relative percentage decrease of >15% was concerning for subclinical cardiotoxicity.

Although the document now advocates for echocardiography as the first line imaging modality of choice for cardiotoxicity surveillance, it also does mention historical proposed surveillance intervals for anthracycline induced cardiotoxicity with MUGA imaging (12):

1. LVEF >50% at baseline
   a. Measurement at 250–300 mg/m²
   b. Measurement at 450 mg/m²
   c. Measurement before each dose above 450 mg/m²
   d. Discontinue therapy if LVEF decreases by ≥10% from baseline and LVEF ≤50%

2. LVEF <50% at baseline
   a. Do not treat if LVEF is <30%
   b. Serial measurement before each dose
   c. Discontinue therapy if LVEF decreases by ≥10% from baseline or LVEF ≤30%

The document does not give recommendations for long term surveillance in cancer survivors.

In a separate document for patients undergoing radiotherapy, the ASE/EACVI Expert Consensus for Multi-Modality Imaging Evaluation of Cardiovascular Complications of Radiotherapy in Adults was released in 2013 (22). Patients at high risk for developing radiation-induced heart disease (RIHD) included the following risk factors:

- Anterior or left chest irradiation location, with one or more of the following risk factors:
  - High cumulative dose of radiation (>30 Gy)
  - Younger patients (<50 years)
  - High dose of radiation fractions (>2 Gy/day)
  - Presence and extent of tumor in or next of the heart
  - Lack of shielding
  - Concomitant chemotherapy (i.e., anthracyclines cause considerably higher risk)
  - Cardiovascular risk factors (i.e., diabetes mellitus, smoking, obesity, moderate hypertension, hypercholesteremia)
  - Preexisting cardiovascular disease.

Because of the complex and extensive effects of chest radiation exposure, including macro- and microvascular injury, valvular dysfunction, progressive myocardial fibrosis, and pericardial disease (38), the document discusses the indications of multiple imaging modalities, including echocardiography, CMR, cardiac computed tomography angiography (CTA), and functional stress testing for specific disease states related to RIHD. However, the frequency and imaging modality of choice in screening for subclinical/clinical RIHD is overall unclear; owing to the relative paucity of evidence, the authors recommend yearly targeted clinical history and physical exam of patients who have received chest radiation exposure. For asymptomatic patients, it was reasonable to perform screening echocardiography to evaluate for overall manifestations of RIHD 5 years after exposure in high-risk patients, and 10 years after exposure in other patients. In high-risk patients, functional

noninvasive stress testing for CAD detection 5–10 years after exposure was reasonable, with reassessment every 5 years.

For other cardiovascular manifestations, including valvular disease, if a cardiac murmur is heard, then echocardiography is indicated with serial imaging as per cardiology guidelines; if neurological symptoms are noted, then carotid ultrasonography is indicated, although frequency of surveillance and when to initiate it for these specific disease states are not known. For suspected pericardial constriction from radiation, CMR was indicated. Workup for suspected angina/ischemia include echocardiography and functional noninvasive stress testing, or invasive testing depending on clinical assessment.

American Society of Nuclear Cardiology

In 2016, the American Society of Nuclear Cardiology (ASNC) published an information statement reviewing the cardiotoxic effects of cancer treatments and a review specifically focused on applications of nuclear cardiology technologies (39). The statement refers to a variety of prior guidelines, including the ESMO Clinical Practice Guidelines and the COG Long Term Follow-Up Guidelines as previously discussed in recommendations on LVEF assessment during and after cancer treatment both in children and adults.

Society of Cardiovascular Angiography and Interventions

In 2016, the Society of Cardiovascular Angiography and Interventions (SCAI) released an expert consensus statement, which provided recommendations on pharmacologic and interventional management of cancer patients with cardiotoxicity, and/or preexisting or acquired atherosclerotic cardiovascular disease (ASCVD) (2). In addition, it also gave expert opinion recommendations on patients receiving specific kinds of radiation therapy that may affect the extracardiac vasculature. Although data on long-term event rates are limited, ABIs and carotid ultrasonography was advised—every 5 years for the latter posttreatment—particularly in patients at elevated ASCVD risk and who received radiation therapy to the neck area (i.e., lymphoma, head and neck cancers). Chemotherapy agents such as cisplatin, nilotinib, and ponatinib were considered to be high risk agents for arterial/venous thrombotic disease. The SCAI document advises consideration of noninvasive imaging modalities such as carotid ultrasound, as well as MRI for cerebrovascular disease and CT aortography for peripheral arterial disease assessment in patients who received agents such as nilotinib and ponatinib.

Similar to the ASE/EACVI expert consensus statements, SCAI recommends that patients who received RT undergo screening echocardiography every 5 years for high-risk patients, and every 10 years for patients with no RIHD risk factors. The document also advocated for consideration of cardiac CT angiography as an alternative to functional exercise stress testing every 5 years after RT, or an additional early evaluation at 2 years if RT was performed at >60 years of age, if the patient had known CAD, or had one or more cardiovascular risk factors.

CONCLUSIONS

There have been many technological advances made in the field of echocardiography, including the advent of 3D imaging, and strain imaging which has allowed for more precise LVEF assessment and less dependence on imaging modalities that required radiation exposure (i.e., MUGA). Echocardiography has largely supplanted MUGA as the test of choice in cardiotoxicity surveillance owing to improvements in imaging quality, as well as being able to provide information on chamber size, valvular function, and the presence of pericardial disease without exposing the patient to ionizing radiation. CMR has now allowed for superior imaging with visualization of pericardial and valvular disease, and there is ongoing interest in developing techniques to assess for subclinical/clinical cardiotoxicity with patterns of gadolinium enhancement in the myocardium. Other advanced imaging modalities, such as cardiac CT angiography, may be useful in selected patients for assessment of atherosclerotic disease but have limited utility in this population. Arterial/venous ultrasounds remain useful in detecting thrombotic complications of cancer and their treatments, as well as sequelae of chemoradiation. However, the frequency and duration of clinical utilization, as well as cost

effectiveness of these imaging modalities, continues to remain a question and an area of ongoing research and interest. Further investigations are warranted in refining the definition of cardiotoxicity, and determining the ideal duration and method of surveillance with the armamentarium of advanced imaging modalities that are available—which will continue to evolve (40).

As cancer treatments continue to develop at a rapid pace, resulting in growing cancer survival rates, precise imaging modalities are critical in detecting preexisting and acquired cardiovascular disease with treatments. It is essential that cardio-oncologists be cognizant of the dynamic nature of multimodality imaging and society-endorsed cardiotoxicity surveillance recommendations for this unique population. In doing so, we can provide the most evidence-based care to cancer patients, ideally enable the continuation of critical cancer treatments, and prevent and/or minimize cardiovascular toxicity in the growing cancer survivor population.

REFERENCES

1. Svilass T, Lefrand JD, Gietema JA, Kamphuisen PA. Long-term arterial complications of chemotherapy in patients with cancer. *Thromb Res.* 2016;140S1:S109–18.
2. Iliescu CA et al. SCAI expert consensus statement: Evaluation, management, and special considerations of cardio-oncology patients in the cardiac catheterization laboratory (Endorsed by the Cardiological Society of India, and Sociedad Latino Americana de Cardiologia Intervencionista). *Catheter Cardiovasc Interv.* 2016;87(5):E202–23.
3. Herrmann J et al. Vascular toxicities of cancer therapies, the old and the new- an evolving avenue. *Circulation.* 2016;133:1272–89.
4. Lennernas B, Albertsson P, Lennernas H, Norrby K. Chemotherapy and antiangiogenesis—drug specific, dose related effects. *Acta Oncol.* 2003;42(4):294–303.
5. Plana, JC et al. Expert consensus for multimodality imaging evaluation of adult patients during and after cancer therapy: A report from the American Society of Echocardiography and the European Association of Cardiovascular Imaging. *J Am Soc Echocardiogr.* 2014;27(9):911–39

6. Dorup I, Levitt G, Sullivan ISK. Prospective longitudinal assessment of late anthracycline cardiotoxicity after childhood cancer: The role of diastolic function. *Heart.* 2004;90(10):1214–6.

7. Thavendiranathan P, Grant AD, Negishi T, Plana JC, Popović ZBMT. Reproducibility of echocardiographic techniques for sequential assessment of left ventricular ejection fraction and volumes: Application to patients undergoing cancer chemotherapy. *J Am Coll Cardiol.* 2013;61(1):77–84.

8. Florido R, Smith KL, Cuomo KK, Russell SD. Cardiotoxicity from human epidermal growth factor receptor-2 (HER2) target therapies. *J Am Heart Assoc.* 2017;6:e006915.

9. Thavendiranathan P, Poulin F, Lim KD, Plana JC, Woo A, Marwick THJ. Use of myocardial strain imaging by echocardiography for the early detection of cardiotoxicity in patients during and after cancer chemotherapy: A systematic review. *J Am Coll Cardiol.* 2014;63(25 Pt A):2751–68.

10. Zamorano JL et al. 2016 ESC position paper on cancer treatments and cardiovascular toxicity developed under the auspices of the ESC Committee for Practice Guidelines: The Task Force for cancer treatments and cardiovascular toxicity of the European Society of Cardiology. *Eur Hear J.* 2016;37(36):2768–801.

11. Sawaya H et al. Assessment of echocardiography and biomarkers for the extended prediction of cardiotoxicity in patients treated with anthracyclines, taxanes, and trastuzumab. *Circ Cardiovasc Imaging.* 2012;5(5):596–603.

12. Schwartz RG, McKenzie WB AJ. Congestive heart failure and left ventricular dysfunction complication doxorubicin therapy: Seven-year experience using serial radionuclide angiocardiography. *Am J Med.* 1987;82:1109–18.

13. van Royen N, Jaffe CC, Krumholz HM, Johnson KM, Lynch PJ, Natale D, Atkinson P, Deman PWF. Comparison and reproducibility of visual echocardiographic and quantitative radionuclide left ventricular ejection fractions. *Am J Cardiol.* 1996;77(10):843–50.

14. Hendel RC et al. ACCF/ACR/SCCT/SCMR/ASNC/NASCI/SCAI/SIR 2006 appropriateness criteria for cardiac computed tomography and cardiac magnetic resonance imaging: A report of the American College of Cardiology Foundation Quality Strategic Directions Committee appropriateness C. *J Am Coll Cardiol.* 2006;48(7):1475–97.

15. FDA Drug Safety Warning. FDA warns that gadolinium-based contrast agents (GBCAs) are retained in the body; requires new class warning. Available from: https://www.fda.gov/Drugs/DrugSafety/ucm589213.htm. Last accessed June 4, 2018.

16. Neilan TG et al. Left ventricular mass in patients with a cardiomyopathy after treatment with anthracyclines. *Am J Cardiol.* 2012;110(11):1679–86.

17. Zagrosek A, Abdel-Aty H, Boye P, Wassmuth R, Messroghli DUW. Cardiac magnetic resonance monitors reversible and irreversible myocardial injury in myocarditis. *JACC Cardiovasc Imaging.* 2009;2:131–8.

18. Neilan TG et al. Myocardial extracellular volume by cardiac magnetic resonance imaging in patients treated with anthracycline-based chemotherapy. *Am J Cardiol.* 2013;111(5):717–22.

19. Fallah-Rad N, Lytwyn M, Fang T, Kirkpatrick IJD. Delayed contrast enhancement cardiac magnetic resonance imaging in trastuzumab induced cardiomyopathy. *J Cardiovasc Magn Reson.* 2008;10(5).

20. Carver JR et al. American society of clinical oncology clinical evidence review on the ongoing care of adult cancer survivors: Cardiac and pulmonary late effects. *J Clin Oncol.* 2007;25(25):3991–4008.

21. Mulrooney DA et al. Coronary artery disease detected by coronary computed tomography angiography in adult survivors of childhood Hodgkin lymphoma. *Cancer.* 2014;120(22):3536–44.

22. Lancellotti P et al. Expert consensus for multimodality imaging evaluation of cardiovascular complications of radiotherapy in adults: A report from the European Association of Cardiovascular Imaging and the American Society of Echocardiography. *Eur Hear J Cardiovasc Imaging.* 2013;14(8):721–40.

23. Nony P et al. In vivo measurement of myocardial oxidative metabolism and blood flow

does not show changes in cancer patients undergoing doxorubicin therapy. *Cancer Chemother Pharmacol.* 2000;45(5):375–80.

24. Borde C, Kand PBS. Enhanced myocardial fluorodeoxyglucose uptake following adriamycin-based therapy: Evidence of early chemotherapeutic cardiotoxicity? *World J Radiol.* 2012;4(5):220–3.

25. Anderson R et al. Relation of coronary artery calcium score to premature coronary artery disease in survivors >15 years of Hodgkin's lymphoma. *Am J Cardiol.* January 15, 2010;105(2):149–52.

26. Ross CTG et al. Is the coronary artery calcium score associated with acute coronary events in breast cancer patients treated with radiotherapy? *Radiother Oncol.* 2018 January;126(1):170–6.

27. Holm Tjessem K et al. Coronary calcium score is 12-year breast cancer survivors after adjuvant radiotherapy with low to moderate heart exposure-Relationship to cardiac radiation dose and cardiovascular risk factors. *Radiother Oncol.* March 2015;114(3):328–34.

28. Cury RC et al. Comprehensive assessment of myocardial perfusion defects, regional wall motion, and left ventricular function by using 64-section multidetector CT. *Radiology.* 2008;248(2):466–75.

29. Detrano R et al. Coronary calcium as a predictor of coronary events in four racial or ethnic groups. *N Engl J Med.* 2008;358(13):1336–45.

30. Pellerito JS, Polak JF. *Introduction to Vascular Ultrasonography.* 6th ed., Elsevier Saunders, 2012.

31. Stein JH, Korcarz CE, Hurst RT et al. Use of carotid ultrasound to identify subclinical vasuclar disease and evaluate cadioascular disease risk: A consensus statement from the American Society of Echocardiography Carotid Intima-Media Thickness Task Force endorsed by the Society of Vascular Medicine. *J Am Soc Echocardiogr* 2008; 21(2):93–111.

32. Jacoby D et al. Carotid intima-media thickness measurement promises to improve cardiovascular risk evaluation in head and neck cancer patients. *Clin Cardiol.* May 2015;38(5):280–4.

33. Children's Oncology Group Long-Term Follow-Up Guidelines. Version 5.0, October 2018. Available from: http://www.survivor-shipguidelines.org/pdf/2018/COG_LTFU_Guidelines_v5.pdf. Last accessed May 27, 2019

34. Armenian SH et al. Recommendations for cardiomyopathy surveillance for survivors of childhood cancer: A report from the International Late Effects of Childhood Cancer Guideline Harmonization Group. *Lancet Oncol.* 2015;16:e123–36.

35. Curigliano G et al. Cardiovascular toxicity induced by chemotherapy, targeted agents and radiotherapy: ESMO clinical practice guidelines. *Ann Oncol.* 2012;23(Suppl 7):vii155–66.

36. Armenian SH et al. Prevention and monitoring of cardiac dysfunction in survivors of adult cancers: American Society of Clinical Oncology Practice Guideline. *J Clin Onc.* 2016;35:893–911.

37. Virani SA et al. Canadian Cardiovascular Society guidelines for evaluation and management of cardiovascular complications of cancer therapy. *Can J Cardiol.* 2016;32:831–41.

38. Veinot JP, Edwards WD. Pathology of radiation-induced heart disease: A surgical and autopsy study of 27 cases. *Hum Pathol.* 1996;27:766–73.

39. Russell RR et al. ASNC information statement: The role and clinical effectiveness of multimodality imaging in the management of cardiac complications of cancer and cancer therapy. *J Nucl Cardiol.* 2016;23(4):856–84.

40. Khouri MG, Douglas PS, Mackey JR, Martin M, Scott JM, Scherrer-Crosbie M. Cancer therapy-induced cardiac toxicity in early breast cancer: Addressing the unresolved issues. *Circulation.* 2012;126:2749–63.

3

Approach to risk stratification in cardio-oncology

CHRISTOPHER B. JOHNSON, GARY SMALL, ANGELINE LAW,
AND HABIBAT GARUBA

PREDICTING LEFT VENTRICULAR DYSFUNCTION FOLLOWING CANCER THERAPY: CLINICAL RISK FACTORS

Case 1

A 50-year-old female has stage III, HER-2 neu positive breast cancer of the left breast. Her past medical history includes hypertension, type II diabetes and a history of coronary disease with a stent inserted in her right coronary artery 3 years ago after presenting with a non-ST segment elevation Myocardial infarction (MI). She is sedentary, but reports no cardiac symptoms during her daily activities. Her cardiovascular exam is notable for systolic hypertension with a blood pressure (BP) of 160/75, abdominal obesity with a waste circumference of 112 cm and body mass index (BMI) of 34.

Her medications include: aspirin 81 mg daily, atorvastatin 80 mg daily, perindopril 4 mg daily, and metformin 1000 mg twice daily. She is treated with three cycles of fluorouracil, epirubicin, cyclophosphamide (FEC) followed by three cycles of taxane-based chemotherapy, cancer surgery, and radiation therapy. Her pretreatment echocardiogram reveals an ejection fraction (EF) of 55%. Her echocardiogram after chemotherapy, prior to starting HER-2 targeted therapy, reveals an EF of 45%, prompting a cardiology referral.

Case 2

A second 50-year-old female also has stage III, HER-2 neu positive breast cancer of the left breast. She has no history of cardiovascular disease, no cardiovascular risk factors, and is an active half marathon runner who follows a vegetarian diet.

Her cardiac exam is normal with a BP of 106/74, a waist circumference of 74 cm and a BMI of 22. She receives treatment with three cycles of FEC followed by three cycles of taxane-based chemotherapy, cancer surgery, and radiation therapy. Her pretreatment echocardiogram reveals an EF of 70%, and her postchemotherapy echocardiogram reports an EF of 60%. After three cycles of trastuzumab, her EF is 40%, prompting interruption of trastuzumab and cardiology referral.

In spite of an ever increasing range of targeted cancer therapies, many adults and children with cancer will receive an anthracycline as part of their oncological treatment. Anthracyclines have long been associated with cardiotoxicity, and their role in causing cardiotoxicity has been extensively studied (1–3). Risk factors for anthracycline induced cardiotoxicity include clinical and cancer treatment related risk factors (Table 3.1) (4–11). Risk calculators familiar to cardiologists and primary care doctors, such as the Framingham risk score, may not reliably estimate the risk of cardiotoxicity in cancer patients (12). However, randomized controlled trial and registry data have been used to predict the risk of cardiotoxicity in cancer patients as depicted in Table 3.2 (13,14).

Returning to our cases, the first patient has underlying coronary disease and multiple cardiac risk factors, including several clinical factors that are known to increase the likelihood of cardiotoxicity after anthracycline exposure. The approach of Romond, which relies only on age and baseline EF to predict risk, estimates a very low risk of cardiotoxicity in spite of her multiple risk factors, a finding that does not match our clinical judgement that this patient has a high risk of cardiotoxicity (13). In contrast, the approach reported by Ezaz (Table 3.2) incorporates several of the variables that have been associated with an increased risk of cardiotoxicity (11,14). When we apply the method described by Ezaz, the first patient receives 6 points (2 for anthracycline, 2 for CAD, 1 for diabetes, and 1 for hypertension), suggesting a 39.5% risk of congestive heart failure (CHF) or cardiotoxicity at 3 years. This fits with our clinical judgment that this is a patient at high risk of cardiotoxicity following cancer therapy. Both risk calculators provide estimates of long-term cardiovascular events,

Table 3.1 Risk factors for anthracycline induced cardiotoxicity

Cancer therapy related	Cumulative lifetime dose
	Radiation therapy to the heart
	Concomitant cancer therapy
Patient related	Extremes of age (<5 or >65 years of age)
	Underlying CAD, AF, cardiomyopathy
	Hypertension
	Renal disease
	Female gender
	Genetic

Abbreviations: CAD, coronary artery disease; AF, atrial fibrillation.

Table 3.2 Cardiotoxicity risk in breast cancer patients treated with trastuzumab

Risk score variable and points	Risk category	Rate of CHF at 3 years
Anthracycline = 2	Low risk (0–3 points)	16.2%
Age ≥80 = 2		
Age 75–79 = 1		
Coronary artery disease = 2	Medium risk (4–5 points)	26.0%
Atrial fibrillation = 2		
Diabetes = 1		
Hypertension = 1	High risk (6+ points)	39.5%
Renal failure = 2		

Source: Romond EH et al. *J Clin Oncol.* 2012;30:3792–9.

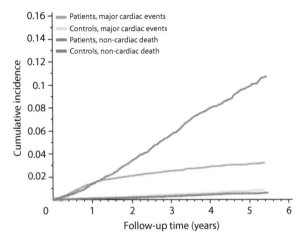

Figure 3.1 Incidence of cardiac events in Ontario breast cancer patients <65 years of age. (From Thavendiranathan P et al. *J Clin Oncol*. July 1, 2016;34[19]:2239–46.)

which is related to the follow-up period used to derive each risk calculator: 3 years of SEER database follow-up for the Ezaz calculator, and 7 years follow-up of a randomized trial for the calculation used by Romond (13). In randomized trials and in real world practice, most of the excess cardiovascular risk attributable to anthracyclines and targeted cancer agents is concentrated in the first one or two years after cancer therapy (Figure 3.1) (15,16). Risk calculators derived from long-term follow-up data are valid tools to help clinicians risk stratify patients for cardiotoxicity risk. Such calculators have the potential to identify patients who may warrant more intensive cardiac monitoring and possibly referral to cardiologists with expertise in cardio-oncology.

Case 2 illustrates the limitation of using clinical variables alone to identify patients at increased risk for cardiotoxicity: The risk is lower for relatively young patients without cardiac disease or risk factors, but low risk is not zero risk. When we apply the Ezaz approach to Case 2, the patient receives 2 points for anthracycline exposure and no other points, suggesting a 16% risk of cardiomyopathy or heart failure at 3 years, with most of this risk concentrated in the first year after cancer therapy exposure. Unfortunately, patients with a low risk clinical profile still experience cardiotoxicity related to their cancer therapy resulting in referral to a cardio-oncology clinic. While our second case has half the risk of the first case, most patients would not accept a 16% risk of cardiomyopathy or heart failure. Most clinical providers monitor cardiac function when

young, healthy patients receive anthracycline cancer therapy, especially when targeted agents are subsequently administered.

CARDIAC BIOMARKERS IN RISK STRATIFICATION

Cardiac biomarkers can detect myocardial injury and predict cardiotoxicity following exposure to anthracycline chemotherapy. The group led by Dr. Cardinale used an intensive schedule of troponin I (TnI) blood tests to detect myocardial injury after high dose chemotherapy, including anthracycline (17). By drawing five blood samples during the first 72 hours after each chemotherapy dose, up to 30% of patients had TnI levels above the detection limit (17). Patients with persistently elevated TnI after chemotherapy had a higher risk of cardiac events related to reduced left ventricular (LV) function (Figure 3.2). Conversely, persistently negative TnIs reliably identified patients at low risk for cardiac events (Figure 3.2). Given their relatively low cost, biomarkers such as TnI are an attractive strategy to detect early myocardial injury following anthracycline exposure, thereby identifying patients who might benefit from cardiac pharmacotherapy to reduce the risk of long-term cardiotoxicity (18). Negative troponins are associated with low cardiotoxicity risk, and may identify patients who do not require intensive cardiac monitoring (17–19).

Positive troponins following oncological treatment are typically low level troponin values, above the lower detection limit, but often below

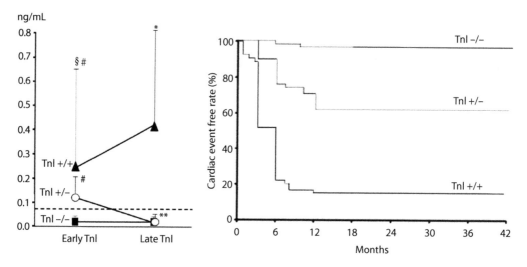

Figure 3.2 Troponins and cardiac events following high dose cancer therapy. (From Cardinale D et al. *Circulation*. June 8, 2004;109[22]:2749–54.)

thresholds generally observed in myocardial infarction in patients presenting with acute coronary syndrome. A number of publications using this approach report clinically valuable predictive ability. However, if the threshold for abnormal is set too low, particularly with very sensitive troponin assays, the utility of this approach in risk stratifying patients may be lost. For example, a recent study detected low level abnormal troponins in 90% of patients after completing a course of dose-dense doxorubicin chemotherapy (20). This is more than three times the rate of abnormal troponin reported in most of the cardio-oncology literature. These data remind us that collaboration with local biochemistry labs is essential to choose cutoffs for troponins that optimize sensitivity and specificity for cardiotoxicity prediction. Once implemented, cutoffs for abnormal troponin may require calibration to ensure clinically useful prediction of cardiotoxicity after cancer therapy exposure.

A second crucial issue is how many troponins should be assayed per patient, per cycle of anthracycline chemotherapy. In a recent trial, 50% of patients only had one, transient troponin abnormality (18). Previous work has demonstrated that transient troponin elevations are worse than never having an elevated troponin, but the highest risk patients are those with persistently abnormal troponins (17). Detection rates for troponin increase if several samples are drawn with each treatment cycle, and detection rates are higher after several

courses of anthracycline (21–23). Troponins may be detected for up to several weeks after an anthracycline has been administered (21).

The final factor to consider in interpreting troponins in the setting of oncology is that troponins can be positive prior to any cancer therapy, in patients without primary cardiac disease and in the absence of a recent or acute cardiac event. Baseline rates of abnormal troponin in oncology populations vary from 3.8% to 4.2% (21–23). How to interpret baseline abnormal troponin values in the context of cardiotoxicity prediction, and whether a baseline troponin should be obtained in all patients, are questions to consider when using troponins to detect cardiotoxicity and to risk stratify patients.

Anthracyclines, not targeted therapies, appear to be the main cause of troponin elevations in oncology patients. A multicenter trial that combined biomarkers and echocardiography noted that the highest average level of TnI is detected soon after anthracycline exposure, and that troponin values decline during subsequent trastuzumab therapy (19). A substudy of HERA with troponin TnI I and troponin T (TnT) measured after each anthracycline cycle and during subsequent trastuzumab, reveals that virtually all positive troponins occur after anthracycline but before any trastuzumab has been administered (24). Very few initial abnormal troponins are detected within the first cycles of trastuzumab. In this study, 14% of patients had an abnormal TnI after completing their course of anthracycline, with only an additional 1.4% of initially TnI negative patients having their first abnormal TnI detected during treatment with trastuzumab, typically within the first few trastuzumab cycles (24). In the same study, 24.5% of patients had an abnormal TnT after anthracycline chemotherapy, and only an additional 6% developed an abnormal TnT during their initial exposure to trastuzumab, again usually within the first several doses of trastuzumab (24). Similar to Cardinale's data, an abnormal troponin after anthracycline but before trastuzumab predicts subsequent cardiotoxicity defined as a drop in EF by 10 units to less than 50, with a hazard ratio (HR) of 4.47 (2.42–8.24, $p < 0.001$) for TnI and HR of 3.59 (1.95–6.58, $p < 0.001$) for TnT (17,18,24). The most convincing evidence that targeted therapies do not result in troponin release, unless there has been prior anthracycline exposure, comes from a substudy of a clinical trial of non-anthracycline cancer therapy (25). Patients with no prior anthracycline exposure had three TnT samples drawn during therapy with either trastuzumab or lapatinib. There was one patient with a baseline abnormal TnT before any cancer treatment, but no new TnT detections occurred over three samples per patient during a course of therapy with trastuzumab or lapatinib (25).

This overview of how TnI and TnT behave after exposure to cancer therapy should guide clinicians in incorporating troponins into cardiotoxicity risk stratification strategies. Table 3.3 summarizes the issues that must be addressed when incorporating troponins into cardiotoxicity detection and risk stratification protocols. Further research is needed to determine optimal timing, number of samples, and cutoffs for troponins. Practical considerations related to local resources and patient convenience typically determine how biomarkers are incorporated into cardiotoxicity risk stratification.

CARDIAC IMAGING IN CARDIOTOXICITY RISK STRATIFICATION: ASSESSMENT OF EJECTION FRACTION

Imaging detection of cardiac dysfunction has a critical role to play in identifying cardiotoxicity, and recent technology may permit very early identification of altered cardiac function following cancer therapy. The first cardiac imaging technology applied to cardiotoxicity monitoring was radionuclide angiography (7). By detecting reductions in EF after anthracyclines using radionuclide angiography, anthracycline therapy could be stopped prior to onset of clinical congestive heart failure (7,8). Definitions of cardiotoxicity based on serial EF changes and absolute EF thresholds were proposed in the context of EF monitoring during anthracycline chemotherapy (26–28). While radionuclide angiography remains a reproducible technique for serial EF monitoring, this technology has largely been replaced by echocardiography, which has the advantage of eliminating exposure to ionizing radiation while obtaining reproducible EF

Table 3.3 Factors to consider when using troponins for early detection of cardiotoxicity

	Specificity: "Rule-in cardiotoxicity"	Sensitivity: "Rule-out cardiotoxicity"	Patient convenience	Cost
Troponin sample late after AC cycle	++++	+	++++	++++
Troponin sample early after AC cycle	++	++++	++++	++++
Multiple troponins/AC cycle	+	++++	+	+
One troponin/AC cycle	++	+	++++	++++
Low threshold for abnormal troponin	+	++++	+	++
High threshold for abnormal troponin	+++	+	++	++

Note: This table illustrates factors that must be considered when designing a cardiotoxicity detection and prediction algorithm using cardiac troponins. The ideal system would use the fewest troponin blood samples drawn at time points and interpreted using thresholds for abnormal that maximize sensitivity & specificity at the lowest cost. Such a system has yet to be established, leaving clinicians to weight the relative importance of each factor in light of local constraints on troponin blood testing. ++++ Very favorable; +++ Favorable; ++ Neutral; + Unfavorable.

Abbreviations: AC, anthracycline chemotherapy.

Table 3.4 Definitions of reversibility of cancer therapy-related cardiac dysfunction (CTRCD)

Reversible	Improvement to within 5% of baseline LVEF
Partially reversible	Improvement by ≥10% from the nadir but still <5% of baseline
Irreversible	Improvement by <10% from the nadir and remaining <5% of baseline
Indeterminate	Patient unavailable for reevaluation

Source: Data from Plana et al. *J Am Soc Echocardiogr.* September 1, 2014 [cited February 19, 2018]; 27(9):911–39.

measurements during cancer therapy (29,30). The recognition of clinical congestive heart failure during treatment with the targeted agent trastuzumab prompted implementation of a schedule of regular EF monitoring in clinical trials, and this monitoring schedule has been adopted into clinical practice today (31).

In addition to detecting ejection fraction drops in order to identify patients at risk for heart failure, definitions of cardiotoxicity are largely based on changes in ejection fraction. In 2014, a consensus statement by the American Society of Echocardiography (ASE) and the European Association of Cardiovascular Imaging (EACI) sought to define cardiotoxicity (32). Cancer therapeutic-related cardiac dysfunction (CRTCD) was defined as a decrease in the left ventricular ejection fraction (LVEF) of greater than 10% to a value <53%, an EF value that is the lower limit of normal (32,33). Repeat cardiac imaging is recommended within 2–3 weeks of the baseline diagnostic study demonstrating the decrease in LVEF, with additional classification based on reversibility, an issue of particular importance for targeted therapies such as trastuzumab (Table 3.4). While different EF thresholds have been reported in various research and clinical settings, the concept that a serial drop in EF to a final value below a threshold appears to identify patients at risk for congestive heart failure, and this appears to hold for any cancer therapy agent that can impair LV systolic function (8,34).

LVEF is the most commonly used parameter to evaluate and monitor LV function with echocardiography. Imaging at baseline is particularly important in patients whose history or clinical presentation suggest underlying LV systolic dysfunction, and in patients with high risk of cardiac events based on traditional risk factors for cardiovascular disease: hypertension, dyslipidemia, cigarette smoking, diabetes, and family history of premature coronary artery disease (CAD) (35).

Baseline evaluations are necessary to compare follow-up studies to facilitate detection of clinically important LVEF changes, particularly as changes in EF are key components in most definitions of cardiotoxicity. Current guidelines recommend calculation of LVEF with modified biplane Simpson's technique (method of disks) by 2D echocardiography (2DE) (36). The use of fractional shortening is discouraged as it only permits assessment of two walls for LVEF calculation, which does not accurately account for regional rather than global myocardial dysfunction, and which may occur with use of certain chemotherapeutic agents and in the presence of CAD. LVEF in the range of 53%–73% is classified as normal (36).

Three-dimensional echocardiography (3DE), where available, may be the most accurate and reproducible echocardiographic modality for monitoring cardiac function during cancer therapy (29,37). 3DE offers the benefit of semi-automated or automated identification of the endocardium rather than manual tracing, does not rely on geometric assumptions, and is less susceptible to differences in acquisition between scans. These advantages make 3DE more reproducible than 2DE for the measurement of LV volumes and in detecting LVEF <50%, and in fact 3DE may approach the accuracy of cardiac magnetic resonance imaging (CMR) in oncology patients (29,37). Noncontrast 3DE has been demonstrated to be highly reproducible with lower intra- and interobserver variability, which is particularly important given the need for serial evaluations in patients at risk of CTRCD (29,30). Utility of 3DE is limited to some extent by cost, but mostly by echo lab and operator expertise in acquiring high-quality images.

Problems with visualization of the endocardial border and attenuation artifacts can occur in breast cancer patients owing to changes post-mastectomy, following breast reconstruction, or from radiation therapy to the chest. This can cause inaccuracy in measurements of LVEF or LV volumes using Simpson's method on 2DE. The use of ultrasonic contrast agents markedly improves endocardial border visualization and is recommended by guidelines when two or more contiguous LV segments are not adequately visualized in noncontrast images 2DE (38–40). In one large prospective study of over 600 patients in a non-oncology setting, the addition of contrast to 2DE studies frequently changed the LVEF measurement, with one-sixth of patients having a contrast EF measurement 10 units different than noncontrast echo EF. In contrast, a prospective study of serial EF monitoring using echo in patients undergoing cancer therapy did not demonstrate an advantage of contrast echo compared to other echo techniques (30). Currently available evidence does not support the addition of contrast in 3DE for measurement of LV volumes or LVEF in patients with cancer (37).

DIASTOLIC DYSFUNCTION AND CARDIOTOXICITY

Assessments of LV diastolic function, including estimates of left atrial filling pressures using Doppler parameters as per current ASE guidelines, are recommended during echocardiographic assessment of LV function (41). During cancer therapy, many variables must be considered in interpreting estimates of LV filling pressure. Changes in preload owing to altered volume status from side effects of chemotherapy (nausea, vomiting, diarrhea, and subsequent dehydration), may be responsible for altered left atrial pressure independent of any cancer therapy-related changes in intrinsic myocardial relaxation. It was previously postulated that LV diastolic dysfunction preceded LV systolic dysfunction in cardiotoxicity from cancer therapy. This concept was largely based on global indexes of diastolic function such as isovolumetric relaxation time (IVRT), peak early (E) and atrial (A) mitral Doppler flow, E/A ratio, and Doppler tissue imaging. However, there is no consistent evidence that these diastolic parameters can predict subsequent cardiotoxicity, likely due to the complex effects of preload and afterload that occur during a given patient's course of cancer therapy (42–44). With the addition of myocardial strain analysis, which is a direct assessment of myocardial contractility, it is now understood that systolic and

diastolic dysfunction occur together. Importantly, changes in strain precede abnormalities in indexes of global LV dysfunction such as ejection fraction, as discussed later in this chapter (45).

In cardio-oncology, as in cardiology, diastolic function evaluation is most valuable in the assessment of patients with symptoms of dyspnea or suspected congestive heart failure. In patients with reduced ejection fraction, severe diastolic dysfunction identifies patients who require prompt cardiology intervention, as severe diastolic dysfunction is associated with a very high cardiac risk (46,47). In older patients, heart failure with preserved ejection fraction is as common as heart failure with reduced ejection fraction, and in such patients, evaluation of diastolic dysfunction using echocardiography can help clinicians investigate symptoms and optimize pharmacotherapy.

While most cardiotoxicity literature focuses on reduced ejection fraction, as older patients are increasingly exposed to cancer therapies, echocardiographic assessment of diastolic dysfunction may become more important. Risk stratification protocols incorporating echo assessment of systolic dysfunction should include identification of severe diastolic dysfunction, as such patients have a high short term risk of cardiac events (46).

ECHOCARDIOGRAPHY: BEYOND EJECTION FRACTION

Echocardiographic assessments in cancer patients should include qualitative and quantitative assessments of the RV, including chamber size, tricuspid annular plane systolic excursion (TAPSE), and Doppler tissue imaging systolic peak velocity of the tricuspid valve (s') (32,33,36). In the setting of suspected pulmonary hypertension as a consequence of chemotherapy (e.g., with dasatanib), it is also important to estimate the RV systolic pressure (RVSP) as a noninvasive screen for pulmonary hypertension. Further studies are needed to adequately determine the frequency and extent of RV involvement in CTRCD, and the prognostic value of RV dysfunction (48).

Valvular heart disease may complicate oncologic therapy as a long-term consequence of radiation treatment, and this is an important issue in cancer survivorship. Short-term valvular complications in cancer patients can include infective endocarditis from chemotherapy-related immunosuppression and subsequent systemic infection, worsening of preexisting valvular dysfunction (e.g., functional mitral regurgitation from LV dysfunction and dilatation), and primary or secondary cardiac tumors (e.g., carcinoid). In addition, nonbacterial thrombotic endocarditis is an important manifestation of disseminated cancer that should be part of the differential diagnosis of valve associated masses. Echocardiographic assessments of valvular stenosis or regurgitation should be performed according to current guideline-based recommendations (49,50). Where there are changes in valvular function, serial assessments may be needed, and intervention of specific for specific valve lesions should be considered according to published guidelines and individualized to the goals of care and prognosis for each patient. While not extensively studied, it is important to emphasize that any moderate or severe left-sided valve lesion will increase LV wall stress. While not specifically addressed in cardio-oncology guidelines, increased LV wall stress owing to moderate or severe left-sided valvular heart disease, when combined with cardiotoxic oncology treatments, likely increases the risk of LV dysfunction. This concept is relevant in echocardiographic assessment of valvular heart disease, since any left-sided valve lesion that is moderate or severe should be approached as an important risk factor for cardiotoxicity from cancer therapy, and such patients should be referred to cardio-oncology.

Pericardial involvement in oncologic patients is common and may be a consequence of chemotherapy, radiation therapy, or malignant metastases to the pericardial space. Pericardial involvement may manifest as pericarditis with or without pericardial effusions and/or constrictive physiology and in some cases progression to cardiac tamponade. Pericarditis may be associated with myocardial involvement/myocarditis. Echocardiography is the modality of choice in pericardial assessment offering the additional benefit of guidance for pericardiocentesis if needed. If effusions are present, they should be quantified and graded by standard methods to allow comparison on future studies. If present, tamponade should also be described according to published standards. The presence of pericardial thickening and constrictive physiology should also be reported according to published guidelines (51).

Stress echocardiography combines 2DE with a physiologic or pharmacologic stressors to detect subsequent wall motion abnormalities or transient changes in regional or global LV function. Stress echo is also useful for assessing myocardial viability as demonstrated by improved LV function or contractility, with application of low-level stress in a region of myocardium with abnormal resting contractility. It is useful in detecting and prognosticating CAD as recommended by guidelines. Stress echocardiography may play a role in cardio-oncology in the following settings: (1) patients undergoing regimens associated with ischemia (fluorouracil, bevacizumab, sorafenib, and sunitinib), especially in patients with intermediate or high pretest probability for CAD; (2) evaluation of subclinical LV dysfunction; (3) evaluation of contractile reserve in patients with CTRCD; and (4) detecting obstructive CAD in patients who have received radiation therapy to the thorax, which accelerates atherosclerosis (32,45,52).

Exercise and dobutamine-stress echo (DSE) have been studied in patients with cancer receiving anthracyclines to detect CTRCD. A study by Civelli et al. prospectively evaluated LV contractile reserve using low-dose DSE in a small cohort of women with breast cancer before each chemotherapy cycle and at 1, 4, and 7 months after cessation of treatment (53). A decrease of 5 points or more in contractile reserve was predictive of later decrease in LVEF to <50% after chemotherapy (53). This, and other approaches to detecting CTRCD, have been largely replaced by newer echo imaging modalities such as strain imaging (54). One potential application of stress echocardiography is in the identification of occult LV dysfunction in adult cancer survivors late after childhood chemotherapy. The current approach in childhood cancer survivors at high risk of long-term cardiomyopathy is lifelong serial echocardiography (55). Stress echo has been evaluated as a method to identify patients with underlying subclinical cardiomyopathy. In contrast to older data suggesting impaired contractile reserve in childhood cancer survivors, more recent work using bicycle stress echocardiography combined with advanced echo imaging including strain, did not demonstrate a reduction in contractile reserve among adult survivors of childhood cancer vs. controls (56,57). Further research is needed to determine if noninvasive imaging can risk stratify adult survivors of childhood cancer.

STRAIN IMAGING AND CARDIOTOXICITY

Strain imaging in echocardiography directly measures myocardial deformation which is useful in detecting subclinical ventricular dysfunction and can prognosticate future ventricular dysfunction in cancer patients (58). Strain is a dimensionless index that describes the total deformation of myocardial tissue as a percentage of the initial length during a cardiac cycle. Strain rate is the rate of stretch or deformation per second. Both can be measured in the longitudinal, radial, and circumferential directions and are less dependent on myocardial load, which is a limitation of other global indexes of systolic and diastolic function. Strain and strain rate can therefore provide information about intrinsic contractile function. Myocardial deformation can be measured either using Doppler tissue imaging (DTI) or speckle-tracking echocardiography (STE). Currently, STE is the favored method because of a lack of angle dependency (32,33).

A systematic review by Thavendiranathan et al. examined 21 studies which evaluated the utility of myocardial deformation measurements in detecting subclinical LV dysfunction in patients treated with chemotherapy (58). The key findings from this analysis are that abnormalities in myocardial deformation preceded decreases in LVEF and persist throughout cancer treatment. While decreases in radial, circumferential, and longitudinal strain can be identified during cardiotoxic cancer therapy, global longitudinal strain (GLS) by STE has emerged as the most feasible and reproducible parameter to detect subclinical LV dysfunction.

GLS should be measured in all patients at baseline where available as well as during chemotherapy in patients receiving agents that can cause CTRCD. A GLS value that falls by 15% (usually 2–3 absolute GLS points) from the baseline is considered abnormal and suggests subclinical cardiotoxicity (32,33). Some centers repeat imaging to confirm abnormal GLS 2–3 weeks after the initial abnormal study. It is important to note that normal reference values for strain differ for each echo manufacturer. This is important, since echo labs using multiple vendors, or patients who receive imaging at different echo labs using different echo machines, may have different GLS results that do not indicate true changes in LV contractility. Ideally, the same type of echo machine should be used for longitudinal follow-up of a given patient, preferably in the same echo lab. A concerted effort should also be made to reduce inter- and intraobserver variability by training sonographers and interpreting physicians in all aspects of GLS acquisition, measurement, and reporting. When incorporating echocardiography into a risk stratification and cardiotoxicity detection scheme, it is recommended to measure and monitor local variability in serial GLS measurements in order to determine what is a true change in GLS using locally available echocardiography, rather than results from published literature. This helps determine appropriate thresholds for a change in GLS on serial imaging that may prompt referral or intervention for an individual patient. Whether used alone or combined with biomarkers and clinical risk factors, strain imaging should play a role in cardiotoxicity risk stratification for patients exposed to anthracyclines alone or in combination with therapies that can potentially reduce myocardial contractility.

RISK ASSESSMENT WITH CARDIAC MRI IN CARDIAC ONCOLOGY

Introduction

With advances in 2D, 3D, and strain imaging using echocardiography, CMR can often be regarded as a luxury or redundant investigation in cardio-oncology (32,33). Recent clinical trials have, however, included CMR as the imaging method of choice to investigate the effects of prophylactic interventions for chemotherapy related cardiotoxicity (59,60). In these studies, CMR was used to assess the effects of prophylactic therapy to influence LV remodeling, LV function, and myocardial tissue characterization after chemotherapy. CMR was chosen in these settings as a result of the reduction in variability in volume and LV ejection fraction measurements achieved by CMR in comparison to echocardiography (echo) or multigated blood pool imaging (MUGA) (37).

Although sensitive and accurate evaluation is important in clinical trials, it is also important in clinical cardio-oncology, as continued cancer treatment often relies on consistent reproducible measurements of cardiac function. The ability of CMR to detect tissue characteristics of edema and fibrosis also may be useful identifying patients with respectively early or late cardiotoxicity (61). In addition, CMR can also be used to evaluate patients in whom echocardiographic assessment of LV function was sub-optima due to poor echo windows, or in cases where there is a discrepancy between echo and MUGA results (37).

Preclinical assessment of cardiotoxicity

A goal of cardiac screening with imaging is the early detection of cardiotoxicity so that increased surveillance, appropriate monitoring, and early institution of heart failure medication can occur (58). There is a time window of approximately 6 months from the detection of CTRCD and the institution of heart failure therapy during which time cardiac dysfunction may be reversible (62). Failure to start therapy during this period is associated with a poor response to therapy and permanent LV impairment.

CMR findings in "early" cardiotoxicity

If early cardiotoxicity is defined as the detection LV functional abnormalities with preserved LV ejection fraction, CMR is able to detect early changes both in performance parameters and in tissue characteristics. Muehlberg demonstrated changes in myocardial tissue characteristics using T1 mapping within 48 hours of receiving the first dose of anthracyclines (63). Those patients who developed reduced T1 relaxation times at this early stage in therapy were subsequently more likely to develop anthracycline mediated cardiomyopathy. In this trial of 30 sarcoma patients who received 360–400 mg/m² of doxorubicin, nine patients developed a reduction in LVEF of >10% at completion of therapy (63). Native T1 time may therefore be a very early preclinical predictor of those patients who will subsequently develop CTRCD. Further larger studies will be needed to confirm these observations.

T2 weighted CMR images can detect myocardial edema; however, there is conflicting evidence as to whether T2 relaxation times are altered by chemotherapy. Grover et al. found that T2 detected edema predicted lower RVEF at 12 months in 46 women receiving anthracycline (59%) or trastuzumab (64). Whereas, others did not observe any differences in T2 weighted images in patients receiving potentially toxic chemotherapy (anthracycline 55%) at 3 months (65).

CMR stain imaging using featured tracking was found to detect subclinical effects of trastuzumab in 41 breast cancer patients (66). In this study, patients were followed by CMR at baseline, 6, 12, and 18 months during trastuzumab therapy. The mean LVEF was reduced (from 60.4% to 57.9%) at 12 months ($p < 0.012$), but remained within the normal range; however, global longitudinal and circumferential strain was reduced in comparison to baseline recordings (66). Similarly, Jolly et al. found that CMR mid LV circumferential strain reduction was present in patients with subclinical reductions in LVEF 3 months after starting potential cardiotoxic chemotherapy (67).

Although the focus of cardiotoxicity is often centered on LV performance, CMR has demonstrated that RV function could be a useful marker of subclinical cardiotoxicity. Barthur demonstrated that RV ejection fraction was temporarily reduced in breast cancer patients receiving trastuzumab and did not correlate with LVEF changes which remained clinically normal through the study (68). RV ejection fraction decreased from 58.3% at baseline to 53.9% at 6 months. The LVEF for the same time points was 60.4% and 58.3%, respectively. It could be argued that the reduction in RVEF was also subclinical and the RV ejection fraction remained within the normal range; however, the implication from the study is that RV function may be effected more than LV function in some cases of CTRCD and should not be overlooked or ignored as a potential preclinical biomarker.

Clinical cardiotoxicity

In cases where cardiotoxicity has occurred, continued monitoring of LVEF or RVEF by CMR may be impractical, especially in cases where there are adequate echocardiographic images. A potential role for CMR in this setting is to evaluate cases where CTRCD is borderline or where the diagnosis is in doubt clinically. In patients receiving chemotherapy who experience LVEF decline, Melendez et al. highlighted the importance of accurate assessment of LV volumes in determining the validity of a proposed LVEF decrease (69). CMR was performed prior to, and 3 months after initiating cardiotoxic chemotherapy in 112 patients (69). LVEF decreased in 26 patients by >10% or to <50% at 3 months. Of those patients with CTRCD, 19% were found to have reductions in LV end diastolic volumes to account for their changes in LVEF. The reduction in LVEF in these patients may therefore be related to changes in volume status rather than an increase in LVESV secondary to reduced myocardial contractility (69).

Cancer survivorship risk of CTRCD and CMR

With successful cancer therapies the number of cancer survivors has increased. Approximately 1% of those who receive anthracyclines, and have a normal LVEF at therapy completion, will develop CTRCD in long-term follow-up (70). Detection of individuals who may be susceptible to latent CTRCD is an important aspect of cancer survivorship care. Annual or biannual echocardiographic assessment is recommended, although the evidence to support this approach is lacking (27). To try and rationalize follow-up, investigators have considered using different CMR biomarkers to identify those at risk.

Adult survivors of pediatric cancers have been shown to have reduced myocardial mass using CMR imaging (63). This may be an important subclinical predictor of latent CTRCD since low LV mass has been shown to be a predictor of adverse cardiac events in patients who received anthracyclines (71). CMR is an attractive method to assess LVEF in adult survivors of pediatric cancer as it does not involve ionizing radiation and many of these patients will have received large doses of radiotherapy during their illness. In addition to the improved accuracy, CMR may reveal prior undiagnosed reductions in LVEF: 11% of patients included in a comparison study had impaired LVEF function measured by CMR, that was not detected by echo. Furthermore approximately 30% of patients in this study without a history of CTRCD were found to have LVEF more than 2 standard deviations below age and gender matched normal data, suggesting the presence of subclinical CTRCD (37).

Tissue characterization in cancer survivors may also help to determine those patients at heightened risk for CTRCD. Late gadolinium enhancement (LGE) imaging is used to detect macroscopic myocardial fibrosis at CMR. In a study of 24 patients who had undergone radiotherapy for esophageal cancer in Japan, 50% had evidence of LGE on CMR performed at a median of 2 years postradiotherapy (72). At the time of the study, these patients had normal LVEF. Larger studies with longer follow-up

are required to determine the significance of radiotherapy-induced LGE.

Myocardial LGE following potentially cardiotoxicity chemotherapy has not been consistently described. Fallah-Rad et al. found that trastuzumab treated breast cancer patients who developed CTRCD had LGE in the mid myocardium of the lateral wall of the LV suggesting that LGE if present may reflect significant cardiotoxicity (73). In a different study of 46 adult survivors of pediatric cancer, all were treated with anthracyclines and had a normal LVEF, LGE was not detected (74). Yet, microscopic diffuse myocardial fibrosis was suggested by postcontrast T1 relaxation reduced values that correlated with low LV mass (74). In this study, CMR derived circumferential strain values were reduced in 45/46 treated with anthracyclines in comparison to normal controls in the presence of normal CMR-derived LVEF (74). Although alternations in T1 relaxation times, LGE and CMR-derived strain parameters might indicate subclinical CTRCD, longer term follow-up of patients with these features will be required to confirm their prognostic significance.

Summary

CMR may appear excessive in an era of advanced echo imaging, yet CMR offers some unique characteristics to assist in the risk stratification of cancer patients exposed to potentially cardiotoxic therapies. All three arenas of risk evaluation in CTRCD can be assisted by CMR, from early detection of subclinical toxicity, to confirmation of suspected LV dysfunction and monitoring of cancer survivors. In view of the expanding use of CMR within cardiac oncology trials, it is likely that the application of CMR will increase in this patient population. Long-term follow-up to confirm the significance of CMR markers of CTRCD risk will be a research priority in the coming years.

PUTTING IT ALL TOGETHER: INTEGRATING APPROACHES TO RISK STRATIFICATION

We have reviewed a variety of strategies to estimate risk of cardiotoxicity from cancer therapy, ranging from clinical risk factors and risk scores, to biomarker based strategies, to cardiac imaging. In isolation, each of these strategies has some utility in predicting risk of cardiotoxicity. Some centers exclusively use one or two of these approaches for estimating cardiotoxicity risk. A promising approach is to combine several strategies to estimate risk of cardiotoxicity. A key multicenter trial in patients with early stage breast cancer combined strain imaging using echocardiography with serial troponins to estimate risk of subsequent cardiotoxicity (19). This approach reliably identified patients at low risk of subsequent cardiotoxicity, with very high negative predictive value for patients whose strain and troponins were normal following sequential anthracycline and trastusumab. Conversely, patients with abnormal strain and or abnormal troponins had a modest increase in their risk for cardiotoxicity. This multicenter trial illustrates the potential of combining biomarkers with cardiac imaging to enhance risk stratification following exposure to cancer therapy (19). The potential to expand on this approach by incorporating clinical risk factors warrants further study. One potential strategy to integrate clinical risk factors, strain imaging, and biomarkers into one protocol is illustrated in Figure 3.3.

RISK STRATIFICATION FOR CARDIOTOXICITY: BEYOND LV DYSFUNCTION

A 64-year-old patient is diagnosed with multiple myeloma and achieves complete remission on a proteasome inhibitor. After 2 years on therapy, he develops severe hypertension refractory to maximum doses of four antihypertensives. Imaging reveals bilateral renal artery stenosis, and he undergoes renal artery angioplasty with perfect angiographic results. Subsequently, his hypertension is well controlled on only two medications. He is referred to cardio-oncology to determine the safety of resuming proteasome inhibitor therapy for his multiple myeloma. His risk factors include hypertension, remote smoking totaling 20 pack years, and dyslipidemia. At the time of his assessment, he has no exertional symptoms, and no history of cardiovascular disease besides his renal artery stenosis with bilateral renal artery angioplasty. Medications at the time of assessment include ASA 81 mg daily, perindopril 8 mg, and indapamide 2.5 mg daily. Physical examination is normal, with a BMI of 23, waist circumference of 80 cm, BP 124/74, no carotid or abdominal bruits, a normal ankle/brachial index, and no extra heart sounds or murmurs.

A 72-year-old male has been treated for locally invasive prostate cancer. Owing to a rising Prostate specific antigen (PSA) more potent androgen deprivation is recommended, but he is reluctant to proceed due to concerns about long-term cardiovascular risks. He has no history of cardiovascular disease, but has risk factors that include type II diabetes, hypertension, and dyslipidemia. He is a lifelong nonsmoker. He reports no exertional

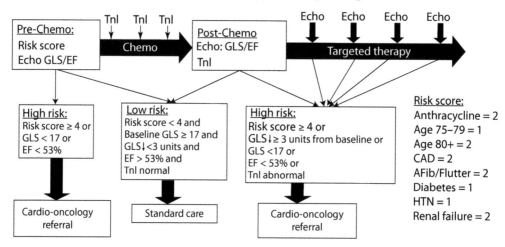

Figure 3.3 Integrated risk stratification for cardiotoxicity. (Includes risk score adapted from Ezaz G et al. *J Am Heart Assoc.* 2014;3:e000472.)

symptoms, but is sedentary. Medications at the time of consultation include metformin 1000 mg PO bid, Perindopril 4 mg PO daily, atorvastatin 80 mg PO daily. Physical exam is notable for obesity with a BMI of 36, waist circumference 134 cm, and BP of 170/80.

These two cases illustrate the wide variety of cancer therapies that are drastically improving cancer survival leading to concerns about long-term cardiovascular health in adult cancer survivors. Newer cancer therapies with potential long-term cardiac risk are increasingly offered to older patients who have underlying cardiovascular risk factors, subclinical cardiovascular disease, and overt cardiovascular diagnoses.

These two cases illustrate the more complex problem of predicting the risk of coronary and noncoronary atherosclerotic events that are associated with some cancer therapies. Unlike serial echocardiograms or biomarkers that detect subclinical cardiotoxicity prior to heart failure in anthracycline-exposed patients, there are currently no acceptable imaging or biomarker based strategies to detect or predict cardiovascular events (e.g., acute coronary syndrome, ischemic stroke or peripheral arterial vascular disease) in patients whose long-term cancer therapies may increase

vascular risk. Rather than protocolized approaches relying on imaging or biomarkers, global cardiovascular risk evaluation and optimization appears to be the most appropriate strategy (35).

A body of evidence is accumulating to suggest that cancer and cardiovascular disease share many lifestyle-related risk factors (75). Particularly in older cancer populations, cardiovascular risk factors and cardiac disease may be present prior to cancer therapy. In addition to direct effects of cancer therapy on the heart, cancer indirectly increases cardiac risk by worsening cardiac risk factors. Many lifestyle risk factors such as lack of exercise and obesity worsen during cancer therapies, and cancer therapies may adversely affect other risk factors such as hypertension, dyslipidemia, and diabetes. In high-risk patients, cancer therapy may be modified to protect patients from cancer therapy-associated cardiotoxicity, potentially resulting in a worse cancer outcomes if less effective cancer treatment is administered. It is well known that cardiac complications of cancer therapy frequently lead to interruption or discontinuation of oncological therapy, leading to worse oncological outcomes. Figure 3.4 summarizes how cardiovascular disease and risk factors interact with cancer and cancer therapy to determine

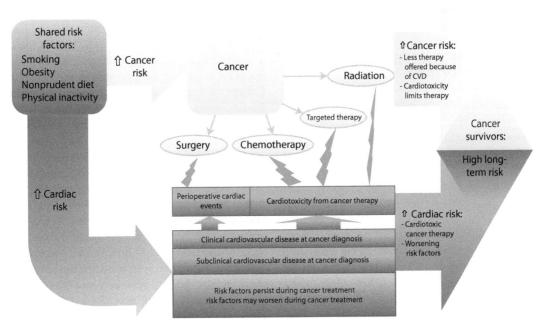

Figure 3.4 Shared risk factors and an approach to cardiovascular risk assessment.

short- and long-term clinical outcomes related to both cancer and cardiovascular disease (75). This framework attempts to link cardiovascular health and cancer, and can be used to identify opportunities to optimize risk factors and cardiovascular health throughout the cancer care continuum: at diagnosis, during cancer therapy, and during long-term cancer survivorship.

At initial diagnosis, attention should focus on optimizing any risk factors and any known cardiovascular disease. Where possible, and subject to constraints imposed by drug–drug and drug–disease interactions, pharmacotherapy for cardiac risk factors and cardiac disease should be continued and optimized, never stopped unless there are specific contraindications based on interactions with cancer drugs or biological effects of cancer therapy (35,75). Following cancer therapy, attention should again focus on supporting optimal lifestyle-related risk factors, and optimal pharmacotherapy for risk factors and cardiovascular disease where appropriate. It must be recognized that optimization of cardiac risk factors and cardiac disease may be beyond the scope of practice for oncology providers. Primary care providers, survivorship programs, rehab programs, and cardio-oncology clinics can support optimization of cardiovascular health. Patient self-care and attention to lifestyle risk factors are important throughout the cancer care continuuum, and in addition to structured rehab programs, can be supported through patient education materials and websites (35,75).

RISK STRATIFICATION AND CANCER SURGERY

A 60-year-old patient is discovered to have a operable primary lung cancer. He reports exertional dyspnea in functional class III with an estimated functional capacity of four metabolic equivalents (METs). His past medical history includes type II diabetes for 20 years, 40 pack years of smoking, hypertension, and dyslipidemia. Medications include long acting insulin, metformin 1000 mg PO bid, atorvastatin 80 mg daily, perindopril 8 mg PO daily, hydrocholorothiazide 25 mg daily, and amlodipine 10 mg daily. Exam reveals HR 70, BP 140/80, normal cardiac exam, a BMI of 32, and a waist circumference of 110 cm. Pulmonary function testing reveals 85% predicted lung function.

A persantine perfusion scan reveals anterior and inferolateral ischemia in addition to transient ischemic dilatation, with preserved LV function. An echocardiogram reveals a normal ejection fraction, moderate (grade II) diastolic dysfunction, but no significant valvular heart disease and no pulmonary hypertension. He is referred to cardiology to determine if he should avoid cancer surgery, relying on radiation therapy and/or chemotherapy to treat his cancer. The alternative option is medical optimization of his coronary disease followed by cancer surgery vs coronary revascularization and cancer surgery, either sequentially or simultaneously.

Cardiologists are familiar with preoperative cardiac assessment prior to noncardiac surgery, a topic that is extensively covered in national guidelines (76–78). This clinical case highlights some important nuances that must be considered when the noncardiac surgery is for cancer treatment. Some cancer surgeries, such as surgery for most breast cancers, have a low risk for cardiac events such that preoperative cardiac assessment may not be indicated. In other cancer surgeries, such as colorectal and thoracic oncological surgery, there is an increased risk of cardiac events such that some patients may require preoperative cardiac testing and optimization. The American College of Cardiology recommends a stepwise approach to determine if cardiac testing is indicated (76). Valid tools are available to precisely estimate precisely operative risk based on clinical factors and to estimate functional capacity, the two key determinants when selecting patients for cardiac testing prior to surgery as suggested by the American College of Cardiology and illustrated in Figure 3.5 (76,79,80). Importantly, cardiac testing is only appropriate if it will modify therapy. In the case of lung cancer, surgical oncology teams may view cardiac testing as part of a patient's staging, in that a high cardiac risk which cannot be mitigated by cardiology intervention may result in a recommendation for nonoperative therapy such as radiation and chemotherapy. In such circumstances, cardiac testing is appropriate since it may alter the assessment of the risks vs. benefits. In cases where cardiac status cannot by optimized, particularly when there are significant pulmonary and other comorbidities, patients may be recommended for nonsurgical cancer therapy. When determining optimal

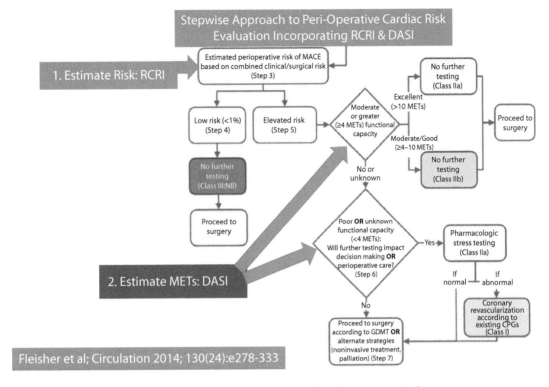

Figure 3.5 Approach to perioperative risk assessment at The Ottawa Hospital.

cancer treatment plans for such high-risk patients, communication between cardiology, anesthesia, cancer surgeons, medical oncology, and radiation oncology is critical.

Cancer patients make up an increasing number of all surgeries, both elective operations to improve prognosis and urgent operations when dealing with surgical complications of cancer. In the VISION trials, approximately one in four patients had active cancer at the time of surgery, and such patients had twice the 30 day adjusted mortality compared to patients without cancer (81,82). As cardiologists approach perioperative cardiac assessment, it is important to recognize the cancer patient as a high risk patient. The mechanism of this excess risk is currently not well understood. The effects of upstream cancer treatment using chemotherapy or radiation, the risk increase associated with multimorbidity and frailty owing to a concomitant cancer diagnosis, or perhaps biological mediators that may increase risk (35,75). Further research in perioperative medicine is needed to better understand factors that make cancer patients high risk, and cardio-oncology research should consider the issue of cancer surgery as a time of particular vulnerability to short-term events.

RISK STRATIFICATION AND CANCER SURVIVORSHIP

A 30-year-old patient who had childhood cancer therapy has undergone regular echocardiographic surveillance in an adult echo lab since the age of 18, with one echo performed every 2 years. On review of the echo database, the ejection fraction has remained in the normal range between 57% and 68% on each of the nine echoes available for review. The patient is referred to cardiology to determine if there are any more definitive assessments that could establish his cardiotoxicity risk to permit him to reduce the frequency of cardiac imaging.

Guidelines published by the Children's Oncology Group recommend that childhood cancer survivors receive serial echocardiographic monitoring with a frequency proportional to the estimated risk of cardiotoxicity (55). Cost-effectiveness analysis suggests that such surveillance is justifiable assuming that pharmacotherapy for reduced cardiac function is effective (27). Accurately risk stratifying patients at the time of initial cancer therapy will facilitate decision making with regards to long term cardiac surveillance. Adult cancer survivorship guidelines endorsed by a variety of imaging and national organizations currently do not endorse long-term serial cardiac testing. It seems intuitive that high-risk patients should have careful clinical follow up to ensure that lifestyle risk factors are addressed, and any non-lifestyle risk factors such as hypertension treated. Whether high-risk patients should undergo long-term serial cardiac imaging or have serial cardiac biomarker testing is uncertain and requires further research. A key first step to determining which, if any, adult cancer survivors need long-term monitoring with cardiac imaging or biomarkers is to risk stratify patients at the time of cancer therapy.

CONCLUSION

We have reviewed a variety of tools that can be useful in risk stratifying patients exposed to cancer therapies. Each varies in cost, complexity, and ease of implementation. Clinical risk stratification requires no technology, but clinicians must devote time and use valid tools in order to identify high-risk patients. Biomarkers and echocardiography require technology and could be more costly than clinical risk stratification, depending on how a particular health system values a clinician's time. Furthermore, cardiac MRI is the most expensive and therefore least available tool relevant to risk stratification. Whether a health system uses some or all of these tools depends on local healthcare resources. Who is responsible for performing risk stratification and reacting to high-risk findings needs to be determined by organizations that provide cancer care. Finally, which tools are applied to risk stratification may vary across the cancer care continuum. While we believe that the best time to risk stratify is at initial cancer therapy, there are many adult survivors of childhood cancer who may benefit from risk stratification. Given the variability and complexity of healthcare systems, we believe that organizations should use combinations of risk stratification strategies that are best suited to their local patient population. Evaluation and dissemination of the results of such schemes is essential if we are to improve our ability to risk stratify patients for cardiotoxicity.

REFERENCES

1. Suter TM, Ewer MS. Cancer drugs and the heart: Importance and management. *Eur Heart J*. 2013;34:1102–11.
2. Bloom MW et al. Cancer therapy–related cardiac dysfunction and heart failure part 1: Definitions, pathophysiology, risk factors, and imaging. *Circ Heart Fail*. 2016;9:e002661.
3. Hamo CE et al. Cancer therapy–related cardiac dysfunction and heart failure part 2: Prevention, treatment, guidelines, and future directions. *Circ Heart Fail*. 2016;9:e002843.
4. Khouri MG et al. Cancer therapy-induced cardiac toxicity in early breast cancer: Addressing the unresolved issues. *Circulation*. 2012;126:2749–63.
5. Lipshultz SE et al. American heart association congenital heart defects committee of the council on cardiovascular disease in the young, council on basic cardiovascular sciences, council on cardiovascular and stroke nursing, council on cardiovascular radiology. Long-term cardiovascular toxicity in children, adolescents, and young adults who receive cancer therapy: Pathophysiology, course, monitoring, management, prevention, and research directions: A scientific statement from the American Heart Association. *Circulation*. 2013;128:1927–95.
6. Eschenhagen T et al. Cardiovascular side effects of cancer therapies: A position statement from the heart failure association of the European society of cardiology. *Eur J Heart Fail*. 2011;13:1–10.
7. Schwartz R et al. Congestive heart failure and left ventricular dysfunction complicating doxorubicin therapy. Seven-year experience using serial radionuclide angiocardiography. *Am J Med*. 1987;82:1109–18.
8. Swain SM, Whaley FS, Ewer MS. Congestive heart failure in patients treated with doxorubicin. *Cancer*. 2003;97:2869–79.
9. Mitani I et al. Doxorubicin cardiotoxicity: Prevention of congestive heart failure with serial cardiac function monitoring with equilibrium radionuclide angiocardiography in the current era. *J Nucl Cardiol*. 2003;10:132–9.
10. Mackey JR et al. Adjuvant docetaxel, doxorubicin, and cyclophosphamide in node-positive breast cancer: 10-year follow-up of the

phase 3 randomised BCIRG 001 trial. *Lancet Oncol.* 2013;14:72–80.

11. Lotrionte M et al. Review and meta-analysis of incidence and clinical predictors of anthracycline cardiotoxicity. *Am J Cardiol.* 2013;112:1980–4.

12. Law W, Johnson C, Rushton M, Dent S. The Framingham risk score underestimates the risk of cardiovascular events in the HER2-positive breast cancer population. *Curr Oncol.* October 2017;24(5):e348–53.

13. Romond EH et al. Seven-year follow-up assessment of cardiac function in NSABP B-31, a randomized trial comparing doxorubicin and cyclophosphamide followed by paclitaxel (ACP) with ACP plus trastuzumab as adjuvant therapy for patients with node-positive, human epidermal growth factor receptor 2–positive breast cancer. *J Clin Oncol.* 2012;30:3792–9.

14. Ezaz G et al. Risk prediction model for heart failure and cardiomyopathy after adjuvant trastuzumab therapy for breast cancer. *J Am Heart Assoc.* 2014;3:e000472.

15. Cardinale D et al. Early detection of anthracycline cardiotoxicity and improvement with heart failure therapy. *Circulation.* June 2, 2015;131(22):1981–8.

16. Thavendiranathan P et al. Breast cancer therapy-related cardiac dysfunction in adult women treated in routine clinical practice: A population based cohort study. *J Clin Oncol.* July 1, 2016;34(19):2239–46.

17. Cardinale D et al. Prognostic value of troponin I in cardiac risk stratification of cancer patients undergoing high-dose chemotherapy. *Circulation.* June 8, 2004;109(22):2749–54.

18. Cardinale D et al. Anthracycline induced cardiotoxicity: A multi-center randomized trial comparing two strategies for guiding prevention with enalapril: The international cardio-oncology society one trial. *Eur J Cancer.* May 2018;94:126–37.

19. Sawaya H et al. Assessment of echocardiography and biomarkers for the extended prediction of cardiotoxicity in patients treated with anthracyclines, taxanes, and trastuzumab. *Circ Cardiovasc Imaging* 2012;5:596–603.

20. Freres P et al. Variations of circulating cardiac biomarkers during and after anthracycline-containing chemotherapy in breast cancer patients. *BMC Cancer* 2018; 18:102.

21. Auner HW et al. Prolonged monitoring of troponin T for the detection of anthracycline cardiotoxicity in adults with hematological malignancies. *Ann Hematol.* 2003;82:218–22.

22. Mokuyasu S et al. High-sensitivity cardiac troponin I detection for 2 types of drug-induced cardiotoxicity in patients with breast cancer. *Breast Cancer.* November 2015;22(6):563–9.

23. Morris PG et al. Troponin I and C-reactive protein are commonly detected in patients with breast cancer treated with dose-dense chemotherapy incorporating trastuzumab and lapatinib. *Clin Cancer Res.* May 15, 2011;17(10):3490–9.

24. Zardavas D et al. Role of troponins I and T and N-terminal prohormone of brain natriuretic peptide in monitoring cardiac safety of patients with early-stage human epidermal growth factor receptor 2–positive breast cancer receiving trastuzumab: A herceptin adjuvant study cardiac marker substudy. *J Clin Oncol.* 2017;35:878–84.

25. Ponde N et al. Cardiac biomarkers for early detection and prediction of trastuzumab and/or lapatinib-induced cardiotoxicity in patients with HER2-positive early-stage breast cancer: A NeoALTTO sub-study (BIG 1-06). *Breast Cancer Res Treat.* April 2018;186(3):631–8.

26. Armenian SH et al. Prevention and monitoring of cardiac dysfunction in survivors of adult cancers: American society of clinical oncology clinical practice guideline. *J Clin Oncol.* March 10, 2017;35(8):893–911.

27. Wong FL et al. Cost-effectiveness of the children's oncology group long-term follow-up screening guidelines for childhood cancer survivors at risk for treatment-related heart failure. *Ann Intern Med.* 2014;160:672–83.

28. Perez EA, Rodeheffer R. Clinical cardiac tolerability of trastuzumab. *J Clin Oncol.* January 2004;22:322–9.

29. Walker J et al. Role of three-dimensional echocardiography in breast cancer: Comparison with two-dimensional echocardiography, multiple-gated acquisition scans, and cardiac magnetic resonance imaging. *J Clin Oncol.* 2010;28:3429–36.

30. Thavendiranathan P et al. Reproducibility of echocardiographic techniques for sequential assessment of left ventricular ejection fraction and volumes. *J Am Coll Cardiol.* 2013;61:77–84.

31. Suter TM et al. Trastuzumab-associated cardiac adverse events in the Herceptin adjuvant trial. *J Clin Oncol.* 2007;25:3859–65.

32. Plana JC et al. Expert consensus for multimodality imaging evaluation of adult patients during and after cancer therapy: A report from the American society of echocardiography and the European association of cardiovascular imaging. *J Am Soc Echocardiogr.* September 1, 2014 [cited February 19, 2018];27(9):911–39.

33. Zamorano JL et al. 2016 ESC position paper on cancer treatments and cardiovascular toxicity developed under the auspices of the esc committee for practice guidelines. *Eur Heart J.* September 21, 2016 [cited February 19, 2018];37(36):2768–801.

34. Tan-Chiu E et al. Assessment of cardiac dysfunction in a randomized trial comparing doxorubicin and cyclophosphamide followed by paclitaxel, with or without trastuzumab as adjuvant therapy in node-positive, human epidermal growth factor receptor 2–overexpressing breast cancer: NSABP B-31. *J Clin Oncol.* 2005;23:7811–9.

35. Virani SA et al. Canadian cardiovascular society guidelines for evaluation and management of cardiovascular complications of cancer therapy. *Can J Cardiol.* July 2016 [cited February 19, 2018];32(7):831–41.

36. Lang RM et al. Recommendations for cardiac chamber quantification by echocardiography in adults: An update from the American society of echocardiography and the European association of cardiovascular imaging. *J Am Soc Echocardiogr* 2015;28:1–39.

37. Armstrong GT et al. Screening adult survivors of childhood cancer for cardiomyopathy: Comparison of echocardiography and cardiac magnetic resonance imaging. *J Clin Oncol.* August 10, 2012 [cited February 19, 2018];30(23):2876–84.

38. Mulvagh SL et al. American Society of Echocardiography consensus statement on the clinical applications of ultrasonic contrast agents in echocardiography. *J Am Soc Echocardiogr.* November 2008 [cited February 26, 2018];21(11):1179–201; quiz 1281.

39. Senior R et al. Contrast echocardiography: Evidence-based recommendations by European Association of Echocardiography. *Eur J Echocardiogr.* August 4, 2008 [cited February 26, 2018];10(2):194–212.

40. Senior R et al. Clinical practice of contrast echocardiography: Recommendation by the European Association of Cardiovascular Imaging (EACVI) 2017. *Eur Hear J – Cardiovasc Imaging.* November 1, 2017 [cited December 22, 2017];18(11):1073–89.

41. Nagueh SF et al. Recommendations for the evaluation of left ventricular diastolic function by echocardiography: An update from the American Society of Echocardiography and the European Association of Cardiovascular Imaging. *J Am Soc Echocardiogr.* April 1, 2016 [cited February 25, 2018];29(4):277–314.

42. Dorup I, Levitt G, Sullivan I, Sorensen K. Prospective longitudinal assessment of late anthracycline cardiotoxicity after childhood cancer: The role of diastolic function. *Heart.* October 1, 2004 [cited February 26, 2018];90(10):1214–6.

43. Stoodley PW et al. Two-dimensional myocardial strain imaging detects changes in left ventricular systolic function immediately after anthracycline chemotherapy. *Eur J Echocardiogr.* December 1, 2011 [cited February 19, 2018];12(12):945–52.

44. Stoddard MF, Seeger J, Liddell NE, Hadley TJ, Sullivan DM, Kupersmith J. Prolongation of isovolumetric relaxation time as assessed by Doppler echocardiography predicts doxorubicin-induced systolic dysfunction in humans. *J Am Coll Cardiol.* July 1992 [cited February 26, 2018];20(1):62–9.

45. Bottinor WJ, Migliore CK, Lenneman CA, Stoddard MF. Echocardiographic assessment of cardiotoxic effects of cancer therapy. *Curr Cardiol Rep.* October 27, 2016 [cited February 22, 2018];18(10):99.

46. Redfield MM et al. Burden of systolic and diastolic ventricular dysfunction in the community: Appreciating the scope of the heart failure epidemic. *JAMA.* 2003;289:194–202.

47. Appleton CP et al. Relation of transmitral flow velocity patterns to left ventricular diastolic function: New insights from a combined hemodynamic and Doppler echocardiographic study. *J Am Coll Cardiol.* 1988;12(2):426–40.

48. Boczar KE et al. Right heart function deteriorates in breast cancer patients undergoing anthracycline based chemotherapy. *Echo Res Pract.* September 2016;3(30):79–84.

49. Zoghbi WA et al. Recommendations for noninvasive evaluation of native valvular regurgitation: A report from the American Society of Echocardiography developed in collaboration with the Society for Cardiovascular Magnetic Resonance. *J Am Soc Echocardiogr.* 2017;30(4):303–71.

50. Baumgartner H et al. Recommendations on the echocardiographic assessment of aortic valve stenosis: A focused update from the European Association of Cardiovascular Imaging and the American Society of Echocardiography. *J Am Soc Echocardiogr.* 2017;30:372–92.

51. Adler Y et al. 2015 ESC guidelines for the diagnosis and management of pericardial diseases: The task force for the diagnosis and management of pericardial diseases of the European Society of Cardiology (ESC). *Eur Heart J.* 2015;36:2921–64.

52. Lancellotti P, Gomez JLZ, Galderisi M. *Anticancer Treatments and Cardiotoxicity: Mechanisms, Diagnostic and Therapeutic Interventions.* First. Lancellotti P, Zamorano J, Galderisi M, eds. Elsevier; 2016. 165 p.

53. Civelli M et al. Early reduction in left ventricular contractile reserve detected by dobutamine stress echo predicts high-dose chemotherapy-induced cardiac toxicity. *Int J Cardiol.* July 28, 2006 [cited February 26, 2018];111(1):120–6.

54. Grosu A, Bombardini T, Senni M, Duino V, Gori M, Picano E. End-systolic pressure/volume relationship during dobutamine stress echo: A prognostically useful non-invasive index of left ventricular contractility. *Eur Heart J.* November 1, 2005 [cited February 26, 2018];26(22):2404–12.

55. Landier W et al. Development of risk-based guidelines for pediatric cancer survivors: The Children's Oncology Group long-term follow-up guidelines from the Children's Oncology Group Late Effects Committee and Nursing Discipline. *J Clin Oncol.* 2004;22:4979–90.

56. Klewer SE et al. Dobutamine stress echocardiogaphy: A sensitive indicator of diminished myocardial function in asymptomatic doxorubicin-treated long-term survivors of childhood cancer. *J Am Coll Cardiol.* 1992; 19(2):394–401.

57. Cifra B et al. Dynamic myocardial response to exercise in childhood cancer survivors treated with anthracyclines. *J Am Soc Echocardiogr.* August 2018;31(8):933–42.

58. Thavendiranathan P, Poulin F, Lim K-D, Plana JC, Woo A, Marwick TH. Use of myocardial strain imaging by echocardiography for the early detection of cardiotoxicity in patients during and after cancer chemotherapy: A systematic review. *J Am Coll Cardiol.* July 1, 2014 [cited February 19, 2018];63(25 Pt A): 2751–68.

59. Heck SL et al. Effect of candesartan and metoprolol on myocardial tissue composition during anthracycline treatment: The PRADA trial. *Eur Heart J Cardiovasc Imaging.* May 1, 2018;19(5):544–52.

60. Pituskin E et al. Multidisciplinary approach to novel therapies in cardio-oncology research (MANTICORE 101-breast): A randomized trial for the prevention of trastuzumab-associated cardiotoxicity. *J Clin Oncol.* March 10, 2017;35(8):870–7.

61. Jordan JH, Todd RM, Vasu S, Hundley WG. Cardiovascular magnetic resonance in the oncology patient. *JACC Cardiovasc Imaging.* August 2018;11(8):1150–72.

62. Cardinale D et al. Anthracycline-induced cardiomyopathy: Clinical relevance and response to pharmacologic therapy. *J Am Coll Cardiol.* January 19, 2010;55(3):213–20.

63. Muehlberg F et al. Native myocardial T1 time can predict development of subsequent anthracycline-induced cardiomyopathy. *ESC Heart Fail.* August 2018;5(4):620–9.

64. Grover S et al. Left and right ventricular effects of anthracycline and trastuzumab chemotherapy: A prospective study using novel cardiac imaging and biochemical markers. *Int J Cardiol.* October 15, 2013; 168(6):5465–7.

65. Jordan JH et al. Longitudinal assessment of concurrent changes in left ventricular ejection fraction and left ventricular myocardial tissue characteristics after administration of cardiotoxic chemotherapies using T1-weighted and T2-weighted cardiovascular magnetic resonance. *Circ Cardiovasc Imaging*. November 2014;7(6):872–9.

66. Ong G et al. Myocardial strain imaging by cardiac magnetic resonance for detection of subclinical myocardial dysfunction in breast cancer patients receiving trastuzumab and chemotherapy. *Int J Cardiol*. January 15, 2018;261:228–33.

67. Jolly MP, Jordan JH, Melendez GC, McNeal GR, D'Agostino RB, Jr., Hundley WG. Automated assessments of circumferential strain from cine CMR correlate with LVEF declines in cancer patients early after receipt of cardio-toxic chemotherapy. *J Cardiovasc Magn Reson*. August 2, 2017;19(1):59.

68. Barthur A et al. Longitudinal assessment of right ventricular structure and function by cardiovascular magnetic resonance in breast cancer patients treated with trastuzumab: A prospective observational study. *J Cardiovasc Magn Reson*. April 10, 2017;19(1):44.

69. Melendez GC et al. Frequency of left ventricular end-diastolic volume-mediated declines in ejection fraction in patients receiving potentially cardiotoxic cancer treatment. *Am J Cardiol*. May 15, 2017;119(10):1637–42.

70. Nathan PC, Amir E, Abdel-Qadir H. Cardiac outcomes in survivors of pediatric and adult cancers. *Can J Cardiol*. July 2016;32(7): 871–80.

71. Neilan TG et al. Left ventricular mass in patients with a cardiomyopathy after treatment with anthracyclines. *Am J Cardiol*. December 1, 2012;110(11):1679–86.

72. Umezawa R et al. MRI findings of radiation-induced myocardial damage in patients with oesophageal cancer. *Clin Radiol*. December 2014;69(12):1273–9.

73. Fallah-Rad N, Lytwyn M, Fang T, Kirkpatrick I, Jassal DS. Delayed contrast enhancement cardiac magnetic resonance imaging in trastuzumab induced cardiomyopathy. *J Cardiovasc Magn Reson*. January 22, 2008;10:5.

74. Toro-Salazar OH, Lee JH, Zellars KN et al. Use of integrated imaging and serum biomarker profiles to identify subclinical dysfunction in pediatric cancer patients treated with anthracyclines. *Cardiooncology*. 2018;4(pii):4. doi: 10.1186/s40959-018-0030-5.

75. Johnson CB, Davis MK, Law A, Sulpher J. Shared risk factors for cardiovascular disease and cancer: Implications for preventive health and clinical care in oncology patients. *Can J Cardiol*. July 2016;32(7):900–7.

76. Fleisher LA, Fleischmann KE, Auerbach AD et al. 2014 ACC/AHA guideline on perioperative cardiovascular evaluation and management of patients undergoing noncardiac surgery. *J Am Coll Cardiol*. 2014, doi: 10.1016/j.jacc.2014.07.944.

77. Duceppe E et al. Canadian cardiovascular society guidelines on perioperative cardiac risk assessment and management for patients undergoing non-cardiac surgery. *Can J Cardiol*. 2017;33:17–32.

78. Kristenson SD et al. 2014 ESC/ESA guidelines on non-cardiac surgery: Cardiovascular assessment and management: The joint task force on non-cardiac surgery: Cardiovascular assessment and management of the European society of cardiology (ESC) and the European society of anaesthesiology (ESA). *Eur Heart J*. September 14, 2014;35(35):2383–431.

79. Lee TH et al. Derivation and prospective validation of a simple index for prediction of cardiac risk of major noncardiac surgery. *Circulation*. September 7, 1999;100(10): 1043–9.

80. Wijeysundera DN et al. Assessment of functional capacity before major non-cardiac surgery: An international, prospective cohort study. *Lancet*. June 30, 2018;391(10140): 2631–40.

81. Devereaux PJ et al. Association between postoperative troponin levels and 30-day mortality among patients undergoing noncardiac surgery. *JAMA*. 2012;307(21):2295–304.

82. Devereaux PJ et al. Association of postoperative high-sensitivity troponin levels with myocardial injury and 30-day mortality among patients undergoing noncardiac surgery. *JAMA*. 2017;317(16):1642–51.

4

Radiotherapy in cancer patients

GIRISH KUNAPAREDDY, ADARSH SIDDA, CHRISTOPHER FLEMING,
CHIRAG SHAH, AND PATRICK COLLIER

INTRODUCTION

For more than a century, the use of radiation therapy has been an integral component in the management of oncological disease, especially breast cancer, Hodgkin's lymphoma, lung cancer, and other malignancies involving the mediastinum and thorax (1). Radiation therapy can be employed as a single treatment modality, simultaneously with systemic therapies, and/or in conjunction with surgery, while potentially improving survival, organ preservation, and quality of life.

Substantial advancements in radiation therapy have allowed for accurate delivery of radiation that maximizes tumor control and survivorship and minimizes total cardiac dose and risk of late cardiovascular complications (2). Blunting this progress is the rising incidence of cardiovascular risk factors within the general population that has an impact on the risk of radiation treatment (3). Nonetheless, with increasing awareness, careful radiation planning, selection of appropriate chemotherapy, and other prevention strategies, cardiac disease from radiation therapy should become less common in the future.

The focus of this chapter is to provide a practical approach for oncologists, cardiologists, and other healthcare providers involved in the management of cancer patients, in order to provide optimal oncologic care before, during, and after radiation therapy. The wide spectrum of pathophysiology that may manifest as radiation-induced heart disease will also be discussed.

CONSIDERATIONS BEFORE STARTING RADIATION THERAPY

Identification of patients at increased risk

Many patient-specific and treatment-specific factors contribute to development of radiation-induced heart disease.

The European Association of Cardiovascular Imaging and the American Society of Echocardiography have suggested that patients who receive anterior or left sided -sided chest radiation in the presence of one or more risk factors should be considered high risk. Risk factors include high cumulative dose of radiation >30 Gy, high dose of radiation fractions >2 Gy/d, younger patients <50 years, presence of the tumor in proximity to the heart, concomitant chemotherapy especially with anthracyclines, lack of shielding, and preexisting cardiovascular disease or cardiovascular risk factors (hypertension, hyperlipidemia, diabetes mellitus, smoking, and obesity) (4). However, these guidelines may need to be updated as data on hypofractionated whole breast irradiation (2.66 Gy/fraction) have failed to demonstrate higher cardiac morbidity and are a standard of care approach (5); additionally, total cumulative dose may no longer correlate with cardiac dose in light of new treatment techniques (2).

The American Society of Clinical Oncology has suggested that the following patients undergoing radiation therapy should be considered high risk: those who receive high-dose radiotherapy ($\geq$30 Gy) where the heart is in the treatment field; and those who receive lower-dose radiotherapy (<30 Gy) where the heart is in the treatment field in combination with lower-dose anthracycline (e.g., doxorubicin at <250 mg/m^2, epirubicin at <600 mg/m^2) (6).

Preventative strategies to minimize risk before initiation of therapy

It is recommended that clinicians should screen for and actively manage modifiable cardiovascular risk factors in all patients receiving potentially cardiotoxic treatments (6). Before initiation of potentially cardiotoxic therapies, clinicians should perform a comprehensive assessment in patients with cancer that includes a history and physical examination, screening for cardiovascular disease risk factors (hypertension, diabetes, dyslipidemia, obesity, and smoking), and an echocardiogram (4,6).

After initial clinical assessment for cardiac risk, cardiology consultation should be considered for patients with high cardiovascular risk, those with symptoms and those with established cardiac disease to initiate or reestablish cardiology follow-up. Evaluation to assess tolerability of the proposed oncological treatment should include review of baseline tests, symptoms, and medications, prior to consideration of the need for further testing and/or treatment. Such a review also offers an opportunity for patient education, with regard to lifestyle/risk factor modifications and reiterating the importance of seeking an early review should a change in clinical condition occur.

For high-risk patients, a multidisciplinary team approach is recommended to assess risks and benefits of treatment plans. Decision-making on what choice regimen to use depends on overall net benefit

of therapy incorporating short- and long-term toxicity, prognosis, and treatment intent (curative vs. palliative), and alternative treatments. In a setting of a malignancy with a higher probability of cure, which would otherwise lead to rapid demise, the threshold to accept higher cardiovascular toxicity would be lower. In contrast, the use of potentially cardiotoxic therapies should be avoided or minimized if established alternatives exist that would not compromise cancer-specific outcomes (6).

CONSIDERATIONS DURING RADIATION THERAPY

This section will discuss the role of radiation therapy in the treatment of more common malignancies of the chest and will highlight current techniques that have been adopted in order to try to reduce cardiac toxicity.

Radiation therapy in breast cancer

In the metastatic setting, radiation has a role in selected cases for local management of the primary or specific metastatic lesions in order to palliate symptoms and prevent cancer-related complications with some evidence suggesting a potential for prolonging survival, although prospective data are lacking (7).

For patients with nonmetastatic disease (the focus of the remainder of this section), radiation therapy is an integral part of the management of patients with early stage and locally advanced breast cancer to eradicate any tumor deposits remaining following surgery (8–10). Postmastectomy radiation therapy has been associated with significant improvements in local recurrence (11). For patients who are candidates for breast-conserving therapy, radiotherapy to the conserved breast halves the rate at which the disease recurs and reduces the breast cancer death rate by about a sixth (12).

Meta-analyses data have shown that radiation therapy produced similar proportional reductions in local recurrence in all women (irrespective of age or tumor characteristics) and in all major trials of radiation therapy vs. not (recent or older; with or without systemic therapy), so the larger the control risk, the larger absolute reductions in local recurrence (11).

Standard whole breast irradiation consists of daily radiation therapy over 5–7 weeks to a total

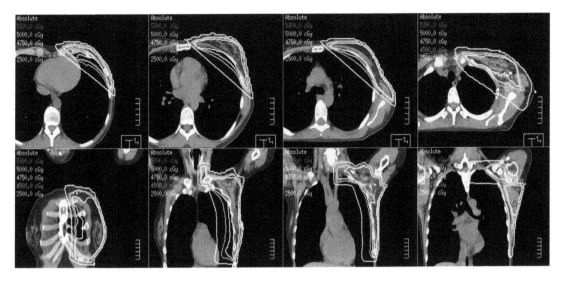

Figure 4.1 Cardiac-sparing 3D conformal radiation therapy in a patient with left-sided breast cancer. Three-dimensional conformal radiation therapy refers to cancer radiation treatment where the radiation beam is shaped to match the tumor mapped from 3D computed tomography scanning to allow more precise treatment of the tumor while avoiding the healthy surrounding tissue and in particular the heart.

dose of 45–66 Gy. More recently, hypofractionated whole breast irradiation allows completion in 3–5 weeks delivering 40 or 42.5 Gy in 15 or 16 fractions respectively (13,14); most patients receive an additional boost to the tumor bed to further reduce the risk of local recurrence (15). In patients with nodal positivity, regional nodal irradiation may be included regardless of axillary surgery performed including the axilla, supraclavicular region as well as the internal mammary nodes (16–18). Limited change in cardiac dose is expected with regional node irradiation with the exception of internal mammary treatment, which may drastically increase heart dose depending on technique utilized.

Given the anatomical location of the heart predominantly on the left side of the chest cavity with the anterior surface of the left ventricle and the distribution of the left anterior descending artery more proximal to the anterior chest wall, left-sided breast cancers have been associated with higher rates of cardiotoxicity than right-sided cancer (19–22). Older radiotherapy regimens were shown to have increased risk of contralateral breast cancer and non-breast cancer mortality mainly from heart disease and lung cancer (11). Such historical data prompted the development of newer radiation therapy techniques aimed at more targeted therapy in order to minimize

long-term off-target toxicities that may attenuate overall survival benefit (Figure 4.1).

While 2D techniques were historically used to deliver radiation therapy, modern planning is computed tomography based allowing for 3D assessment of targets and organs at risk (23). Additionally, modern techniques to deliver external beam radiotherapy use tangential fields to treat the whole breast while minimizing cardiac and pulmonary dose and therefore potential toxicity (23).

Other strategies have been incorporated into breast cancer radiation therapy techniques to reduce cardiac dose (23). These include adjusting the timing of delivery of radiation therapy with the respiratory cycle, intensity-modulated radiotherapy, prone patient positioning, proton beam therapy, and accelerated partial breast irradiation; these will be discussed in the following section.

During the inspiratory phase of the respiratory cycle, there is a corresponding expansion of the thoracic cavity, with simultaneous displacement of the heart away from the anterior chest wall. By providing the treatment during a deep inspiration breath hold, when the heart achieves the ideal distance away from the chest wall, the radiation dose to the heart can be substantially reduced (24–26). A recent systematic review found that early postradiation perfusion defects evident after

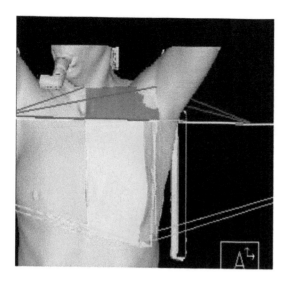

Figure 4.2 Cardiac-sparing active breathing control in a patient with left-sided breast cancer. Active breathing control involves attaching a breathing device to the patient's mouth to ensure that radiation is applied during deep inspiration when the heart is further away from the tumor to limit the radiation dose.

incidental irradiation of the heart in cases of left breast/chest wall radiation therapy were absent in studies that used cardiac sparing techniques (such as deep inspiration) (27). As such, deep inspiration breath hold represents the technique with the strongest data supporting its use in cardiac sparing approaches (Figure 4.2).

Intensity-modulated radiotherapy takes advantage of advances in linear accelerator technology (multileaf collimator) and has seen increased utilization in the treatment of breast cancer, especially in left-sided cancers (25,28). This technique has shown better dose homogeneity in the breast with reduced cardiac doses during treatment of left-sided cancers, in both intact and postmastectomy settings (29), compared to 3D conformal radiation therapy (23). Several studies have also shown that this technique specifically reduces dose to the coronary arteries and the left ventricle compared to conventional methods (30). When combined with breath holding and prone positioning, this technique can further reduce total cardiac dose (31). However, intensity-modulated radiotherapy may increase the cost of therapy while not having been shown to consistently reduce heart dose as compared to opposed-tangent 3D radiotherapy plans with deep inspiration breath hold (32).

Patients undergoing radiation therapy are typically treated in the supine position; however, prone positioning may be useful in patients with large, pendulous breasts by allowing the breast to fall away from the chest wall and the heart, reducing total cardiac dose (33–36). Nevertheless, there are conflicting data regarding the practical value of the prone positioning technique. A recent study demonstrated that this technique reduced cardiac doses in 19 out of 30 patients, but increased cardiac dose in 8 of the 30 patients (37). Another study showed essentially no difference between prone and supine positions when radiation was administered via intensity-modulated radiotherapy (31). These discrepancies could be due to barriers in reproducibility of this technique owing to operator dependent variation (38). Additionally, a recent study comparing prone to breath hold found improved cardiac sparing with breath hold as compared to prone radiotherapy with respect to mean heart and left anterior descending arterial doses (39).

Proton beam irradiation takes advantage of the unique properties of protons over photons. The proton energy can be tailored to attain Bragg's peak at the target site, with minimal residual radiation around or beyond it. This approach has been suggested to reduce the cardiac radiation doses (40,41). This allows for larger doses per fraction and accelerated hypofractionation over smaller target tissue. Limitations of this technique are higher costs, the availability of the devices at institutions, larger skin doses, and the need for large studies to validate its use. Additionally, it is unclear if the marginal advantage in cardiac dose compared with opposed-tangent 3D radiotherapy plans with deep inspiration breath hold is clinically meaningful in light of the higher costs and limited data.

Accelerated partial breast irradiation involves radiation limited to the lumpectomy with a margin, while sparing the rest of the breast and axilla, used for early stage tumors including patients aged >50, with lymph node and margin negative tumors less than <3 cm. This technique has been found to provide equivalent local-regional control along with a better side effect profile, including cardiac toxicity, as compared to whole breast radiotherapy, although location and technique play important roles in cardiac dose and need to be considered (42–45).

Radiation therapy in Hodgkin's lymphoma

Radiation therapy was the definitive treatment for Hodgkin's lymphoma for many years. However, with the advent of newer chemotherapy agents and advances in radiation techniques, the treatment of Hodgkin's lymphoma has evolved considerably, with majority of the patients receiving multimodality therapy with excellent clinical outcomes (46).

Historically, extended field radiation therapy was widely used to deliver radiation to the affected lymph nodes as well as to adjacent uninvolved nodes, entailing broader coverage but with a larger dose to normal tissues (47). Additionally, doses exceeding 40 Gy were routinely utilized. Improvements in radiation therapy with respect to technique, dose, and radiation fields have resulted in lesser toxicity without compromising survival rates (48,49).

Smaller radiation fields (involved field radiation therapy) have led to focus on involved regions such as the mediastinum. More recently, even smaller target fields, such as involved site radiation therapy (ISRT) and involved node radiation therapy (INRT), have come to the forefront of therapy and are currently the preferred radiation technique for most patients (2,50). ISRT and INRT fields provide radiation to only the involved areas, with a small margin of healthy tissue, but may require detailed imaging studies to guide treatment. Additionally, lower doses of radiation are now used in conjunction with systemic therapy (51). It is therefore important to recognize that the data regarding cardiac toxicity with older radiotherapy paradigms may no longer be representative of current practice. For patients with early stage classical Hodgkin's lymphoma, the radiation therapy dose is 30 Gy if complete remission is observed after systemic therapy, and can be lowered to 20 Gy with favorable prognostic factors (52). However, if the patient has residual disease then increasing the dose to the clinical target volume would be considered. Additionally, new techniques, including Intensity-modulated radiation therapy (IMRT) and proton therapy, can reduce cardiac dose in mediastinal lymphomas.

Radiation therapy in lung cancer

The two primary forms of lungs cancers are small cell lung cancer (SCLC) and non-small cell lung cancer (NSCLC) with radiation therapy being standard of care in the management of both.

SCLC is divided into limited stage and extensive stage. Radiation therapy in combination with chemotherapy is often utilized in limited stage presentations (53). Accelerated hyperfractionation with twice daily fractions given over 3 weeks for a total of 45 Gy or daily 2 y fraction to a total dose of 60–70 Gy is a standard regimen. Extensive stage SCLC is primarily treated with chemotherapy. In patients who show complete or partial response to chemotherapy, thoracic radiation therapy may be pursued for management of residual disease. While traditional techniques often lead to higher heart doses, modern techniques, including IMRT, reduce the dose to the lungs and heart, potentially reducing cardiac toxicity; however, it is important to recognize that median survival with SCLC is lower than most breast cancers and as such the potential benefits of cardiac sparing approaches may be more limited.

Stage I and Stage II NSCLCs are generally treated with surgical resection. Radiation therapy with stereotactic body radiation therapy (SBRT) or more conventional methods are an option for non-surgical candidates, with growing data supporting their role for operable patients as well (54). Stage III disease can be treated using a combined modality approach that may include chemotherapy, radiation and surgery, chemoradiation alone, or sequential chemotherapy and radiation depending on patient performance status and comorbidities (55). A typical radiation dose for Stage III disease is 60 Gy in 30 daily fractions. Radiation Therapy Oncology Group (RTOG) 0617 has shown that using higher doses of radiation therapy with concurrent chemotherapy did not result in better outcomes than 60 Gy in Sage III NSCLC (56). Moreover, use of IMRT was associated with lower cardiac doses compared to 3D conformal radiation therapy in patients with locally advanced NSCLC (57).

Radiation therapy in esophageal (squamous cell cancer)

Patients with T1N0 esophageal cancer usually undergo surgical resection without any neoadjuvant therapy (58). The approach to T2N0 cancers is controversial due to discrepancies in staging, and varies by histological type, but in practice follows that of higher stage disease given very poor concordance of clinical and pathological staging. Prospective studies have demonstrated that combined modality therapy with neoadjuvant chemoradiation, followed by surgery, represents the standard of care in the treatment of T3N0, T4N0, and node positive esophageal cancer (58,59). The radiation dosage used for the combined modality therapy was 50–50.4 Gy administered in 25–28 daily fractions; however, data from the CROSS trial demonstrated the feasibility of 41.4 Gy in 23 fractions (60). Owing to proximity to the heart, cardiac doses can be high with radiation therapy in esophageal cancer; however, techniques including IMRT can be utilized to reduce cardiac doses as can proton therapy (61).

RADIATION-INDUCED HEART DISEASE

Radiation-induced heart disease is considered a pancarditis, meaning all cardiovascular tissues (including the coronary arteries, capillaries, myocardium, valves, pericardium, and the conduction system) are prone to fibroinflammatory pathological changes following radiation exposure that ultimately may result in a heart failure syndrome (Figure 4.3).

With contemporary practice, acute toxicity from radiotherapy is rarely seen. This is primarily due to better patient selection and more importantly, from advances in treatment planning and delivery.

Acute pericarditis usually occurs within the first few weeks of radiation therapy. Pericarditis, the most common cardiac complication historically, is now seldom observed on account of newer techniques incorporating cardioprotective methods, including lowered radiation doses, more efficient targeting, and incorporation of shielding blocks (62). Acute pericarditis is generally self-limiting, with half of the patients recovering with rest alone, while others are treated with nonsteroidal anti-inflammatory drugs, colchicine, and possibly the addition of diuretics. Increased vascular permeability accounts for extravasation of protein-rich fluid leading to pericardial effusions. Pericardial effusions may be seen in the acute setting but usually accumulate gradually, without sudden cardiovascular compromise. If hemodynamic instability from effusions does occur, it needs to be rapidly relieved with a needle pericardiocentesis or surgical window.

For the remainder of this section, we will discuss latent toxic effects on cardiovascular tissues. Again, it is important to reiterate that much of these data arise from older studies, with lower radiation exposures expected with modern radiation therapy.

With regard to the pericardium, chronic pericardial remodeling can occur months to years after

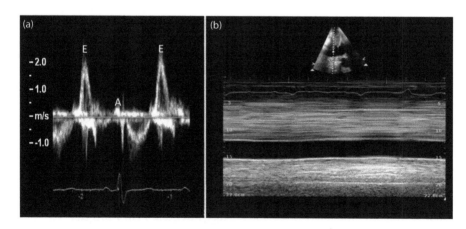

Figure 4.3 Elevated filling pressures in radiation-induced heart disease. Panel (a) shows pulsed wave Doppler of mitral inflow showing high E wave velocity, diminutive A wave velocity, a high (>2) E/A wave velocity ratio, and a rapid E wave deceleration time, collectively indicating high left ventricular filling pressures, which in radiation-induced pancarditis may be due to restrictive cardiomyopathy, constrictive pericarditis, severe mitral regurgitation and/or advanced diastolic dysfunction. Panel (b) shows an M-mode view of the inferior vena cava, which is dilated and plethoric (does not reduce in size with inspiration), indicative of elevated right atrial pressure.

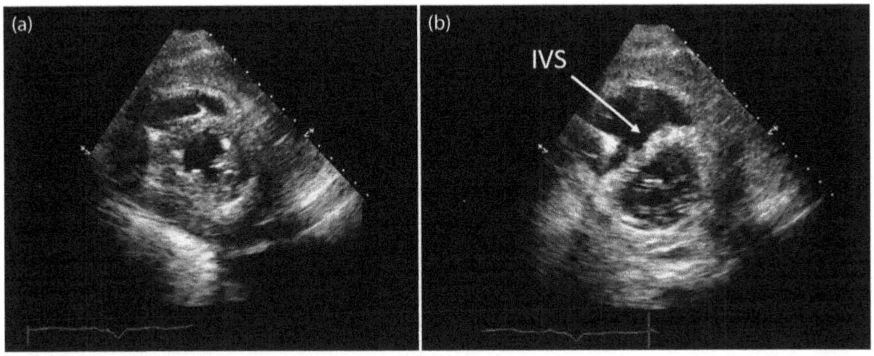

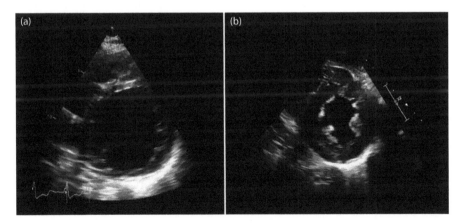

Figure 4.4 Abnormal interventricular septal motion in radiation-induced heart disease. Radiation-induced constrictive pericarditis results in abnormal interventricular septal motion involving a cardio-phasic septal bounce (caused by abrupt cessation of diastolic inflow due to pericardial constraint) and respiro-phasic shifting (related to interventricular dependence where one ventricle can only fill at the expense of the other). Such a relative leftward inspiratory shift is seen in Panel (b) vs. Panel (a).

initial radiotherapy, characterized by recurrent inflammation, fibrosis, and calcification that may eventually result in constrictive pericarditis (Figure 4.4). Pericardiectomy can be considered for very symptomatic patients, but in this setting surgery is associated with very high morbidity and mortality.

Cardiomyopathy may result from interstitial fibrosis when excessive collagen deposition occurs within the interstitium, thereby causing mainly restrictive disease and diastolic dysfunction (63–65). Radiation results in pro-inflammatory free radical formation and augments fibroblastic activity by facilitating the release of growth factor 2 and transforming growth factor beta leading to cell

death and systolic heart failure (66). Higher radiation doses along with the potential interaction of anthracycline toxicity can cause additional cell necrosis. Heart failure caused by cardiotoxic therapies exhibits the same clinical features and treatment options as other causes of heart failure in the general population (Figure 4.5) (67).

Radiotherapy can lead to micro- and macroangiopathy of the coronary arteries, with oxidative damage from free radical generation, causing endothelial injury and increased vascular permeability (68). Endothelial injury hastens atherosclerotic changes with its characteristic inflammation, lipid-rich plaque formation, vascular remodeling,

Figure 4.5 Cardiomyopathy in radiation-induced heart disease. Dilated cardiomyopathy (Panel [a]) with reduced left ventricular ejection fraction can occur in the setting of radiation exposure particularly in those who received concomitant cardiotoxic chemotherapy such as anthracyclines. Restrictive cardiomyopathy (Panel [b]) with preserved left ventricular ejection fraction can also occur, which is characterized by left ventricular hypertrophy, fibrosis, and increased stiffness.

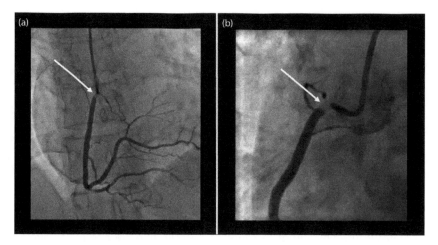

Figure 4.6 Ostial coronary artery disease in radiation-induced heart disease. Coronary angiography showing ostial right coronary artery disease (white arrow) in a patient with prior radiation exposure. The contrast-filled catheter within the ascending aorta and aortic root is seen above the coronary artery. Panel A is right anterior oblique view. Panel B is zoomed left anterior oblique view.

and intraluminal thrombosis, leading to coronary artery disease and tissue ischemia (69). Radiation can cause a significant overall reduction in the number of capillaries perfusing the myocardium, accentuating ischemia (70).

Historically, accelerated coronary artery disease has been the most fatal complication from radiotherapy to the thorax. The risk increases 10 years after initial radiation therapy and continues to gradually increase with time (71). A study looking at postradiation therapy cardiovascular risk in patients with Hodgkin's lymphoma found a greater than 10% risk for development of symptomatic coronary artery

disease 9–13 years after radiation therapy (72). There is a higher propensity for injury to the vessels located over the radiation field with a predisposition for ostial involvement (Figure 4.6). As such, there is a higher incidences of severe left main coronary artery disease and ostial lesions of the right coronary and left anterior descending arteries compared to the other coronary vasculature (72).

Radiation may also affect valve tissue—classically affecting multiple valves in mixed ways (causing a mixture of both stenosis and regurgitation) due to fibrocalcific remodeling (Figure 4.7). Greater incidence of aortic and mitral valve pathology

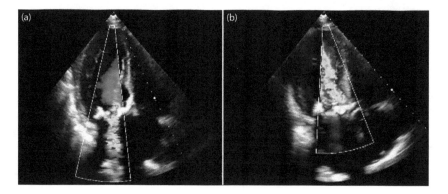

Figure 4.7 Radiation exposure is associated with mixed lesions in multiple valves. Panel (a) shows turbulent systolic flow of mitral regurgitation while Panel (b) shows turbulent diastolic flow of confluent mitral stenosis and aortic regurgitation. This patient was also found to have calcific aortic stenosis and tricuspid regurgitation. Ultimately, this patient went on to have aortic and mitral valve replacement and tricuspid valve repair.

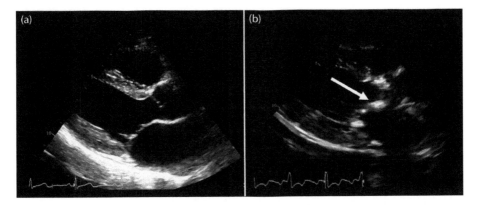

Figure 4.8 Thickened aorto-mitral curtain in radiation valve disease. A characteristic and prognostic echo finding in valvular disease in the setting of prior radiation exposure is thickening of the aorto-mitral curtain (white arrow, Panel [b]) vs. a normal heart (Panel [a]).

compared to tricuspid and pulmonic valves independent of relative dose distribution of radiation therapy has been noted, likely attributed to the higher-pressure gradients across the left side of the heart (73).

A specific pathognomonic finding on echocardiography indicative of prior radiation exposure is prominent thickening of the aorto-mitral curtain where the anterior mitral valve leaflet approaches the left/nonaortic commissure (Figure 4.8) (74). The degree of thickening seen is prognostic and has been shown to be an independent predictor of mortality in patients with radiation-induced heart disease (75).

A total radiation dose above 35 Gy significantly increases the risk for the development of severe valvulopathy requiring surgery, compared to patients who received less than 30 Gy (76). Regurgitation is typically the preliminary valvulopathy, with stenosis occurring years thereafter (77). In one study, clinically asymptomatic valve disease was diagnosed at an average of 11.5 years postradiation, compared to symptomatic valve disease diagnosed at 16.5 years, signifying a mean 5-year interval prior to symptom development (73). Surgical valve replacement is superior to reparative procedures in management of these patients (78). Although currently not part of standard surgical risk stratification scores, prior mediastinal radiation therapy confers significantly worse longer-term survival for patients undergoing valve surgery vs. a matched cohort (79). It may be prudent to delay surgery until patients develop symptoms. More rigorous preoperative testing may help detect concomitant

pulmonary hypertension (via right heart catheterization), pulmonary fibrosis (via pulmonary function testing with assessment of diffusion capacity), cardiac fibrosis (via magnetic resonance imaging-based techniques), critical chest entry anatomy and extensive calcific remodeling (via noncontrast CT) (Figures 4.9 and 4.10). Reoperation risk is particularly high so that the use of transcatheter aortic valve replacement should be considered in otherwise poor surgical candidates (80).

The conduction system is quite radiation-sensitive and electrophysiological disturbances may stem from fibrotic remodeling as a result of direct radiation injury. Such conduction abnormalities include right and left bundle branch blocks, varying degrees of heart blocks including complete heart block, sick sinus syndrome, supraventricular arrhythmias, ventricular tachycardia, and prolonged QTc (81). Ventricular ectopy is more commonly seen, likely from ventricular fibrosis. Clinically, right bundle branch blocks are likely to be observed more than left bundle branch blocks, as the right bundle is located more anteriorly, with higher exposure to radiation (82). Though most patients are asymptomatic, the presenting features can include palpitations, dizziness, syncope, and even sudden death (83).

CONSIDERATIONS AFTER RADIATION THERAPY

Current guidelines recommend a careful annual history and physical exam for all survivors of cancer previously treated with potentially cardiotoxic

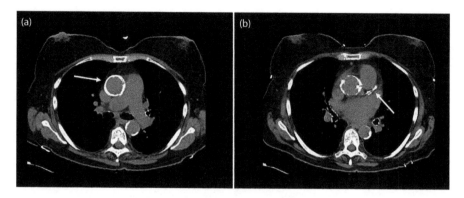

Figure 4.9 Calcification in radiation-induced heart disease. Porcelain aorta refers to calcium deposited in the aortic wall circumferentially as shown by computed tomography in Panel (a). Associated calcification of the ostial left main coronary artery is shown in Panel (b).

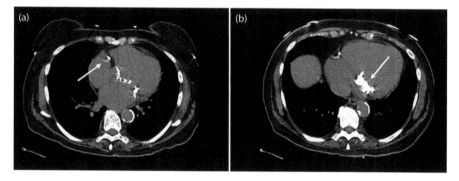

Figure 4.10 Calcification in radiation-induced heart disease. Calcification of the proximal right coronary artery disease by computed tomography is shown in Panel (a). Associated dense mitral annular calcification is shown in Panel (b).

therapies (4). A heart-healthy lifestyle, including the role of diet and exercise, should be promoted as part of long-term follow-up care (6).

For patients with symptoms concerning for cardiac dysfunction following completion of potentially cardiotoxic therapies, recommended initial care includes serum cardiac biomarkers (troponins, natriuretic peptides) and echocardiogram (with preferable consideration of cardiac magnetic resonance imaging if suboptimal echocardiogram) for diagnostic workup with referral to a cardiologist based on findings (6).

For asymptomatic patients considered to be at increased risk of developing cardiac dysfunction, similar imaging tests may be performed between 6 and 12 months after completion of cancer-directed therapy with referral to cardiology for further assessment and management if cardiac dysfunction is identified (6).

Given the potential for a prolonged latent period following radiation therapy prior to the development of symptoms, survivors should be advised to seek medical attention if there is a change in their symptom status and to inform their caregivers of their prior treatments (4).

Patients with significant prior radiation exposure should be given special consideration and considered as a unique population, particularly given the potential risk of harm arising because current standard preoperative risk testing grossly underestimates risk of cardiotoxicity, and because risks with interventions are significantly increased compared to the general population. It is hoped that better patient and physician awareness of these issues may lead to a more comprehensive preoperative assessment, improved informed consent, and a better selected surgical population.

CONCLUSIONS

Radiation therapy remains an important part of treatment for breast cancer as well as for other malignancies of the thorax. With increased survivorship comes additional emphasis on efforts to minimize, in particular, longer-term cardiac toxicity. Advances in radiation technology, techniques, dosimetry, precautions, and patient selection have led to reductions in cardiac radiation dose. Given the latency in cardiac sequelae with radiation exposure, the benefits of modern radiation therapy protocols will likely be observed over the next several years.

REFERENCES

1. Heidenreich PA et al. Screening for coronary artery disease after mediastinal irradiation for Hodgkin's disease. *J Clin Oncol.* 2007;25(1):43–9.
2. Specht L et al. Modern radiation therapy for Hodgkin lymphoma: Field and dose guidelines from the international lymphoma radiation oncology group (ILROG). *Int J Radiat Oncol Biol Phys.* 2014;89(4):854–62.
3. Darby SC et al. Risk of ischemic heart disease in women after radiotherapy for breast cancer. *N Engl J Med.* 2013;368(11):987–98.
4. Lancellotti P et al. Expert consensus for multi-modality imaging evaluation of cardiovascular complications of radiotherapy in adults: A report from the European Association of Cardiovascular Imaging and the American Society of Echocardiography. *J Am Soc Echocardiogr.* 2013;26(9):1013–32.
5. Chan EK et al. Adjuvant hypofractionated versus conventional whole breast radiation therapy for early-stage breast cancer: Long-term hospital-related morbidity from cardiac causes. *Int J Radiat Oncol Biol Phys.* 2014;88(4):786–92.
6. Armenian SH et al. Prevention and monitoring of cardiac dysfunction in survivors of adult cancers: American Society of Clinical Oncology clinical practice guideline. *J Clin Oncol.* 2017;35(8):893–911.
7. Pagani O et al. International guidelines for management of metastatic breast cancer: Can metastatic breast cancer be cured? *J Natl Cancer Inst.* 2010;102(7):456–63.
8. Agarwal S et al. Effect of breast conservation therapy vs mastectomy on disease-specific survival for early-stage breast cancer. *JAMA Surg.* 2014;149(3):267–74.
9. Fisher B et al. Twenty-year follow-up of a randomized trial comparing total mastectomy, lumpectomy, and lumpectomy plus irradiation for the treatment of invasive breast cancer. *N Engl J Med.* 2002;347(16):1233–41.
10. Litiere S et al. Breast conserving therapy versus mastectomy for stage I-II breast cancer: 20 year follow-up of the EORTC. 10801 phase 3 randomised trial. *Lancet Oncol.* 2012;13(4):412–9.
11. Clarke M et al. Effects of radiotherapy and of differences in the extent of surgery for early breast cancer on local recurrence and 15-year survival: An overview of the randomised trials. *Lancet* 2005;366(9503):2087–106.
12. Darby S et al. Effect of radiotherapy after breast-conserving surgery on 10-year recurrence and 15-year breast cancer death: Meta-analysis of individual patient data for 10,801 women in 17 randomised trials. *Lancet* 2011;378(9804):1707–16.
13. Smith BD et al. Fractionation for whole breast irradiation: An American society for radiation oncology (ASTRO) evidence-based guideline. *Int J Radiat Oncol Biol Phys.* 2011;81(1):59–68.
14. Whelan TJ et al. Long-term results of hypofractionated radiation therapy for breast cancer. *N Engl J Med.* 2010;362(6):513–20.
15. Kindts I et al. Tumour bed boost radiotherapy for women after breast-conserving surgery. *Cochrane Database Syst Rev.* 2017;11:CD011987.
16. Donker M et al. Radiotherapy or surgery of the axilla after a positive sentinel node in breast cancer (EORTC. 10981–22023 AMAROS): A randomised, multicentre, open-label, phase 3 non-inferiority trial. *Lancet Oncol.* 2014;15(12):1303–10.
17. Giuliano AE et al. Effect of axillary dissection vs no axillary dissection on 10-year overall survival among women with invasive breast cancer and sentinel node metastasis: The ACOSOG Z0011 (Alliance) randomized clinical trial. *JAMA.* 2017;318(10):918–26.
18. Poortmans PM et al. Internal mammary and medial supraclavicular irradiation in breast cancer. *N Engl J Med.* 2015;373(4):317–27.

19. Taylor CW et al. Cardiac exposures in breast cancer radiotherapy: 1950s–1990s. *Int J Radiat Oncol Biol Phys.* 2007;69(5):1484–95.

20. Darby SC et al. Long-term mortality from heart disease and lung cancer after radiotherapy for early breast cancer: Prospective cohort study of about 300,000 women in US SEER cancer registries. *Lancet Oncol.* 2005;6(8):557–65.

21. McGale P et al. Incidence of heart disease in 35,000 women treated with radiotherapy for breast cancer in Denmark and Sweden. *Radiother Oncol.* 2011;100(2):167–75.

22. Rehammar JC et al. Risk of heart disease in relation to radiotherapy and chemotherapy with anthracyclines among 19,464 breast cancer patients in Denmark. 1977–2005. *Radiother Oncol.* 2017;123(2):299–305.

23. Shah C et al. Cardiac dose sparing and avoidance techniques in breast cancer radiotherapy. *Radiother Oncol.* 2014;112(1):9–16.

24. Freedman GMLL, Cardiac-sparing radiation therapy for breast cancer. *Appl Rad Oncol.* September 12, 2016:6–11.

25. Shah C et al. Use of intensity modulated radiation therapy to reduce acute and chronic toxicities of breast cancer patients treated with traditional and accelerated whole breast irradiation. *Pract Radiat Oncol.* 2012;2(4):e45–51.

26. Nissen, HD and AL Appelt, Improved heart, lung and target dose with deep inspiration breath hold in a large clinical series of breast cancer patients. *Radiother Oncol.* 2013;106(1):28–32.

27. Kaidar-Person O et al. Early cardiac perfusion defects after left-sided radiation therapy for breast cancer: Is there a volume response? *Breast Cancer Res Treat.* 2017;164(2):253–62.

28. Arthur DW, Morris MM, Vicini FA. Breast cancer: New radiation treatment options. *Oncology (Williston Park)* 2004;18(13):1621–9; discussion 1629–30, 1636–38.

29. Li JG et al. Breast-conserving radiation therapy using combined electron and intensity-modulated radiotherapy technique. *Radiother Oncol.* 2000;56(1):65–71.

30. Lohr F et al. Potential effect of robust and simple IMRT approach for left-sided breast cancer on cardiac mortality. *Int J Radiat Oncol Biol Phys.* 2009;74(1):73–80.

31. Mulliez T et al. Whole breast radiotherapy in prone and supine position: Is there a place for multi-beam IMRT? *Radiat Oncol.* 2013;8:151.

32. Sripathi LK et al. Cardiac dose reduction with deep-inspiratory breath hold technique of radiotherapy for left-sided breast cancer. *J Med Phys.* 2017;42(3):123–7.

33. Chen JL et al. Prone breast forward intensity-modulated radiotherapy for Asian women with early left breast cancer: Factors for cardiac sparing and clinical outcomes. *J Radiat Res.* 2013;54(5):899–908.

34. Fernandez-Lizarbe E et al. Pilot study of feasibility and dosimetric comparison of prone versus supine breast radiotherapy. *Clin Transl Oncol.* 2013;15(6):450–9.

35. Merchant TE, McCormick B. Prone position breast irradiation. *Int J Radiat Oncol Biol Phys.* 1994;30(1):197–203.

36. Chino JP and LB Marks, Prone positioning causes the heart to be displaced anteriorly within the thorax: Implications for breast cancer treatment. *Int J Radiat Oncol Biol Phys.* 2008;70(3):916–20.

37. Kirby AM et al. Prone versus supine positioning for whole and partial-breast radiotherapy: A comparison of non-target tissue dosimetry. *Radiother Oncol.* 2010;96(2):178–84.

38. Huppert N et al. The role of a prone setup in breast radiation therapy. *Front Oncol.* 2011;1:31.

39. Bartlett FR et al. The UK HeartSpare study (Stage IB): Randomised comparison of a voluntary breath-hold technique and prone radiotherapy after breast conserving surgery. *Radiother Oncol.* 2015;114(1):66–72.

40. Patel SA et al. Postmastectomy radiation therapy technique and cardiopulmonary sparing: A dosimetric comparative analysis between photons and protons with free breathing versus deep inspiration breath hold. *Pract Radiat Oncol.* 2017;7(6):e377–84.

41. Tommasino F et al. Model-based approach for quantitative estimates of skin, heart, and lung toxicity risk for left-side photon and proton irradiation after breast-conserving surgery. *Acta Oncol.* 2017;56(5):730–6.

42. Lettmaier S et al. Radiation exposure of the heart, lung and skin by radiation therapy

for breast cancer: A dosimetric comparison between partial breast irradiation using multi-catheter brachytherapy and whole breast tele-therapy. *Radiother Oncol.* 2011;100(2):189–94.

43. Polgar C et al. Breast-conserving therapy with partial or whole breast irradiation: Ten-year results of the Budapest randomized trial. *Radiother Oncol.* 2013;108(2):197–202.

44. Shah C et al. Treatment efficacy with accel-erated partial breast irradiation (APBI): Final analysis of the American society of breast surgeons MammoSite® breast brachy-therapy registry trial. *Ann Surg Oncol.* 2013;20(10):3279–85.

45. Strnad V et al. 5-year results of accelerated partial breast irradiation using sole interstitial multicatheter brachytherapy versus whole-breast irradiation with boost after breast-conserving surgery for low-risk invasive and in-situ carcinoma of the female breast: A ran-domised, phase 3, non-inferiority trial. *Lancet* 2016;387(10015):229–38.

46. Bonadonna G et al. Hodgkin's disease: The Milan Cancer Institute experience with MOPP and ABVD. *Recent Results Cancer Res.* 1989;117:169–74.

47. Witkowska M, Majchrzak A, Smolewski P. The role of radiotherapy in Hodgkin's lymphoma: What has been achieved during the last 50 years? *Biomed Res Int.* 2015;2015:485071.

48. Engert A et al. Involved-field radiotherapy is equally effective and less toxic compared with extended-field radiotherapy after four cycles of chemotherapy in patients with early-stage unfavorable Hodgkin's lymphoma: Results of the HD8 trial of the German Hodgkin's lymphoma study group. *J Clin Oncol.* 2003;21(19):3601–8.

49. Sasse S et al. Long-term follow-up of contemporary treatment in early-stage Hodgkin lymphoma: Updated analyses of the German Hodgkin Study Group HD7, HD8, HD10, and HD11 trials. *J Clin Oncol.* 2017;35(18):1999–2007.

50. Girinsky T et al. Involved-node radiotherapy (INRT) in patients with early Hodgkin lym-phoma: Concepts and guidelines. *Radiother Oncol.* 2006;79(3):270–7.

51. Ferme C et al. Chemotherapy plus involved-field radiation in early-stage Hodgkin's dis-ease. *N Engl J Med.* 2007;357(19):1916–27.

52. Engert A et al. Reduced treatment inten-sity in patients with early-stage Hodgkin's lymphoma. *N Engl J Med.* 2010;363(7):640–52.

53. Kalemkerian GP, Chemotherapy for small-cell lung cancer. *Lancet Oncol.* 2014;15(1):13–4.

54. Guckenberger M et al. Definition of ste-reotactic body radiotherapy: Principles and practice for the treatment of stage I non-small cell lung cancer. *Strahlenther Onkol.* 2014;190(1):26–33.

55. Willers H et al. ACR appropriateness crite-ria® induction and adjuvant therapy for N2 non-small-cell lung cancer. *Am J Clin Oncol.* 2015;38(2):197–205.

56. Bradley JD et al. Standard-dose versus high-dose conformal radiotherapy with concur-rent and consolidation carboplatin plus paclitaxel with or without cetuximab for patients with stage IIIA or IIIB non-small-cell lung cancer (RTOG. 0617): A randomised, two-by-two factorial phase 3 study. *Lancet Oncol.* 2015;16(2):187–99.

57. Chun SG et al. Impact of intensity-modu-lated radiation therapy technique for locally advanced non-small-cell lung cancer: A sec-ondary analysis of the NRG Oncology RTOG. 0617 randomized clinical trial. *J Clin Oncol.* 2017;35(1):56–62.

58. Jang R, Darling G, Wong RK. Multimodality approaches for the curative treatment of esophageal cancer. *J Natl Compr Canc Netw.* 2015;13(2):229–38.

59. van Hagen P et al. Preoperative chemoradio-therapy for esophageal or junctional cancer. *N Engl J Med.* 2012;366(22):2074–84.

60. Shapiro J et al. Neoadjuvant chemoradio-therapy plus surgery versus surgery alone for oesophageal or junctional cancer (CROSS): Long-term results of a randomised controlled trial. *Lancet Oncol.* 2015;16(9):1090–8.

61. Shiraishi Y et al. Dosimetric comparison to the heart and cardiac substructure in a large cohort of esophageal cancer patients treated with proton beam therapy or Intensity-modulated radiation therapy. *Radiother Oncol.* 2017;125(1):48–54.

62. van Rijswijk S et al. Mini-review on cardiac complications after mediastinal irradia-tion for Hodgkin lymphoma. *Neth J Med.* 2008;66(6):234–7.

63. Sridharan V et al. Cardiac inflammation after local irradiation is influenced by the kallikrein-kinin system. *Cancer Res.* 2012;72(19):4984–92.

64. Heidenreich PA et al. Diastolic dysfunction after mediastinal irradiation. *Am Heart J.* 2005;150(5):977–82.

65. Iarussi D et al. Evaluation of left ventricular function in long-term survivors of childhood Hodgkin disease. *Pediatr Blood Cancer* 2005;45(5):700–5.

66. Adams MJ et al. Radiation-associated cardiovascular disease: Manifestations and management. *Semin Radiat Oncol.* 2003;13(3):346–56.

67. Tsai HR et al. Left ventricular function assessed by two-dimensional speckle tracking echocardiography in long-term survivors of Hodgkin's lymphoma treated by mediastinal radiotherapy with or without anthracycline therapy. *Am J Cardiol.* 2011;107(3):472–7.

68. Nilsson G et al. Distribution of coronary artery stenosis after radiation for breast cancer. *J Clin Oncol.* 2012;30(4):380–6.

69. McEniery PT et al. Clinical and angiographic features of coronary artery disease after chest irradiation. *Am J Cardiol.* 1987;60(13):1020–4.

70. Walaszczyk A et al. Heart irradiation reduces microvascular density and accumulation of HSPA1 in mice. *Strahlenther Onkol.* 2018;194(3):235–42.

71. Madan R et al. Radiation induced heart disease: Pathogenesis, management and review literature. *J Egypt Natl Canc Inst.* 2015;27(4):187–93.

72. Jaworski C et al. Cardiac complications of thoracic irradiation. *J Am Coll Cardiol.* 2013;61(23):2319–28.

73. Yusuf SW, Sami S, Daher IN. Radiation-induced heart disease: A clinical update. *Cardiol Res Pract.* 2011;2011:317659.

74. Hering D, Faber L, Horstkotte D. Echocardiographic features of radiation-associated valvular disease. *Am J Cardiol.* 2003;92(2):226–30.

75. Desai MY et al. Increased aorto-mitral curtain thickness independently predicts mortality in patients with radiation-associated cardiac disease undergoing cardiac surgery. *Ann Thorac Surg.* 2014;97(4):1348–55.

76. Galper SL et al. Clinically significant cardiac disease in patients with Hodgkin lymphoma treated with mediastinal irradiation. *Blood.* 2011;117(2):412–8.

77. Wethal T et al. Valvular dysfunction and left ventricular changes in Hodgkin's lymphoma survivors. A longitudinal study. *Br J Cancer.* 2009;101(4):575–81.

78. Crestanello JA et al. Mitral and tricuspid valve repair in patients with previous mediastinal radiation therapy. *Ann Thorac Surg.* 2004;78(3):826–31; discussion 826–31.

79. Donnellan E et al. Long-term outcomes of patients with mediastinal radiation-associated severe aortic stenosis and subsequent surgical aortic valve replacement: A matched cohort study. *J Am Heart Assoc.* 2017;6(5).

80. Latib A et al. Percutaneous valve replacement in a young adult for radiation-induced aortic stenosis. *J Cardiovasc Med (Hagerstown)* 2012;13(6):397–8.

81. Heidenreich PA et al. Asymptomatic cardiac disease following mediastinal irradiation. *J Am Coll Cardiol.* 2003;42(4):743–9.

82. Totterman KJ, Pesonen E, Siltanen P. Radiation-related chronic heart disease. *Chest.* 1983;83(6):875–8.

83. Lee MS, Finch W, Mahmud E. Cardiovascular complications of radiotherapy. *Am J Cardiol.* 2013;112(10):1688–96.

5

Overview of changes in cancer treatment strategies

GRACE TANG AND CHRISTINE BREZDEN-MASLEY

INTRODUCTION

Improvements in oncologic therapeutic agents have resulted in a significant reduction in morbidity and mortality in cancer patients over the last several decades (1). However, cardiac-related adverse events are common complications and their prevention remains an important challenge for those with or surviving cancer. Table 5.1 outlines several cancer therapies and their associated cardiac side effects (2). Prior to initiation of therapy, baseline assessment is crucial to identify patients who are at risk for cardiotoxicity (3). Medical history of previous cardiovascular disease, cytotoxic treatments, radiotherapy, or abnormal baseline imaging results may warrant alternative cancer treatment options or administration of cardioprotective medications such as angiotensin-converting enzyme (ACE) inhibitors and beta-blockers (BBs) (2,4,5). Factors such as demographics and lifestyle (e.g., smoking, alcohol, obesity) should also be taken into account during initial risk assessment (1). As per European Society for Medical Oncology (ESMO) guidelines, modifications for blood pressure control, lipid level reduction, and smoking cessation can also reduce the risk of cardiac events (6,7). Cardiac monitoring (e.g., electrocardiography [ECG], echocardiography

[echo], multiple-gated acquisition [MUGA], or cardiac magnetic resonance imaging [MRI]) and blood pressure measurements should be performed at baseline screening and after treatment initiation for early detection of rhythmic alterations, a sign of cardiac overload (4). An example of an algorithm for monitoring of cardiotoxicity is shown in Figure 5.1 (6). As the use of cardiotoxic treatments increases, dramatic improvements have been made to reduce the incidence of cardiotoxicity for various cancer treatments. This chapter will provide a brief overview of the evolution of cancer treatment as it pertains to mitigating the effects of cardiotoxic anticancer therapies.

CHEMOTHERAPEUTICS

Anthracyclines

Anthracycline therapy has played a prominent role in the treatment of a wide variety of solid and hematologic malignancies since its introduction in the 1960s (8,9). The four most common anthracyclines are doxorubicin, daunorubicin, epirubicin, and idarubicin (9,10). Approximately 32% of breast cancer patients (11) and 57%–70% of elderly lymphoma (12,13) patients are treated

Table 5.1 Summary of common antineoplastic agents and relevant cardiotoxicities

Systemic therapy class		Incidence					
Drug name	Indication(s)[a]	Arrhythmia	Long QTc	Systolic dysfunction	Hypertension	Myocardial ischemia	Thromboembolism
Anthracycline							
Daunorubicin	Leukemia	++/+++	✓	+	−	−	−
Doxorubicin	Breast, lymphoma	+/++	✓	++/+++	−	−	✓
Doxorubicin (liposomal)	Sarcoma	+	✓	−	−	+/++/+++	−
Epirubicin	Breast, gastric	−	✓	+/++	−	−	✓
Idarubicin	Leukemia	++/+++	✓	++/+++	−	−	✓
Mitoxantrone	Leukemia	++/+++	✓	++/+++	++	++	−
Alkylating agent							
Cisplatin	Bladder, HNC, lung, ovarian	✓	✓	✓	✓	✓	++
Cyclophosphamide	Heme cancer	−	−	✓	−	−	+
Ifosfamide	Cervical, sarcoma	✓	−	+++	−	−	+
Antimicrotubule agent							
Docetaxel	Breast, lung	+/++	✓	++	++	++	✓
Nab-paclitaxel	Breast, pancreas	+/++	✓	−	−	−	+
Paclitaxel	Breast, lung	++	✓	+	−	+	−
Antimetabolite							
Capecitabine	Colorectal, breast	✓	✓	✓	−	++	+/++
5-Fluorouracil	Gastrointestinal	✓	✓	+	−	++/+++	✓

(Continued)

Table 5.1 (Continued) Summary of common antineoplastic agents and relevant cardiotoxicities

| Systemic therapy class | | Incidence | | | | | |
Drug name	Indication(s)[a]	Arrhythmia	Long QTc	Systolic dysfunction	Hypertension	Myocardial ischemia	Thromboembolism
Hormone therapy							
Abiraterone acetate	Prostate	++	–	++	++/+++	++	–
Anastrozole	Breast	–	–	–	++/+++	++	++
Exemestane	Breast	–	–	–	++	++	+
Letrozole	Breast	–	–	–	++	++/+++	++
Tamoxifen	Breast	–	✓	–	++/+++	++	++
Monoclonal antibody-based targeted therapy							
Bevacizumab	Colorectal	++	✓	+/++	++/+++	+/++	++/+++
Brentuximab	Lymphoma	–	–	–	–	+	++
Cetuximab	Colorectal, HNC	++	–	✓	++	✓	+/++
Ipilimumab	Melanoma	–	–	–	–	–	–
Panitumumab	Colorectal	✓	–	–	++	++	+
Pertuzumab	Breast	–	–	++	–	–	–
Rituximab	Heme cancer	✓	–	–	++	++	++/+++
Trastuzumab	Breast, gastric	++	–	++/+++	++	–	+/++
Small-molecule targeted therapy							
Bortezomib	Multiple myeloma	+	–	+/++	+	+	+
Dasatinib (TKI)	Leukemia	++/+++	+/++	++	++	++	+/++
Erlotinib (TKI)	Lung	✓	✓	–	–	++	++
Gefitinib (TKI)	Lung	✓	✓	–	–	+/++	✓
Imatinib (TKI)	CML	–	–	+/++	–	+++	+
Lapatinib (TKI)	Breast	✓	+++	++	–	–	–
Nilotinib (TKI)	CML	++	++	++	++	✓	+

(Continued)

Table 5.1 (Continued) Summary of common antineoplastic agents and relevant cardiotoxicities

Systemic therapy class		Incidence					
Drug name	Indication(s)[a]	Arrhythmia	Long QTc	Systolic dysfunction	Hypertension	Myocardial ischemia	Thromboembolism
Pazopanib (TKI)	RCC	–	–	+	+++	+/++	++
Sorafenib (TKI)	RCC, HCC	+	✓	+	+++	++	++
Sunitinib (TKI)	GIST, RCC	+	+	++/+++	+++	++	+/++
Vemurafenib (TKI)	Melanoma	++	✓	+	++	++	++
Miscellaneous							
Everolimus	RCC	–	–	++	++	–	+
Lenalidomide	Myeloma	+/++	+	++	++	++	++/+++
Temsirolimus	RCC	–	✓	–	++	+++	++

Source: Truong J et al. *Can J Cardiol.* 2014 August 1;30(8):869–78.

Note: +++ represents >10%; ++ represents 1%–10%; + represents <1% or rare; ✓ represents observed but precise incidence not well established; and – represents not well-recognized complication with no/minimal data.

Abbreviations: CML, chronic myeloid leukemia; GIST, gastrointestinal stromal tumor; HCC, hepatocellular carcinoma; Heme, hematological; HNC, head and neck cancer; RCC, renal cell carcinoma; TKI, tyrosine kinase inhibitor.

[a] Selected examples.

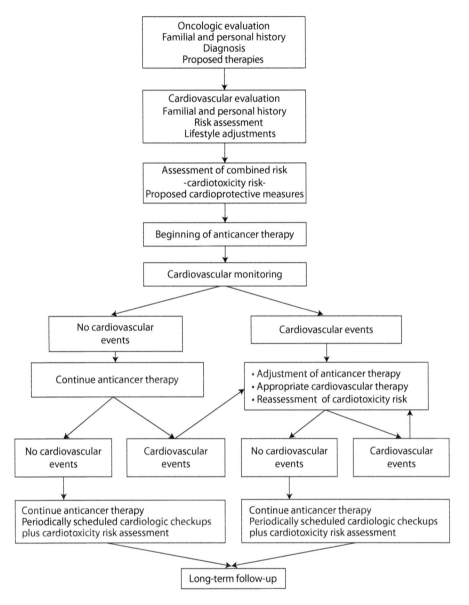

Figure 5.1 Algorithm for monitoring of cardiotoxicity. (From Berardi R et al. *Crit Rev Oncol Hematol.* 2013;88(1):75–86.)

with an anthracycline-based regimen (10). It is well documented in the literature that cumulative anthracycline dose is linked to irreversible cardiac dysfunction, left ventricle dysfunction, and heart failure (3,9). A meta-analysis of 55 published randomized control trials (RCTs) reported a significantly greater risk of clinical cardiotoxicity with anthracycline regimens compared to regimens without (odds ratio [OR]: 5.43, 95% confidence interval [CI] 2.34–12.62) (14). Anthracycline-related cardiotoxicity can present acutely and/or

have a chronic effect, which can occur months, years, or decades after completion of therapy (1).

Preventative management of anthracycline-induced cardiotoxicity is classified into two approaches: (1) reduce cardiotoxic potency; and (2) use a cardioprotective agent concurrently with treatment (15).

One way cardiotoxicity is reduced is by replacing bolus administration with slow infusions over 24–96 hours (8). Pharmacodynamic and pharmacokinetic studies in animal models have reported that increasing infusion duration reduces cardiotoxicity without compromising the oncologic efficacy of anthracycline therapy (8,16). While anthracycline activity is correlated with total plasma (i.e., area under the curve [AUC]), cardiotoxicity is correlated with peak plasma level of the anthracycline (C_{max}) (17). As such, slow infusions do not significantly affect the AUC, but diminish the C_{max} and anthracycline accumulation in the heart (8,17). In sarcoma and lymphoma patients, slow continuous doxorubicin infusions between 48 and 72 hours are often used (16).

Infusions longer than 96 hours are associated with higher incidence of stomatitis, as well as a need for a prolonged infusion pump and an indwelling catheter (16). Notably, the benefit of slower infusions may be counterbalanced by patients' discomfort due to prolonged hospitalization, myelotoxicity, mucositis, and alopecia (8). For children with acute lymphoblastic leukemia (ALL), there are no advantages to substituting bolus administration with continuous doxorubicin infusion (8,9,16,18).

Another preventative strategy is using liposomal encapsulation to reduce cardiotoxicity from anthracyclines. By modifying pharmacokinetic and tissue distribution, the risk of cardiotoxicity diminishes without decreasing tumoricidal efficacy (19,20). Liposomal encapsulated doxorubicin has been shown to limit diffusion through the endothelial lining of the cardiac microvasculature (8,9,19). Although liposomal encapsulated doxorubicin is associated with lower rates of heart failure and subclinical changes in left ventricular function, it is costly and there are limited approved clinical indications due to lack of RCT data (21). The U.S. Food and Drug Administration (FDA) has only approved its use in ovarian cancer, acquired immune deficiency syndrome-related Kaposi's sarcoma, and multiple myeloma after failure of at least one prior therapy (8,9,16,22).

Currently, dexrazoxane (DRZ) is the only FDA-approved cardioprotective agent for anthracycline-induced cardiotoxicity (23). Following infusion, DRZ is taken up rapidly by the myocardium and competes with ATP-binding sites on topoisomerase IIβ (23). Studies in pediatric and adult cancer patients have reported DRZ as a cardioprotective agent (24,25). However, the clinical use of DRZ is limited by a report of possible interference with anthracycline's antitumor efficacy in metastatic breast cancer (26). Additional concerns regarding the potential risk of secondary malignancies in childhood lymphoma have led to its restricted use (27). American Society of Clinical Oncology (ASCO) guidelines recommend DRZ only in one clinical indication: for metastatic breast cancer patients who have received >300 mg/m² of doxorubicin and may benefit from continued treatment (28). Table 5.2 summarizes primary prevention strategies for anthracycline-induced cardiotoxicity (8).

Nonanthracyclines

While less common than anthracycline-induced cardiotoxicity, other chemotherapeutic agents used to treat cancer are also associated with cardiotoxicity.

5-FLUOROUACIL/CAPECITABINE

The antimetabolite 5-flourouracil (5-FU) is used alone or in combination with other regimens for a variety of cancers, including breast, gastrointestinal, head, and neck (29). Capecitabine, its oral prodrug, is used for colorectal and metastatic breast cancer (3,29). Large retrospective studies have suggested an incidence between 1.3 and 4.3% for symptomatic cardiotoxicities in patients receiving these agents (1,29). However, this may be underestimated due to differences in the definition of cardiotoxicity and treatment schedules across studies (29). A systematic review of 30 studies found that the most common cardiac side effects of 5-FU and capecitabine are chest pain, palpitations, dyspnea, and hypotension (29). Serious complications are present in 0%–2% of patients and include myocardial infarction, cardiogenic shock, and cardiac arrest (29). Continuous infusion is associated with a higher risk of cardiotoxicities compared to bolus administration (30). The mechanism of 5FU-induced cardiotoxicity is not completely understood; however, possible explanations include coronary thrombosis, arteritis, vasospasm, direct toxic effects on the heart, interaction with the coagulation system, and autoimmune responses (1,31).

Patients receiving 5-FU regimen should be observed closely, and treatment should be discontinued if cardiac symptoms develop (30). A rechallenge of 5-FU should occur if there is no alternative therapy, and should be performed in the setting of aggressive prophylaxis and close monitoring (30).

TAXANES

Taxanes, such as paclitaxel and docetaxel, are commonly used in a variety of cancers and in combination

Table 5.2 Primary prevention strategies of anthracycline-induced cardiotoxicity

Strategy	Mechanism of protection	Clinical benefit	Disadvantages/limitations
Slow infusions	Lowered C_{max}	Preservation of anthracycline activity, with reduced cardiac exposure to and penetration by anthracyclines	The patient undergoes prolonged hospitalization and discomfort from prolonged exposure; a lack of long-term cardiac protection in some pediatric settings; a reported accumulation of DNA-oxidized bases in normal cells
Liposomal formulations	Limited diffusions through the endothelial lining of the cardiac microvasculature	Preservation of antitumor activity and improved cardiac tolerability	Limited approved indications
Dexrazoxane	Iron chelation and mitigation of ROS-mediated damage; inhibition of topoisomerase IIβ	Prevention of cardiotoxicity in both child and adult cancer patients	Clinicians should weigh the cardioprotective effect of dexrazoxane against the possible risk of adverse effects for each individual patient

Source: Menna P, Salvatorelli E. Chemotherapy. 2017;62(3):159–68; van Dalen EC et al. Cardioprotective interventions for cancer patients receiving anthracyclines. Cochrane Database of Systematic Reviews. 2011;(6).
Abbreviations: ROS, reactive oxygen species; DNA, deoxyribonucleic acid.

with anthracyclines (3,32). Acute asymptomatic bradycardia has been reported in up to 30% of patients, while serious complications are less frequent (32–34). An early case series reported a 5% incidence of serious arrhythmias, ventricular tachycardia, and cardiac ischemia in patients who received paclitaxel (33). Proposed mechanisms of action for rhythmic disturbances include damage to the cell's organelles and histamine-induced response (33).

Preventative strategies include slow infusion of doxorubicin and paclitaxel, or increased time (24 hours) between doxorubicin and paclitaxel infusions (35,36). The cumulative dose of doxorubicin when combined with paclitaxel should not exceed 360 mg/m^2 (37).

Monoclonal antibodies

TRASTUZUMAB

Trastuzumab is a humanized monoclonal antibody that targets the extracellular membrane of human epidermal growth factor receptor 2 (HER2) (38). Since its introduction, trastuzumab has dramatically improved the survival of HER2-positive (HER2+) breast cancer patients and is used in the neoadjuvant, adjuvant, and metastatic settings (1,38). Trastuzumab-induced cardiotoxicity is well documented in the literature. Incidence of cardiotoxicity in RCTs is generally low (38); however, they are likely underestimated, as "real world" studies have reported up to a 53% incidence in the metastatic breast cancer population (3,39). ESMO and Canadian working group guidelines recommend specific screening and management of cardiotoxicity and follow-up during treatment (15,40,41).

Pharmacologic cardioprotective strategies during trastuzumab treatment are currently being explored to prevent future toxicity (38). A large population-based study of elderly women (>66 years old) reported that ACE inhibitors/BBs showed favorable effects in preventing cardiotoxicity (42). When used in combination with trastuzumab and anthracycline therapy, ACE inhibitors/BBs were associated with a 23% decreased risk of cardiotoxicity and a 21% decreased risk of all-cause mortality (42). The study also reported that those who had earlier treatment with ACE inhibitors/BBs (≤6 months after initiation of trastuzumab/anthracycline) and longer duration of use (>6 months) have a lower risk of cardiotoxicity and all-cause mortality compared to those not exposed (42).

In the double-blinded, placebo-controlled MANITORE study, HER2+ early breast cancer patients were randomized to treatment with perindopril, bisoprolol, or placebo (1:1:1) during trastuzumab therapy (43). Patients on bisoprolol experienced successful prevention in left ventricular ejection fraction (LVEF) drops and fewer treatment interruptions compared to perindopril or placebo arms (43). However, these pharmacotherapies did not prevent trastuzumab-mediated left ventricular remodeling, a possible early marker of cardiotoxicity (38,43). The PRADA study compared candesartan and metoprolol in combination or alone against placebo in early breast cancer patients treated with adjuvant anthracycline and trastuzumab (38,44). Concomitant administration of candesartan significantly reduced the decline in LVEF that occurred during adjuvant therapy compared to placebo ($p = 0.026$).

Although results of the MANITORE and PRADA studies suggest promising benefits from administering prophylactic cardioprotective agents, the small sample size and wide exclusion criteria must be taken into consideration. Therefore, these results do not provide a solid basis of clinical decision-making, and larger studies are recommended.

ANTIANGIOGENESIS ANTIBODIES

Bevacizumab

Bevacizumab is a humanized monoclonal antibody against the VEGF-A ligand, which works by preventing its interaction with vascular endothelial growth factor (VEGF) receptor-2, inhibiting endothelial proliferation, and downgrading angiogenesis (4,6). It is used for a variety of treatments for many advanced solid tumors including colorectal, non-small cell lung, breast, and ovarian cancers (45–48). Bevacizumab is associated with a spectrum of adverse events such as arterial hypertension, heart failure, pulmonary hemorrhage, gastrointestinal bleeding, pulmonary edema, and venous and arterial thromboembolic events (4,6,49). A meta-analysis of breast cancer patients treated with bevacizumab showed an increased risk of grade III/IV congestive heart failure (CHF; relative risk [RR] 4.74, 95% CI: 1.66–11.18), with an

incidence of 1.6% (1,50). In clinical trials, incidence of severe hypertension occurred in up to 14.8% of patients while incidence of heart failure occurred in 1.5% (4,48,51).

ESMO guidelines suggest standard antihypertensive medications should be considered, and close blood pressure monitoring is recommended with the objective of maintaining blood pressure <140/90 mm Hg (6,41,45). Bevacizumab therapy should be discontinued in patients who develop severe arterial thrombotic events (ATEs) during treatment (6). ESMO guidelines for reducing cardiotoxicity, such as blood pressure control and lifestyle modifications, should be followed as preventative strategies for patients on bevacizumab (6,7).

Ramucirumab

Ramucirumab is a human immunoglobin G1 monoclonal antibody that blocks the VEGF receptor 2 (52,53). It is approved for the treatment of gastric, non-small cell lung, and colorectal cancer (52). Clinical trials have reported CHF, hypertension, and ATEs including myocardial infarction and cerebral ischemia (53–55). In the metastatic gastric cancer REGARD trial, incidence of hypertension was higher in patients receiving ramucirumab compared to those on placebo (16% vs. 8%) (54).

Management of cardiotoxic events includes permanent discontinuation for those who experience severe ATE, and antihypertensive treatment. ASCO guidelines on preventative strategies to minimize potentially cardiotoxic cancer treatment recommend monitoring of blood pressure and controlling preexisting hypertension prior to starting treatment (5).

Small molecules

TYROSINE KINASE INHIBITORS

Small molecule tyrosine kinase inhibitors (TKIs) are an effective therapeutic option for several hematological and solid malignancies that increase survival and delay tumor progression (56,57). Common TKIs include lapatinib, imatinib, afatinib, sunitinib, sorafenib, pazopanib, vandetanib, and nilotinib (6,56–58). TKIs interfere with kinase activity and are characterized by their targeted action (1,59). In the literature, reports of hypertension, heart failure, left ventricular dysfunction and QTc prolongation have been described in clinical trials (56,60). The incidence of cardiac events for TKIs ranges from 1.5% to 11% for left ventricular dysfunction, 2.7%–3.0% for ischemia, and 5.0%–43% for hypertension (6,61). A systematic review reported the risk of developing QTc prolongation with TKIs ranged between 0%–22.7% with severe prolongation (QTc >500 ms) reported in 0%–5.2% of patients (62).

In addition to the preventative and management strategies described earlier for hypertension and heart failure, special considerations should be noted for QTc prolongation (56). Compared to other cardiotoxic effects, it is difficult to assess the development of abnormal arrhythmias from QTc prolongation (58,63,64). The degree of prolonged QTc interval does not reliably correlate with the incidence of torsades de pointes (TdP) and sudden death (56,58,63). A detailed risk assessment for history of QT interval prolongation, preexisting cardiovascular disease, history of TdP, abnormal arrhythmias, and heart failure should be conducted prior to treatment initiation (56). Electrolyte concentrations should be measured at baseline and corrected prior to TKI therapy (56). Different types of TKIs require different ECG and electrolyte monitoring during treatment and after dose adjustments; potassium and magnesium

levels should be supplemented as needed (56). Medical reconciliation is essential to avoid potential drug interactions with other QTc-prolonging drugs including antiarrhythmic, antibiotic, and antifungal agents (56,62). Table 5.3 summarizes strategies to minimize cancer therapy-related QTc prolongation and risk of TdP (62,65).

CYCLIN-DEPENDENT KINASE 4/6 INHIBITORS

Cyclin-dependent kinase (CDK) 4/6 inhibitors are molecules that prevent the formation of active kinase complex by inhibiting their activity to slow the progression of cancer (58,66). Currently, three CDK 4/6 inhibitors (ribociclib, palbociclib, and abemaciclib) are approved for the treatment of advanced breast cancer (58,66). Limited data are available on the cardiac safety of CDK4/6 inhibitors; however, clinical trials have reported potential increase in QTc interval specific to ribociclib (3,58). In the phase III MONALEESA-2 trial, an increase of >60 ms from baseline was reported in 2.7% patients in the ribociclib with letrozole group (3,58,67). In subsequent phase III MONALEESA-7 and MONALEESA-3 trials, an increase >60 ms from baseline was reported in 10% in the ribociclib plus endocrine therapy group, and 6.5% in

---

Table 5.3 Summary of strategies to minimize cancer therapy-related QTc prolongation and risk of TdP

1. Avoid use of QTc-prolongation drugs in patients with pretreatment QTc >450 ms
2. Discontinue QTc-prolongation drug(s) if QTc interval prolongs to >500 or >550 ms if a baseline widening of QRS is present (>120 ms secondary to pacing or bundle branch block)
3. Reduce dose or discontinue QTc-prolonging drug(s) if the QTc increases ≥60 ms from pretreatment value
4. Maintain electrolytes' (serum potassium, magnesium, and calcium) concentration within normal range
5. Avoid important known drug interactions
6. Adjust doses of renally eliminated QTc-prolonging drugs in patients with acute kidney injury or chronic kidney disease
7. Avoid rapid intravenous administration of QTc-prolonging drugs'
8. Administration of >1 drug with the potential to prolong the QT interval should be avoided
9. Avoid use of QTc-prolonging drugs in patients with a history of drug-induced TdP or those who have previously been resuscitated from an episode of SCD
10. Avoid use of QTc interval–prolonging drugs in patients who have been diagnosed as having one of the congenital long QT syndromes
11. The frequency of ECG monitoring will depend on on-going therapy, drugs concentrations, and dose changes of QTc prolonging therapy

---

Source: Porta-Sánchez A et al. *J Am Heart Assoc.* 2017;6(12):1–18, Tisdale JE. *Can Pharm J.* 2016;149(3):139–52.
Abbreviations: QTc, corrected QT; SCD, sudden cardiac death; TdP, torsades de pointes.

the ribociclib plus fulvestrant group, respectively (68,69). In the MONALEESA-3 trial, three patients in the ribociclib plus fulvestrant arm discontinued study treatment owing to a prolonged QTc interval (69). In the phase III PALOMA-3 trial, one patient experienced reversible QTc prolongation in the palbociclib plus fulvestrant arm (58,70). One patient of the palbocicilib arm in the phase II PALOMA-1 trial was diagnosed with coronary arterial disease (3,71).

Preventative and management strategies for QTc prolongation in CDK4/6 inhibitors are similar to those described for TKIs. Baseline risk assessment (i.e., history of cardiac disease, QTc prolongation), close monitoring, and correction of electrolyte abnormalities are recommended for ribociclib (58). ECG and electrolyte monitoring at baseline and during treatment are also recommended.

PROTEASOME INHIBITORS

Proteasome inhibitors such as bortezomib and carfilzomib are cornerstone therapies for management of multiple myeloma (MM) (72,73). These agents target the 26S proteasome, causing accumulation of protein byproducts within plasma cells and subsequent apoptosis (72–75). Bortezomib is typically used in the first-line setting while carfilzomib is used as second-line therapy in the relapsed setting (72).

While relatively rare, proteasome inhibitors are associated with cardiac toxicities including heart failure and hypertension (72,73,76,77). In a meta-analysis of clinical trials comparing bortezomib to control medication, MM patients had an increased risk of cardiotoxicity compared to other tumor types in all grades (4.3% vs. 2.3%, $p < 0.001$) and high-grade toxicity (2.5% vs. 1.8%, $p = 0.004$) (73,78). Cardiotoxicity was defined as LVEF decline or dysfunction, cardiac failure, cardiomyopathy, cardiac arrest or cardiac arrhythmia, and classified using the National Cancer Institute's common terminology criteria for adverse events (78). In the phase III ENDEAVOR trial, there was a higher proportion of grade III or higher cardiac failure (4.75% vs. 1.75%) and grade III hypertension (9% vs. 3%) in the carfilzomib and dexamethasone group compared to the bortezomib and dexamethasone group (73,76). Furthermore, in the phase III ASPIRE trial, patients in the carfilzomib, lenalidomide, and dexamethasone group had a significantly higher incidence of grade III or higher

cardiac failure (3.8% vs. 1.8%) and grade III hypertension (4.3% vs. 1.8%) compared to the lenalidomide and dexamethasone group (73,77).

At baseline, MM patients have a 54–74% risk of cardiovascular disease owing to advanced age at diagnosis (median 62 years), autologous stem cell transplantation, and disease-specific complications such as cardiac amyloidosis (72,79–82). Therefore, careful monitoring and a detailed history for cardiovascular risk factors and prior chemotherapy exposure (with particular attention to anthracyclines) are suggested (73). While there are no standard practice guidelines, Chari and Hajje published a set of recommendations for patients exposed to carfilzomib (83). In brief, screening echocardiograms should be obtained for all patients over the age of 60, with a history of amyloidosis, or other cardiovascular risk factors and repeated every two to three cycles (83). Carfilzomib should be administered slowly over 30 minutes instead of the 2–10 minutes indicated (83). In the event of suspected toxicity, carfilzomib should be withheld until complication resolves to below grade II and rechallenged at the last used or reduced dose (83).

Immunotherapy

The role of immunotherapies in oncology has substantially improved the management and survival of several advanced-stage malignancies (84). Adoptive cell therapy (ACT) and immune checkpoint inhibitors (ICIs) have been described to induce cardiac toxicities such as left ventricular dysfunction and CHF (85). Although current literature remains limited to case reports and early clinical trials, strategies are proposed to prevent and manage potentially fatal complications.

ADOPTIVE T CELL THERAPY

ACT-associated cardiotoxicities are mostly related to the context of cytokine release syndrome (CRS) (85). The effects of CRS can result in hemodynamic instability, left ventricular dysfunction, hypotension, QTc prolongation, arrhythmias, tachycardia, and cardiopulmonary arrest (85–87). The overall incidence of CRS in ACT remains unknown and is currently limited to case reports (85).

Compared to the costly direct cytokine level assays, daily monitoring of C-reactive protein (CRP) levels can be used to identify patients with

CRS (87). Strategies proposed by Brudno et al. suggest obtaining ECG, serum troponin, and echo for patients who do develop hypotension (88). Other strategies include transfer to an intensive care unit to maintain adequate perfusion and treatment of any significant arrhythmias. Tocilizumab and glucocorticoids should be considered as first-line and second-line therapy in the event of cardiotoxicity, respectively (85,88).

IMMUNE CHECKPOINT INHIBITORS

Complications from ICI-related cardiotoxicity are highly variable and include elevated cardiac biomarkers in the absence of symptoms such as nausea, cardiogenic shock, CHF, arrhythmias, conduction abnormalities, and pericarditis (85,89,90). Studies have observed that patients may be concurrently diagnosed with other immune-related adverse events such as myositis autoimmune thyroiditis and hypophysitis with cardiotoxicity (85,89). From the limited literature, ipilimumab and/or nivolumab-induced myocarditis was reported in 0.09% of patients and 0.3% for combination therapy (85,91,92). Notably, the incidence may be underestimated as cardiac screening is not routinely performed in immunotherapy studies (84,85).

ECG monitoring and troponin levels (if treated with combination immunotherapy) at baseline during diagnostic workup are recommended by ASCO guidelines (85,89,93). Further monitoring using imaging tests can be ordered, such as cardiac MRI and transthoracic echo, in the event that ICI cardiotoxicity is suspected (85,93). Proposed treatment of ICI-cardiotoxicity involves glucocorticoids, intravenous methylprednisolone, or oral prednisone and potentially the addition of mycophenolate, infliximab, or antithymocyte globin (85,93,94). ASCO guidelines recommend a hospital admission patient and a cardiology consult to manage the patient's cardiac symptoms (93).

RADIATION THERAPY

Radiation therapy is an essential and effective treatment modality for several solid and hematological malignancies (95–97). Cardiotoxicity related to radiation therapy is well studied and remains the most common nonmalignant cause of morbidity and mortality in survivors (1,96,98). Cardiotoxic manifestations during or after radiation therapy

Table 5.4 Cardiac-sparing techniques

Technique	Cardiac-sparing mechanism
Breath hold	With inspiration, distance from chest wall to the heart increases
Prone position	Breast falls away from chest wall
	Increases distance from the heart to radiation therapy beam
Intensity-modulated radiation therapy	Computerized leaves and dose planning algorithms allow for shaping of radiation field to limit cardiac dose

Source: Shah C et al. Radiother Oncol. 2014;112(1):9–16.

can include valvular dysfunction, atherosclerosis, fibrosis, arrhythmias, pericarditis, CHF, left ventricle dysfunction, and myocardial infarctions (1,32,96,99,100). Methods of cardiac dose protection and/or avoidance techniques are described in detail in Chapter 4 and are briefly summarized in Table 5.4 (96,101).

Supportive medications in cardiology

5-HT$_3$ RECEPTOR ANTAGONISTS

5-HT$_3$ receptor antagonists (5-HT$_3$ RAs) or serotonin blockers are typically used to control chemotherapy-induced nausea and vomiting (102). While clinical studies are limited, QTc prolongation has been identified in 5-HT$_3$ RAs such as ondansetron and dolasetron and arrhythmias from granisetron (102,103). Elderly patients (>70 years old) are at greater risk due to polypharmacy and use of cardiotoxic therapeutics (103).

Preventative and management strategies are similar to TKIs and include ECG and electrolyte screening prior to treatment for those who are at high risk (104). For ondansetron, QTc prolongation is dose-dependent, therefore dosages are restricted to reduce the risk in older adults (105). Adoption of cardio-gentle antiemetics (e.g., palonosetron, granisetron transdermal release) are recommended for those with higher cardiovascular risk to reduce the burden of arrhythmic events (103).

STEROIDS

Corticosteroids such as dexamethasone are prescribed for nausea and hypersensitivity during chemotherapy treatment (e.g., taxanes) (103,106). Studies and case reports have reported an association between high doses of corticosteroids and cardiac events such as atrial fibrillation and hypertension (103,107). This observation was noted in hematological malignancies and suggests that high doses of corticosteroids might mediate potassium outflow from cells, thereby inducing arrhythmias (103,108).

EMERGING CARDIAC MONITORING METHODOLOGIES

In addition to standard cardiac monitoring techniques, new and accurate methods to detect early cardiotoxicity include tissue Doppler imaging (TDI) and myocardial strain imaging (109). A study in children with acute lymphocytic leukemia (ALL) treated with low cumulative dose of doxorubicin (100 mg/m²), concluded that TDI detected cardiac changes earlier than conventional echo and better delineated diastolic function (109,110). Strain imaging and tissue velocity index have been proposed to detect preclinical changes in left ventricular systolic function up to 3 months prior to detection of LVEF in echoes (110,111). However, future studies with larger sample sizes are warranted.

Serum cardiac biomarkers such as troponin and B-type natriuretic peptides are recommended by ASCO guidelines for surveillance in conjunction with routine imaging (5). New biomarkers such as high-sensitivity cardiac troponin I, C-reactive protein, growth differentiation factor 15, and N-terminal pro-B-type natriuretic peptide have been studied in breast cancer patients receiving anthracycline and trastuzumab therapy (109,112–114). However, the studies concluded that further validation is needed before routine clinical use.

CARDIOPROTECTIVE TREATMENTS

As previously discussed earlier in this chapter, ACE inhibitors and beta blockers (BBs) may play a role in prophylactic prevention or treatment of cardiotoxicity. A meta-analysis by Kalam et al. reported that prophylactic treatment with BBs, statins, or angiotensin antagonists has a similar efficacy in reducing cardiotoxicity to prevent heart failure (115). A more recent meta-analysis of six randomized control trial (RCTs) in BBs and/or angiotensin antagonists as cardioprotective agents found better preservation of LVEF, particularly in patients who were exposed to a higher cumulative dose of anthracyclines (116). Both meta-analyses have some limitations and should be interpreted cautiously, as both these studies suffer from patient and treatment heterogeneity. Nonetheless, ASCO

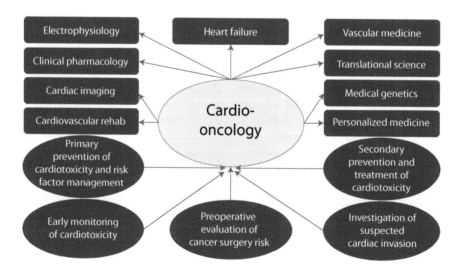

Figure 5.2 The role of a cardio-oncology service. (From Han X et al. *NPJ Precis Oncol.* 2017;1(1):31; available from: http://www.nature.com/articles/s41698-017-0034-x.)

guidelines do not recommend the use of primary prophylactic cardiac medications owing to small sample size, lack of clinical efficacy, and use of nonrandomized study designs (5).

At present, these therapies are indicated when patients experience heart failure symptoms or a drop in LVEF (2,109). Referral to a cardiologist for routine clinical heart failure (stage B) management is the standard of care. Management strategies may include ACE inhibitors, BBs, diuretics, and implantable defibrillators (15,109,117).

MULTIDISCIPLINARY APPROACH TO CARDIO-ONCOLOGY

There is an increasing focus on the cardiac health of patients who are undergoing or have survived cardiotoxic treatments (118). The field of cardio-oncology promotes optimal cancer treatment with a focus on limiting collateral cardiac damage (118,119). Along with the collaboration between cardiologists and oncologists, imaging specialists, clinical pharmacologists, nursing support, researchers, and educators are needed in this complex field (1). Cardio-oncology clinics allow clinicians to assess and prescribe appropriate therapeutic management if cardiac risk factors are present or if cardiotoxicity is identified (1). Figure 5.2 shows the role of a cardio-oncology service and common referrals (1). The creation of a specific cardio-oncology training program has been proposed by several experts to further advance this important therapeutic discipline (118).

CONCLUSION

This chapter summarizes the current landscape of cardiotoxic anticancer therapies, and how cancer treatment strategies have evolved in order to reduce the risk of cardiotoxic events in cancer patients. Today, there are established cardio-oncology societies and networks (e.g., the Canadian Cardiac Oncology Network [CCON]; the Global Cardio-Oncology Summit [GCOS] and the International Cardio-Oncology Society [ICOS]) dedicated to bring together healthcare professionals. As the number of patients treated with cardiotoxic agents increases, it is imperative that we prevent cancer patients and survivors from becoming cardiac patients. As newer complex targeted therapies are

aiming to cure cancer, we also need to ensure we are protecting their hearts.

REFERENCES

1. Han X, Zhou Y, Liu W. Precision cardio-oncology: Understanding the cardiotoxicity of cancer therapy. *NPJ Precis Oncol.* 2017; 1(1):31.
2. Truong J, Yan AT, Cramarossa G, Chan KKW. Chemotherapy-induced cardiotoxicity: Detection, prevention, and management. *Can J Cardiol.* 2014 August 1; 30(8):869–78.
3. Martel S, Maurer C, Lambertini M, Pondé N, De Azambuja E. Breast cancer treatment-induced cardiotoxicity. *Expert Opin Drug Saf.* 2017;16(9):1021–38.
4. Giordano G et al. Cancer drug related cardiotoxicity during breast cancer treatment. *Expert Opin Drug Saf.* 2016;15(8):1063–74.
5. Armenian SH et al. Prevention and monitoring of cardiac dysfunction in survivors of adult cancers: American Society of Clinical Oncology clinical practice guideline. *J Clin Oncol.* 2017;35(8):893–911.
6. Berardi R et al. State of the art for cardiotoxicity due to chemotherapy and to targeted therapies: A literature review. *Crit Rev Oncol Hematol.* 2013;88(1):75–86.
7. Bovelli D, Plataniotis G, Roila F. Cardiotoxicity of chemotherapeutic agents and radiotherapy-related heart disease: ESMO clinical practice guidelines. *Ann Oncol.* 2010;21 (SUPPL. 5):277–82.
8. Menna P, Salvatorelli E. Primary prevention strategies for anthracycline cardiotoxicity: A brief overview. *Chemotherapy.* 2017;62(3): 159–68.
9. Henriksen PA. Anthracycline cardiotoxicity: An update on mechanisms, monitoring and prevention. *Heart.* 2018;104(12):971–7.
10. McGowan JV, Chung R, Maulik A, Piotrowska I, Walker JM, Yellon DM. Anthracycline chemotherapy and cardiotoxicity. *Cardiovasc Drugs Ther.* 2017;31(1):63–75.
11. Giordano SH, Lin YL, Kuo YF, Hortobagyi GN, Goodwin JS. Decline in the use of anthracyclines for breast cancer. *J Clin Oncol.* 2012; 30(18):2232–9.
12. Nabhan C et al. Disease characteristics, treatment patterns, prognosis, outcomes

and lymphoma-related mortality in elderly follicular lymphoma in the United States. *Br J Haematol*. 2015;170(1):85–95.

13. Chihara D et al. Management strategies and outcomes for very elderly patients with diffuse large B-cell lymphoma. *Cancer* 2016; 122(20):3145–51.

14. Smith LA et al. Cardiotoxicity of anthracycline agents for the treatment of cancer: Systematic review and meta-analysis of randomised controlled trials. *BMC Cancer* 2010;10.

15. Mackey JR et al. Cardiac management during adjuvant trastuzumab therapy: Recommendations of the Canadian Trastuzumab working group. *Curr Oncol*. 2008 January;15(1):24–35.

16. Vejpongsa P, Yeh ETH. Prevention of anthracycline-induced cardiotoxicity: Challenges and opportunities. *J Am Coll Cardiol*. 2014; 64(9):938–45.

17. Minotti G. Anthracyclines: Molecular advances and pharmacologic developments in antitumor activity and cardiotoxicity. *Pharmacol Rev*. 2004;56(2):185–229.

18. Lipshultz SE et al. Continuous versus bolus infusion of doxorubicin in children with all: Long-term cardiac outcomes. *Pediatrics*. 2012;130(6):1003–11.

19. Gabizon AA. Pegylated liposomal doxorubicin: Metamorphosis of an old drug into a new form of chemotherapy. *Cancer Invest*. 2001 January 1;19(4):424–36. Available from: www.dekker.com

20. Gabizon AA. Stealth liposomes and tumor targeting: One step further in the quest for the magic bullet stealth liposomes and tumor targeting: One step further in the quest for the magic bullet. *Clin Cancer Res*. 2001 February;7:223–5.

21. van Dalen EC, Michiels EMC, Caron HN, Kremer LCM. Different anthracycline derivates for reducing cardiotoxicity in cancer patients. *Cochrane Database Syst Rev*. 2010;2010(5).

22. Salvatorelli E et al. The concomitant management of cancer therapy and cardiac therapy. *Biochim Biophys Acta – Biomembr*. 2015;1848(10):2727–37.

23. Yi LL et al. Topoisomerase IIβ-mediated DNA double-strand breaks: Implications in doxorubicin cardiotoxicity and prevention by dexrazoxane. *Cancer Res*. 2007;67(18): 8839–46.

24. Abdel-Qadir H et al. Interventions for preventing cardiomyopathy due to anthracyclines: A Bayesian network meta-analysis. *Ann Oncol*. 2017;28(3):628–33.

25. Speyer JL, Green MD, Zeleniuch-Jacquotte A, Wernz JC, Rey M, Sanger J, Kramer E, Ferrans V, Hochster H, Meyers M. ICRF-187 permits longer treatment with doxorubicin in women with breast cancer. *J Clin Oncol*. 1992 January 10;10(1):117–27.

26. Swain BSM et al. Cardioprotection with dexrazoxane for doxorubicin-containing therapy in advanced breast cancer. *J Clin Oncol*. 1997;15(4):1318–32.

27. Tebbi CK et al. Dexrazoxane-associated risk for acute myeloid leukemia/myelodysplastic syndrome and other secondary malignancies in pediatric Hodgkin's disease. *J Clin Oncol*. 2007;25(5):493–500.

28. Schuchter LM, Hensley ML, Meropol NJ, Winer EP. Update of recommendations for the use of chemotherapy and radiotherapy protectants: Clinical practice guidelines of the American Society of Clinical Oncology. *J Clin Oncol*. 2002;20(12):2895–903.

29. Polk A, Vaage-Nilsen M, Vistisen K, Nielsen DL. Cardiotoxicity in cancer patients treated with 5-fluorouracil or capecitabine: A systematic review of incidence, manifestations and predisposing factors. *Cancer Treat Rev*. 2013;39(8):974–84.

30. Saif MW, Shah MM, Shah AR. Fluoropyrimidine-associated cardiotoxicity: Revisited. *Expert Opin Drug Saf*. 2009;8(2):191–202.

31. Kosmas C et al. Cardiotoxicity of fluoropyrimidines in different schedules of administration: A prospective study. *J Cancer Res Clin Oncol*. 2008;134(1):75–82.

32. Healey Bird BRJ, Swain SM. Cardiac toxicity in breast cancer survivors: Review of potential cardiac problems. *Clin Cancer Res*. 2008;14(1):14–24.

33. Rowinsky EK, McGuire WP, Guarnieri T, Fisherman JS, Christian MC, Donehower RC. Cardiac disturbances during the administration of taxol. *J Clin Oncol*. 1991;9(9):1704–12.

34. Arbuck SG et al. A reassessment of cardiac toxicity associated with Taxol. *J Natl Cancer Inst Monogr*. 1993;(15):117–30.

35. Holmes FA et al. Paclitaxel by 24-hour infusion with doxorubicin by 48-hour infusion as initial therapy for metastatic breast cancer: Phase I results. *Ann Oncol.* 1999;10(4):403–11.

36. Jassem J et al. Doxorubicin and paclitaxel versus fluorouracil, doxorubicin, and cyclophosphamide as first-line therapy for women with metastatic breast cancer: Final results of a randomized phase III multicenter trial. *J Clin Oncol.* 2001 March;19(6):1707–15.

37. Giordano SH et al. A detailed evaluation of cardiac toxicity: A phase II study of doxorubicin and one- or three-hour-infusion paclitaxel in patients with metastatic breast cancer. *Clin Cancer Res.* 2002 November;8(11):3360–8.

38. Pondé NF, Lambertini M, de Azambuja E. Twenty years of anti-HER2 therapy-associated cardiotoxicity. *ESMO Open.* 2016;1(4):e000073.

39. Grazziotin L, Picon P. Observational study of trastuzumab-related cardiotoxicity in early and metastatic breast cancer. *J Oncol Pharm Pract.* 2016; Available from: http://opp.sagepub.com/cgi/doi/10.1177/1078155216639755

40. Zamorano JL et al. 2016 European society of cardiology position paper on cancer treatments and cardiovascular toxicity. *Eur Heart J.* 2016;37(36):2768–801.

41. Curigliano G et al. Cardiovascular toxicity induced by chemotherapy, targeted agents and radiotherapy: ESMO clinical practice guidelines. *Ann Oncol.* 2012;23(SUPPL. 7).

42. Wittayanukorn S, Qian J, Westrick SC, Billor N, Johnson B, Hansen RA. Prevention of Trastuzumab and anthracycline-induced cardiotoxicity using angiotensin-converting enzyme inhibitors or β-blockers in older adults with breast cancer. *Am J Clin Oncol.* 2018 September 1;41(9):909–18.

43. Pituskin E et al. Multidisciplinary approach to novel therapies in cardio-oncology research (MANTICORE 101-Breast): A randomized trial for the prevention of trastuzumab-associated cardiotoxicity. *J Clin Oncol.* 2017;35(8):870–7.

44. Gulati G et al. Prevention of cardiac dysfunction during adjuvant breast cancer therapy (PRADA): A 2 × 2 factorial, randomized, placebo-controlled, double-blind clinical trial of candesartan and metoprolol. *Eur Heart J.* 2016;37(21):1671–80.

45. Economopoulou P, Kotsakis A, Kapiris I, Kentepozidis N. Cancer therapy and cardiovascular risk: Focus on bevacizumab. *Cancer Manag Res.* 2015;7:133–43.

46. Giantonio BJ et al. Bevacizumab in combination with oxaliplatin, fluorouracil, and leucovorin (FOLFOX4) for previously treated metastatic colorectal cancer: Results from the Eastern Cooperative oncology group study E3200. *J Clin Oncol.* 2007;25(12):1539–44.

47. Rini BI et al. Phase III trial of bevacizumab plus interferon alfa versus interferon alfa monotherapy in patients with metastatic renal cell carcinoma: Final results of CALGB 90206. *J Clin Oncol.* 2010;28(13):2137–43.

48. Miller K et al. Paclitaxel plus Bevacizumab versus paclitaxel alone for metastatic breast cancer. *N Engl J Med.* 2007;357(26):2666–76.

49. Giordano G et al. Targeting angiogenesis and tumor microenvironment in metastatic colorectal cancer: Role of Aflibercept. *Gastroenterol Res Pract.* 2014;2014.

50. Choueiri TK et al. Congestive heart failure risk in patients with breast cancer treated with bevacizumab. *J Clin Oncol.* 2011;29(6):632–8.

51. Robert NJ et al. RIBBON-1: Randomized, double-blind, placebo-controlled, phase III trial of chemotherapy with or without bevacizumab for first-line treatment of human epidermal growth factor receptor 2-negative, locally recurrent or metastatic breast cancer. *J Clin Oncol.* 2011 April;29(10):1252–60.

52. Olszanski AJ et al. Electrocardiographic characterization of ramucirumab on the corrected QT interval in a phase II study of patients with advanced solid tumors. *Oncologist.* 2016;21(4):402–403f.

53. Eli Lilly Canada Inc. CYRAMZA® product monograph. Toronto, Ontario; July 16, 2015. Available from: http://www.ipcc.ch/publications_and_data/publications_and_data_reports.shtml

54. Fuchs CS et al. Ramucirumab monotherapy for previously treated advanced gastric or gastro-oesophageal junction adenocarcinoma (REGARD): An international, randomised, multicentre, placebo-controlled, phase 3 trial. *Lancet.* 2014;383(9911):31–9.

55. Wilke H et al. Ramucirumab plus paclitaxel versus placebo plus paclitaxel in patients with previously treated advanced gastric or gastro-oesophageal junction adenocarcinoma (RAINBOW): A double-blind, randomised phase 3 trial. *Lancet Oncol.* 2014;15(11):1224–35.

56. Lenihan DJ, Kowey PR. Overview and management of cardiac adverse events associated with tyrosine kinase inhibitors. *Oncologist.* 2013;18(8):900–8.

57. Orphanos GS, Ioannidis GN, Ardavanis AG. Cardiotoxicity induced by tyrosine kinase inhibitors. *Acta Oncol (Madr).* 2009;48(7):964–70.

58. Coppola C, Rienzo A, Piscopo G, Barbieri A, Arra C, Maurea N. Management of QT prolongation induced by anti-cancer drugs: Target therapy and old agents. Different algorithms for different drugs. *Cancer Treat Rev.* 2018;63:135–43.

59. Bronte G et al. Conquests and perspectives of cardio-oncology in the field of tumor angiogenesis-targeting tyrosine kinase inhibitor-based therapy. *Expert Opin Drug Saf.* 2015;14(2):253–67.

60. Yeh ETH, Bickford CL. Cardiovascular complications of cancer therapy. *J Am Coll Cardiol.* 2009;53(24):2231–47.

61. Crone SA et al. ErbB2 is essential in the prevention of dilated cardiomyopathy. *Nat Med.* 2002;8(5):459–65.

62. Porta-Sánchez A et al. Incidence, diagnosis, and management of QT prolongation induced by cancer therapies: A systematic review. *J Am Heart Assoc.* 2017;6(12):1–18.

63. Brell JM. Prolonged QTc interval in cancer therapeutic drug development: Defining arrhythmic risk in malignancy. *Prog Cardiovasc Dis.* 2010;53(2):164–72.

64. Nielsen J, Graff C, Kanters JK, Toft E, Taylor D, Meyer JM. Assessing QT interval prolongation and its associated risks with antipsychotics. *CNS Drugs.* 2011 June;25(6):473–90.

65. Tisdale JE. Drug-induced QT interval prolongation and torsades de pointes: Role of the pharmacist in risk assessment, prevention and management. *Can Pharm J.* 2016;149(3):139–52.

66. Xu H et al. Recent advances of highly selective CDK4/6 inhibitors in breast cancer. *J Hematol Oncol.* 2017;10(1):97.

67. Sonke GS et al. Ribociclib with letrozole vs letrozole alone in elderly patients with hormone receptor-positive, HER2-negative breast cancer in the randomized MONALEESA-2 trial. *Breast Cancer Res Treat.* 2017;167(3):1–11.

68. Tripathy D et al. Ribociclib plus endocrine therapy for premenopausal women with hormone-receptor-positive, advanced breast cancer (MONALEESA-7): A randomised phase 3 trial. *Lancet Oncol.* 2018;19(7):904–15.

69. Slamon DJ et al. Phase III randomized study of ribociclib and fulvestrant in hormone receptor–positive, human epidermal growth factor receptor 2–negative advanced breast cancer: MONALEESA-3. *J Clin Oncol.* 2018;36(24):JCO.2018.78.990.

70. Cristofanilli M et al. Fulvestrant plus palbociclib versus fulvestrant plus placebo for treatment of hormone-receptor-positive, HER2-negative metastatic breast cancer that progressed on previous endocrine therapy (PALOMA-3): Final analysis of the multicentre, double-blind, phas. *Lancet Oncol.* 2016;17(4):425–39.

71. Finn RS et al. The cyclin-dependent kinase 4/6 inhibitor palbociclib in combination with letrozole versus letrozole alone as first-line treatment of oestrogen receptor-positive, HER2-negative, advanced breast cancer (PALOMA-1/TRIO-18): A randomised phase 2 study. *Lancet Oncol.* 2015;16(1):25–35.

72. Chen JH, Lenihan DJ, Phillips SE, Harrell SL, Cornell RF. Cardiac events during treatment with proteasome inhibitor therapy for multiple myeloma. *Cardio-Oncology.* 2017;3(1):4.

73. Cole DC, Frishman WH. Cardiovascular complications of proteasome inhibitors used in multiple myeloma. *Cardiol Rev.* 2018;26(3):122–9.

74. Demo SD et al. Antitumor activity of PR-171, a novel irreversible inhibitor of the proteasome. *Cancer Res.* 2007 July;67(13):6383–91.

75. Kuhn DJ et al. Potent activity of carfilzomib, a novel, irreversible inhibitor of the ubiquitin-proteasome pathway, against preclinical models of multiple myeloma. *Blood.* 2007 November;110(9):3281–90.

76. Dimopoulos MA et al. Carfilzomib and dexamethasone versus bortezomib and dexamethasone for patients with relapsed or refractory multiple myeloma (ENDEAVOR): A randomised, phase 3, open-label, multicentre study. *Lancet Oncol.* 2016 January;17(1):27–38.

77. Stewart AK et al. Carfilzomib, lenalidomide, and dexamethasone for relapsed multiple myeloma. *N Engl J Med.* 2015;372(2):142–52.

78. Xiao Y, Yin J, Wei J, Shang Z. Incidence and risk of cardiotoxicity associated with bortezomib in the treatment of cancer: A systematic review and meta-analysis. *PLOS ONE.* 2014;9(1).

79. Raab MS, Podar K, Breitkreutz I, Richardson PG, Anderson KC. Multiple myeloma. *Lancet* 2009 July;374(9686):324–39.

80. Siegel D et al. Integrated safety profile of single-agent carfilzomib: Experience from 526 patients enrolled in 4 phase II clinical studies. *Haematologica* 2013 November;98(11): 1753–61.

81. Atrash S et al. Cardiac complications in relapsed and refractory multiple myeloma patients treated with carfilzomib. *Blood Cancer J.* United States; 2015;5:e272.

82. Li W et al. Cardiovascular and thrombotic complications of novel multiple myeloma therapies: A review. *JAMA Oncol.* 2017 July;3(7): 980–8.

83. Chari A, Hajje D. Case series discussion of cardiac and vascular events following carfilzomib treatment: Possible mechanism, screening, and monitoring. *BMC Cancer* 2014;14(1):1–9.

84. Varricchi G et al. Cardiotoxicity of immune checkpoint inhibitors. *ESMO Open.* 2017;2(4):e000247.

85. Asnani A. Cardiotoxicity of immunotherapy: Incidence, diagnosis, and management. *Curr Oncol Rep.* 2018 June 1;20(6):44.

86. Lee DW et al. T cells expressing CD19 chimeric antigen receptors for acute lymphoblastic leukaemia in children and young adults: A phase 1 dose-escalation trial. *Lancet].* 2015; 385(9967):517–28.

87. Davila ML et al. Efficacy and toxicity management of 19-28z CAR T cell therapy in B cell acute lymphoblastic leukemia. *Sci Transl Med.* 2014;6(224):224ra25–224ra25.

88. Brudno JN, Kochenderfer JN. Toxicities of chimeric antigen receptor T cells: Recognition and management. *Blood.* 2016 June 30; 127(26):3321–30.

89. Escudier M et al. Clinical features, management, and outcomes of immune checkpoint inhibitor–related cardiotoxicity. *Circulation.* 2017;136(21):2085–7.

90. Yun S, Vincelette ND, Mansour I, Hariri D, Motamed S. Late onset ipilimumab-induced pericarditis and pericardial effusion: A rare but life threatening complication. *Case Rep Oncol Med.* 2015;2015(Figure 2): 1–5. Available from: http://www.hindawi.com/journals/crionm/2015/794842/

91. Cheng F, Loscalzo J. Autoimmune cardiotoxicity of cancer immunotherapy. *Trends Immunol.* 2017;38(2):77–8.

92. Johnson DB et al. Fulminant myocarditis with combination immune checkpoint blockade. *N Engl J Med.* 2016;375(18):1749–55.

93. Brahmer JR et al. Management of immune-related adverse events in patients treated with immune checkpoint inhibitor therapy: American society of clinical oncology clinical practice guideline. *J Clin Oncol.* 2018;4: JCO.2017.77.638.

94. Norwood TG et al. Smoldering myocarditis following immune checkpoint blockade. *J Immunother Cancer.* 2017;5(1):4–9.

95. Raghunathan D, Khilji MI, Hassan SA, Yusuf SW. Radiation-induced cardiovascular disease. *Curr Atheroscler Rep.* 2017;19(5). (no[22]).

96. Shah C et al. Cardiac dose sparing and avoidance techniques in breast cancer radiotherapy. *Radiother Oncol.* 2014;112(1):9–16.

97. Taylor CW, Zhe W, Macaulay E, Jagsi R, Duane F, Darby SC. Exposure of the heart in breast cancer radiation therapy: A systematic review of heart doses published during 2003 to 2013. *Int J Radiat Oncol Biol Phys.* 2015;93(4):845–53.

98. Cuomo JR, Sharma GK, Conger PD, Weintraub NL. Novel concepts in radiation-induced cardiovascular disease. *World J Cardiol.* 2016;8(9):504.

99. Filopei J, Frishman W. Radiation-induced heart disease. *Cardiol Rev.* 2012;20(4):184–8.

100. Duma MN, Molls M, Trott KR. From heart to heart for breast cancer patients—cardiovascular toxicities in breast cancer radiotherapy. *Strahlentherapie und Onkol.* 2014;190(1):5–7.

101. Ahmed SH, Moussa Sherif D-E, Fouad Y, Kelany M, Abdel-Rahman O. Principles of a risk evaluation and mitigation strategy (REMS) for breast cancer patients receiving potentially cardiotoxic adjuvant treatments. *Expert Opin Drug Saf.* 2016;15(7):911–23.

102. Keefe DL. Trastuzumab-associated cardiotoxicity. *Cancer.* October 1, 2002 [cited July 17, 2014];95(7):1592–600.

103. Barni S, Petrelli F, Cabiddu M. Cardiotoxicity of antiemetic drugs in oncology: An overview of the current state of the art. *Crit Rev Oncol Hematol.* 2016;102:125–34.

104. Freedman SB, Uleryk E, Rumantir M, Finkelstein Y. Ondansetron and the risk of cardiac arrhythmias: A systematic review and postmarketing analysis. *Ann Emerg Med .* 2014;64(1):19–25.e6.

105. Government of Canada. 2014. Zofran (ondansetron)—Dosage and Administration of Intravenous Ondansetron in Geriatrics (>65 years of age)—For Health Professionals. Retrieved from http://healthycanadians.gc.ca/recall-alert-rappel-avis/hc-sc/2014/39943a-eng.php. Date accessed May 2018.

106. Picard M, Castells MC. Re-visiting hypersensitivity reactions to taxanes: A comprehensive review. *Clin Rev Allergy Immunol.* 2015;49(2):177–91.

107. Thompson JF, Chalmers DH, Wood RF, Kirkham SR, Morris PJ. Sudden death following high-dose intravenous methylprednisolone. *Transplantation.* 1983;36:594–6.

108. van der Hooft CS et al. Corticosteroids and the risk of atrial fibrillation. *J Am Med Assoc.* 2006;165:1016–20.

109. Fanous I, Dillon P. Cancer treatment-related cardiac toxicity: Prevention, assessment and management. *Med Oncol.* 2016;33(8):1–11.

110. Bayram C et al. Evaluation of cardiotoxicity by tissue Doppler imaging in childhood leukemia survivors treated with low-dose anthracycline. *Pediatr Cardiol.* 2015;36(4):862–6.

111. Fallah-Rad N et al. The utility of cardiac biomarkers, tissue velocity and strain imaging, and cardiac magnetic resonance imaging in predicting early left ventricular dysfunction in patients with human epidermal growth factor receptor II positive breast cancer treated with adjuvant trastuzumab therapy. *J Am Coll Cardiol.* 2011;57(22):2263–70.

112. Katsurada K, Ichida M, Sakuragi M, Takehara M, Hozumi Y, Kario K. High-sensitivity troponin T as a marker to predict cardiotoxicity in breast cancer patients with adjuvant trastuzumab therapy. *Springerplus.* 2014;3(1):1–7.

113. De Iuliis F et al. Serum biomarkers evaluation to predict chemotherapy-induced cardiotoxicity in breast cancer patients. *Tumor Biol.* 2016;37(3):3379–87.

114. Putt M et al. Longitudinal changes in multiple biomarkers are associated with cardiotoxicity in breast cancer patients treated with Doxorubicin, Taxanes, and Trastuzumab. *Clin Chem.* 2015 September;61(9):1164–72.

115. Kalam K, Marwick TH. Role of cardioprotective therapy for prevention of cardiotoxicity with chemotherapy: A systematic review and meta-analysis. *Eur J Cancer.* 2013;49(13):2900–9.

116. Yun S, Vincelette ND, Abraham I. Cardioprotective role of β-blockers and angiotensin antagonists in early-onset anthracyclines-induced cardiotoxicity in adult patients: A systematic review and meta-analysis. *Postgrad Med J.* 2015;91(1081):627–33.

117. Yancy CW et al. 2013 ACCF/AHA guideline for the management of heart failure: A report of the American College of Cardiology Foundation/American Heart Association task force on practice guidelines. *J Am Coll Cardiol.* 2013;62(16):e147–239.

118. Lenihan DJ et al. Cardio-oncology training: A proposal from the International Cardio-Oncology Society and Canadian Cardiac Oncology Network for a new multidisciplinary specialty. *J Card Fail.* 2016;22(6):465–71.

119. Tajiri K, Aonuma K, Sekine I. Cardio-oncology: A multidisciplinary approach for detection, prevention and management of cardiac dysfunction in cancer patients. *Jpn J Clin Oncol.* 2017;47(8):678–82.

120. van Dalen EC, Caron HN, Dickinson HO, Kremer LC. Cardioprotective interventions for cancer patients receiving anthracyclines. *Cochrane Database of Systematic Reviews.* 2011;(6).

6

Overview of current guidelines

FELICITY LEE AND GIRISH DWIVEDI

INTRODUCTION

Advances in cancer detection and treatment strategies have resulted in a major improvement in survival rates. Currently, there are over 14 million cancer survivors in the USA and close to 30 million cancer survivors worldwide (1,2). As a result, the focus has now turned to the detection, prevention, and management of cancer treatment-related toxicities. In particular, cardiotoxicity is now recognized as a leading cause of morbidity and mortality among cancer survivors.

This chapter aims to provide an overview of the current major societal guidelines and recommendations within the field of cardio-oncology. These include the (a) definition of cancer therapeutics related cardiac dysfunction (CTRCD); (b) diagnosis of CTRCD with a multimodality imaging approach and serum biomarkers; (c) identification of patients at high risk of cardiotoxicity; (d) prevention of cardiotoxicity; (e) monitoring of cardiotoxicity; and (f) treatment of cardiotoxicity. Guidelines and position statements reviewed include the 2016 European Society of Cardiology (ESC) Position Paper (3); the 2016 American Society of Clinical Oncology (ASCO) Practice Guidelines (4); the 2016 Canadian Cardiovascular Society (CCS) Guidelines (5); the 2014 Report from the American

Society of Echocardiography (ASE) and the European Association of Cardiovascular Imaging (EACVI) (6); and the 2012 European Society of Medical Oncology (ESMO) Clinical Practice Guidelines (7). The guidelines aim to provide some consensus on the general management of patients with cardiotoxicity. Minor discrepancies exist owing to differences in each society's focus and target audience.

Recommendations are created using the ASCO GuideLines Into DEcision Support (GLIDES) methodology (4). The type of recommendation is classified as "evidence-based," "formal consensus," "informal consensus," or "no recommendation." The strength of each recommendation is rated as "strong," "medium," or "weak" based on the evidence of a true net effect, consistency of results, concerns about study quality and the extent of agreement among panelists (4).

DEFINITION OF CTRCD

Cardiotoxicity as a result of cancer treatment (chemotherapy, radiotherapy, and/or immunotherapy) has various manifestations, including myocardial dysfunction and heart failure, coronary artery disease, valvular heart disease, arrhythmias including QT interval prolongation, arterial hypertension, thromboembolic disease, peripheral vascular disease, pulmonary hypertension, and pericardial disease (3).

The American College of Cardiology and American Heart Association further categorizes heart failure into the following stages. Stage A patients do not have structural heart disease or symptoms of heart failure, but are at high risk for heart failure. Stage B patients have structural heart disease but no signs or symptoms of heart failure. Stage C patients have structural heart disease with prior or current symptoms of heart failure, and stage D patients have refractory heart failure requiring specialized interventions (8).

The ASE/EACVI and ESC define CTRCD as a decrease in left ventricular (LV) ejection fraction (EF) by >10 percentage points, to a value <53% based on echocardiography (3,6). The ESC also identifies patients with cardiotoxicity if there is a >10 percentage points decrease in left ventricular ejection fraction (LVEF) with a value <50% as identified on nuclear cardiac imaging with a multigated acquisition scan (MUGA). This decrease in EF should be confirmed by repeated cardiac imaging 2–3 weeks following the baseline diagnostic study (3).

The ASE/EACVI further classifies CTRCD into either those associated with anthracycline or trastuzumab use. Anthracycline-related CRTCD is cumulative, dose-dependent, and often progressive and irreversible at the cell level (6). On the other hand, trastuzumab-related CRTCD is dose-independent, does not lead to cell death, and is often reversible (6).

DIAGNOSIS OF CARDIOTOXICITY

Imaging

Serial measurement of LV function, in particular LVEF, is the most commonly applied modality used to detect cardiotoxicity. Transthoracic echocardiography (TTE) is typically the method of choice due to its availability and reproducibility. TTE also has additional advantages; there is no radiation exposure to the patient and the right ventricle, valves, and pericardium can be assessed (4–6). Cardiac magnetic resonance imaging (MRI) or a MUGA scan can be used if TTE is not technically feasible or available.

TTE

LV systolic function

According to joint recommendations from the ASE/EACVI, the method of choice for LV volumes quantification and LVEF calculation is the modified

biplane Simpson's technique by 2D echocardiography, with an LVEF $\geq$55% as a normal reference range (6,9). Calculation of LVEF should be also combined with assessment of the wall motion score index, which is based on a 16-segment model of the left ventricle (9). When two contiguous LV segments are not well visualized on noncontrast apical images, the use of myocardial contrast agents are recommended to better delineate the endocardial border (6,10,11). Three-dimensional (3D) echocardiography has been shown to be more accurate than 2D echocardiography in the measurement of LV volumes (12). The ASE recommends 3D echocardiography as the preferred technique for monitoring LV function and detecting CTRCD (5,6). However, it is recommended that calculation of LVEF by the biplane Simpson's method also be included in the echocardiographic report to allow comparison with previous studies. Any changes in LVEF should be confirmed on repeat imaging 2–3 weeks after the initial study.

LV diastolic function

A comprehensive assessment of LV diastolic function including grading of diastolic function and an estimate of LV filling pressures should be performed in addition to the assessment of LV systolic function (13). Although abnormal diastolic parameters may reflect subclinical LV dysfunction, it has not been found to be prognostic of cardiotoxicity and its clinical significance remains uncertain (6).

LV strain

Myocardial deformation (strain) can be measured using doppler tissue imaging or 2D speckle tracking echocardiography (STE). Global longitudinal strain (GLS) via 2D STE has been widely studied and is the optimal parameter of deformation for the early detection of subclinical LV dysfunction (14). Other indices of strain such as radial and circumferential strain and strain rate are still under investigation and do not have any current clinical implications (6,15). It is recommended that the same vendor's machine and software version be used, and sonographers and interpreting physicians have adequate training to reduce both intra- and interobserver and test-retest variability (6,16,17).

MUGA

Evaluation of LV systolic function with MUGA has been shown to be accurate and reproducible. As a 3D imaging technique, MUGA is superior to 2D echocardiography and the values obtained by MUGA also had better correlation with other 3D imaging modalities such as 3D echocardiography and cardiac MRI (6,18,19). However, the disadvantages of using MUGA for serial assessments of LV function include radiation exposure and its limited ability to assess cardiac structure and hemodynamics (7). As such, MUGA is often used as an adjunct rather than a substitute for echocardiography.

CARDIAC MRI

Cardiac MRI is a useful tool in assessing cardiac structure and function and is the reference standard in the evaluation of left and right ventricular volumes and LVEF (20,21). The ASE/EACVI recommend that cardiac MRI be used as an additional tool in situations where discontinuation or change of chemotherapy regimens secondary to CTRCD is being considered (6,22). This may be due to technical limitations or poor quality of echocardiographic images or when the LVEF by 2D/3D echocardiography is controversial or unreliable (4–7). In addition, cardiac MRI can evaluate the pericardium and detect scarring and myocardial fibrosis (3). The use of advanced techniques such as T1 and T2 mapping and extracellular volume fraction quantification can assist in tissue characterization, evaluation of cardiac masses, and identification of infiltrative diseases (3). Disadvantages of this imaging modality include cost, its limited availability, and its dependence on patient compliance (ability to breath-hold and not being claustrophobic) (6,22).

Serum biomarkers

Cardiac biomarkers may have a role in the detection of subclinical LV dysfunction (3,6). Although an abnormal result may indicate an increased risk of cardiotoxicity, it is insufficient to warrant cessation or interruption of chemotherapy treatment. Owing to variations in normal references and the use of different assays, the role of serum biomarkers in routine surveillance and the significance of subtle rises in assay levels is unknown. The timing of biomarker testing in relation to administration of chemotherapy is also uncertain. The two most commonly used biomarkers are serum troponin and serum brain-type natriuretic peptide (BNP).

TROPONIN

Cardiac troponins are the gold standard biomarkers for the diagnosis of myocardial injury (23). In patients treated with anthracycline chemotherapy, increased levels of troponin can be used to identify patients who are at risk of developing CTRCD (24). A persistent troponin rise is associated with an increase in the severity of CRTCD and number of cardiac events compared to a transient rise (24).

BNP

Elevations in BNP are more reflective of abnormal filling pressures and may be less consistent in the detection of subclinical LV dysfunction. No definite association between BNP and LV dysfunction has been ascertained yet (25,26).

Recommendations

Please refer to Table 6.1.

IDENTIFICATION OF THE HIGH-RISK POPULATION

The prevalence and mortality related to cardiovascular (CV) disease has been shown to be significantly higher in both short- and long-term cancer survivors compared to noncancer survivors (27). Preexisting CV risk factors in this population compounded with the cancer diagnosis and cardiotoxic effects of cancer therapy reduce an individual's CV reserve, predisposing them to cardiac disease along with its associated morbidity and mortality (5,28).

ASCO recommends that patients with cancer treated with high-dose anthracycline (e.g., doxorubicin $\geq$250 mg/m^2 or epirubicin $\geq$600 mg/m^2); high-dose radiotherapy (radiotherapy $\geq$30 Gy with the heart in the treatment field); or lower-dose anthracycline in combination with lower-dose radiotherapy should be considered at increased risk of developing cardiac dysfunction (4,29–31). Patients treated with lower-dose anthracycline or trastuzumab alone, but in the presence of multiple CV risk factors (smoking, hypertension, diabetes, dyslipidemia, and obesity); older age ($\geq$60 years) at cancer treatment; or compromised cardiac function (e.g., borderline low LVEF 50%–55%, history of myocardial infarction, $\geq$moderate valvular heart disease) at any time before or during

Table 6.1 A summary of recommendations for the diagnosis of cardiotoxicity including the type of recommendation and the strength of recommendation, created by ASCO using the GLIDES methodology

Recommendations	Type	Strength
Echocardiography is the standard imaging modality of choice for assessment of cardiac structure and function (ASE/EACVI)	Evidence-based	Strong
If echocardiography is not available or technically feasible, MUGA scan or cardiac MRI can be used, with preference given to cardiac MRI (ASCO, ASE/EACVI)	Evidence-based	Moderate
MUGA scan can reduce interobserver variability, but has the disadvantage of limited data on cardiac structure and function and increased radiation exposure. Cardiac MRI is another alternative imaging modality, especially when cessation of treatment is being considered, but its use is limited by reduced availability, cost, and patient factors (claustrophobia, metalwork) (ASCO, ASE/EACVI, ESMO)	Evidence-based	Moderate
The same imaging modality and method should be utilized to determine LVEF before, during, and after completion of cancer therapy (CCS, ASE/EACVI). 3D echocardiography is the preferred technique in monitoring LV function and detecting CTRCD (CCS, ASE/EACVI)	Formal consensus	Moderate
2D STE (GLS) and serum biomarkers, in particular troponin, are useful tools for detecting subclinical LV dysfunction but their significance is still unknown (ESC, ASCO, CCS, ASE/EACVI, ESMO)	Formal consensus	Moderate

treatment are also considered at increased risk of developing cardiac dysfunction (4,32–35).

Recommendations

Please refer to Table 6.2.

PREVENTION OF CARDIOTOXICITY

Chemotherapy

The ESC and ASCO recommend various strategies to prevent the development of LV dysfunction and heart failure with high dose anthracycline use (3,4). This includes reducing the cumulative dose, use of a continuous infusion to decrease peak plasma levels, and use of analogues (epirubicin, pixantrone) or liposomal formulations (36–39). The use of dexrazoxane, an iron-chelating agent as a cardio-protectant is recommended only for patients with metastatic breast cancer who have already received more than 300 mg/m^2 of doxorubicin (4,37–39). Prophylactic use of angiotensin-converting enzyme

(ACE) inhibitors, beta-blockers or angiotensin receptor blockers (ARBs) in the prevention of anthracycline-induced cardiotoxicity remains controversial. This is an area of active investigation, but there have been limited studies, most of which have small sample sizes, different endpoints, and inconclusive data (38,39). Cardiotoxicity can also be minimized with the introduction of a drug-free interval between anthracycline and trastuzumab use (7).

Optimization of cardiovascular risk factors is also paramount prior to exposure to cardiotoxic agents. This includes management of hypertension, metabolic disorders, preexisting heart failure, and other cardiac conditions (e.g., angina), as well as counseling regarding smoking cessation, weight loss, and physical activity (3–5,7).

Radiotherapy

Techniques that reduce both the volume and dose of incidental cardiac irradiation should be utilized. These include deep inspiration breath holding or respiratory gating, multiple or rotational sources

Table 6.2 A summary of recommendations for the identification of patients at high risk of cardiotoxicity including the type of recommendation and the strength of recommendation, created by ASCO using the GLIDES methodology

Recommendations	Type	Strength
All patients receiving potentially cardiotoxic treatments should undergo a baseline comprehensive assessment including history and physical examination, and screening for cardiovascular disease risk factors (ESC, ASCO, CCS, ESMO)	Informal consensus and evidence-based	Strong
A thorough diagnostic evaluation of traditional cardiovascular risk factors if present (hypertension, diabetes, dyslipidaemia, obesity) should be undertaken. Patients should be educated on lifestyle modifications and, if indicated, be commenced on appropriate pharmacologic treatment (ESC, ASCO, CCS, ESMO)	Informal consensus and evidence-based	Strong
Hypertension should be identified and treated accordingly, with a goal of less than 140/90 mm Hg for most patients and 125–130/80 mm Hg for those with preexisting diabetes and chronic kidney disease. ACE inhibitors or angiotensin receptor blockers (ARBs), beta blockers, and dihydropyridine calcium channel blockers are the preferred antihypertensive drugs. Nondihydropyridine calcium channel blocks should be avoided due to drug interactions (ESC, CCS)	Evidence-based	Strong
A standard 12-lead ECG should be recorded for all patients and QT time (QTc) should be corrected for heart rate with Bazett's formula ($QTc = QT/\sqrt{RR}$). Caution should be undertaken in view of potential drug interactions when prescribing supportive medications that can prolong QT time during cancer treatment (e.g., antiemetics, analgesics, antibiotics, and antidepressants). If the QTC is >500 ms, metabolic and electrolyte disturbances should be identified and corrected and use of concomitant QT-prolonging drugs be minimized (ESC, CCS, ESMO)	Informal consensus	Moderate
Evaluation of left ventricular ejection fraction prior to commencement of potentially cardiotoxic cancer treatment is necessary. Periodic assessment during and after treatment is recommended especially in symptomatic patients (ESC, ASCO, CCS, ASE/EACVI, ESMO)	Formal consensus and evidence-based	Strong

of radiation beams, and intensity-modulated radiation beams using multileaf collimators (3–5,40–43).

Recommendations

Please refer to Table 6.3.

MONITORING OF CARDIOTOXICITY

The ESC, ASCO, CCS, and ASE/EACVI guidelines recommend baseline evaluation of LVEF, GLS, and troponin prior to initiation of agents associated with CTRCD (6). According to ESC/ASE/EACVI, patients receiving anthracyclines should have repeat measurements performed at completion of therapy and 6 months later for doses <240 g/m² (3,6,29,44). Once this dose is exceeded, repeat assessment is recommended before each additional 50 mg/m² (6). In patients receiving trastuzumab, repeat measurements are to be performed every 3 months during therapy, and once after completion of therapy (3,6). Any abnormality (LVEF <53%, GLS <lower limit of

Table 6.3 A summary of recommendations for the prevention of cardiotoxicity including the type of recommendation and the strength of recommendation, created by ASCO using the GLIDES methodology

Recommendations	Type	Strength
Cardioprotective measures such as the use of continuous infusions or liposomal formulation of doxorubicin and the use of the cardioprotectant dexrazoxane should be considered in patients at high risk of cardiotoxicity (ESC, ASCO, ESMO)	Evidence-based	Moderate
ACE inhibitors, ARBs, and/or beta blockers can be considered to reduce the risk of cardiotoxicity in patients deemed at high risk of cancer treatment-related LV dysfunction (ESC, CCS, ESMO)	Formal consensus and evidence-based	Weak
Modern radiotherapy techniques (3D conformal or intensity-modulated radiotherapy), use of lower radiation doses and tailored radiation fields should be utilized during planning mediastinal and chest radiation to reduce the risk of short- and long-term cardiotoxicity (ESC, ASCO, CCS, ESMO)	Informal consensus and evidence-based	Weak

normal or positive troponin) or the development of signs and symptoms of heart failure should prompt further evaluation and a cardiology consultation (6,24,45,46).

The ESMO guidelines outline two pathways for cardiac monitoring (7). The first involves cardiac imaging only, and the second involves a combination of both serum troponin and cardiac imaging after baseline cardiac evaluation and echocardiography (7). In the former, an echocardiogram is performed at baseline, 3, 6, and 9, months during treatment, and then at 12 and 18 months after the initiation of treatment. In the latter, a serum troponin is performed after each chemotherapy cycle (7). Troponin-negative patients would then have yearly echocardiograms. ASCO guidelines have a more generalized approach and state that the frequency of surveillance should be determined by healthcare providers based on clinical judgment and patient circumstances (4).

The ASE/EACVI/ESC guidelines also recommend use of GLS for the identification of subclinical LV dysfunction. If baseline strain is available, a relative percentage decrease of >15% compared with baseline is likely to be of clinical significance whereas a decrease of <8% is not. The abnormal GLS value should be confirmed on a repeat study performed 2–3 weeks after the initial abnormal study (3,6,46).

The ESC and ASE/EACVI guidelines recommend that in patients who have received high doses of chest irradiation (>30 Gy), screening with stress testing, echocardiography, perfusion imaging, and/or coronary calcium scoring by computed tomography should be considered, starting 10–15 years after initial cancer treatment and continuing for the lifetime of the patient (3,47). This is especially encouraged in patients with preexisting risk factors for cardiovascular disease (6,47).

Recommendations

Please refer to Table 6.4.

TREATMENT OF CARDIOTOXICITY

Heart failure and LV dysfunction

There are still significant variations in management among the major societies. Other causes of cardiomyopathy should be accounted for (5).

ANTHRAYCYCLINE-INDUCED CARDIOTOXICITY

The ESC guidelines state that patients with a significant decline in LVEF (decrease of more than 10%) to an LVEF <50% should be commenced on ACE inhibitors (or ARBs) and beta blockers to prevent further LV dysfunction (3). These medications should be considered in both patients with

Table 6.4 A summary of recommendations for the monitoring of cardiotoxicity including the type of recommendation and the strength of recommendation, created by ASCO using the GLIDES methodology

Recommendations	Type	Strength
Baseline evaluation of LVEF, GLS, and troponin should be undertaken prior to initiation of agents associated with CTRCD (ESC, ASCO, CCS, ASE/EACVI)	Evidence-based	Moderate
Serial assessments with cardiac imaging and/or serum biomarkers are recommended during treatment and after completion of therapy (ESC, ASCO, CCS, ASE/EACVI, ESMO)	Evidence-based	Moderate
In patients who receive high doses of chest irradiation, screening with noninvasive imaging should be considered 10–15 years after initial treatment (ESC, ASE/EACVI)	Evidence-based	Weak

symptomatic heart failure or asymptomatic cardiac dysfunction. For patients with a decline in LVEF by >10% to an LVEF >50%, repeated assessment of LVEF shortly after and during cancer treatment is recommended (3).

According to ESMO, troponin-positive patients should be started on an ACE inhibitor to prevent LVEF reduction, with an echocardiogram performed at the end of chemotherapy and every 3 months afterward (7). If symptomatic LV dysfunction is detected (LVEF <40%), cessation of chemotherapy and initiation of appropriate heart failure therapy with ACE inhibitors and beta blockers is recommended (7). If the LVEF is >40% but <50%, a reassessment is necessary in 3 weeks. If this is confirmed, cessation of chemotherapy, initiation of appropriate heart failure pharmacotherapy, and more frequent follow-up is recommended (7). In patients with symptomatic heart failure without a decline in LVEF, chemotherapy can still be continued and an individualized approach is necessary. For an asymptomatic decline in LVEF <40% or an LVEF reduction of ≥15% from baseline to LVEF <50%, anthracycline therapy should be withheld, heart failure pharmacotherapy initiated, and a risk-benefit discussion between the patient, oncologist, and cardiologist is recommended (7). A choice to continue therapy may be made for individual patients, particularly those who are being treated for curative intent or for whom other appropriate options are not available. For an asymptomatic decline in LVEF <50% but >40%, anthracycline therapy can be continued. Initiation of ACE inhibitors and beta blockers in addition to more frequent echocardiography and clinical review is recommended (7).

TRASTUZUMAB-INDUCED CARDIOTOXICITY

The ASCO/ESC/CCS adhere to the following recommendations for the management of trastuzumab-induced cardiotoxicity. If LVEF decreases to <45% or >10% from baseline to a value between 45 and 49%, trastuzumab should be withheld and a repeat LVEF measurement should be performed in 3 weeks (3–5,28). On serial assessment, if the LVEF is restored to >49%, trastuzumab can be reinitiated. If the LVEF is between 45%–49%, trastuzumab may be continued but an ACE inhibitor should be initiated. If the LVEF remains ≤44%, trastuzumab should be stopped with initiation of standard heart failure pharmacotherapy (ACE inhibitors and beta blockers) (3–5,28). Trastuzumab-related cardiotoxicity is reversible and often responsive to standard medical treatment for heart failure and discontinuation of the causative agent (28,48).

The ESMO Clinical Practice Guidelines have a more simplified algorithm. Patients with symptomatic heart failure and LVEF <40% should be treated with an ACE inhibitor in combination with a beta blocker (7). An ACE inhibitor should also be considered for symptomatic patients if the LVEF is between 40% and 50% (7). In asymptomatic patients with an LVEF <40%, ACE inhibitors should be used (7). Beta blockers can also be considered for this subgroup, especially in the setting of previous myocardial infarction (7).

The concurrent use of high dose anthracyclines and trastuzumab should be avoided; however, at a limited dose (≤180 mg/m^2 of doxorubicin), simultaneous trastuzumab is a potentially safe option (49). The combination of trastuzumab with taxanes, endocrine therapy, or radiation therapy does not carry a significant risk of cardiac toxicity (50,51).

Hypertension

Vascular endothelial growth factor (VEGF) inhibitors are associated with the onset of hypertension as well as destabilization of previously controlled hypertension (5,7,52–54). In patients starting VEGF inhibitors, blood pressure (BP) should be obtained at ≥ 2 clinic visits. Once hypertension is identified (>140/90 mm Hg), the goals of managing hypertension are to reduce the short-term risk of its related morbidities while maintaining effective antiangiogenic therapy for optimal cancer treatment as per the ESC/CCS/ESMO guidelines (3,5,7,55).

Other medications (such as nonsteroidal anti-inflammatory drugs and steroids) that contribute to hypertension should be factored into each patient's management (3–5). According to ESC/ASCO/CCS guidelines, ACE inhibitors, ARBs, vasodilatory beta blockers, and dihydropyridine calcium channel blockers are the preferred antihypertensive drugs (3–5,56). Nondihydropyridine calcium channel blockers are avoided due to their inhibition of cytochrome P450 3A4 and resultant risk of drug interactions. Renal function can affect the choice of antihypertensive agents and should be assessed at baseline and during treatment. After initiation of treatment with an antihypertensive agent, weekly monitoring of blood pressure is recommended during the first cycle of therapy and then every 2–3 weeks for the duration of cancer therapy (5).

Coronary artery disease

Fluoropyrimidines such as 5-fluorouracil (5-FU) and its oral form capecitabine can induce myocardial ischemia via mechanisms of coronary vasospasm and endothelial injury (57). The ESMO guidelines recommend baseline electrocardiogram (ECG) evaluation prior to initiation of therapy (7). According to the CCS guidelines, the temporal relationship between drug administration and chest pain onset is also important to establish (5). If symptoms occur during 5-FU administration, the infusion should be ceased (5). Cardiac monitoring, ECG and troponins should then be performed (5).

Sublingual glyceryl trinitrate and opiate therapy can be administered if symptoms do not resolve upon cessation of chemotherapy (58). In the event of troponin elevation, initiation of acute coronary syndrome management should be undertaken (59). The CCS guidelines also state that the decision to pursue further investigations should involve discussion between the treating oncologist and cardiologist. In the event that revascularization via percutaneous coronary intervention is required, the requirement for longer-term dual antiplatelet therapy in the setting of anticipated thrombocytopenia from cancer treatment should be considered (5). The ESC/CCS guidelines state that drug rechallenge is not routinely recommended, but can be considered if no alternate treatment is available. In this situation, close cardiac monitoring, safer administrative regimens (dose reduction or bolus instead of infusion), and prophylactic therapy (nitrates and calcium channel blockers) may reduce symptom recurrence (3–5,60).

Arrhythmias

Atrial fibrillation is the most common supraventricular arrhythmia among cancer patients and does not warrant interruption or discontinuation of cancer treatment (3,5). Modifiable risk factors including electrolyte disturbances, sepsis, and thyroid disorders should be identified and corrected. The CCS guidelines state that longer-term management decisions need to be individualized and relate to a rate vs. rhythm control strategy and the need for oral anticoagulation for stroke prevention (61). Use of a beta-blocker or nondihydropyridine calcium channel blocker can help with rate control (3). Digoxin is useful in patients with coexisting heart failure or LV systolic dysfunction (3). The role of anticoagulation should be based on the patient's thromboembolic and bleeding risk. While cancer often results in a prothrombotic state, cancer treatments can cause significant cytopenias, limiting treatment options. There are three types of anticoagulation choices that can be considered if the platelet count is >50,000/mm^3, namely therapeutic low molecular weight heparin (LMWH), warfarin, and the novel oral anticoagulants (NOAC) (3). The ESC/CCS guidelines recommend LMWH as a reasonable short-term measure, and it is particularly useful in bridging patients who require surgery (3,5). Warfarin has multiple drug interactions and it should be used with

Table 6.5 A summary of recommendations for the treatment of patients with cardiotoxicity including the type of recommendation and the strength of recommendation, created by ASCO using the GLIDES methodology

Recommendations	Type	Strength
Significant changes in LVEF necessitate confirmation with repeat imaging within 2–3 weeks. A significant decline in LVEF warrants institution of heart failure treatment (ACE inhibitors/ARBs and beta blockers) (ESC, ASCO, CCS, ESMO)	Evidence-based	Strong
The decision to withhold or discontinue cancer therapy should be made by the oncologist in close collaboration with a cardiologist after considering the risks and benefits of continuation of therapy (ASCO)	Informal consensus	Weak
A target BP of <140/90 mm Hg (or lower in those with diabetes or proteinuria) should be maintained (ESC, CCS)	Evidence-based	Strong
Patients who experience symptoms to suggest myocardial ischaemia during cancer therapy should be investigated with serial ECGs and troponins. Alternative antineoplastic treatment should be considered (ESC, CCS, ESMO)	Informal consensus	Moderate
Patients who have a QTc interval exceeding 500 ms during treatment should have reversible causes of QT prolongation identified and corrected. Exposure to other QT-prolonging drugs should be minimized (ESC, CCS)	Informal consensus	Weak

caution. There is limited data on the use of NOACs in cancer patients with atrial fibrillation; however, a meta-analysis has suggested that these drugs are safe among cancer patients requiring treatment of venous thromboembolism (62).

QT interval prolongation is seen predominantly in patients on tyrosine kinase inhibitors and arsenic trioxide (3,63–65). The ESC/CCS guidelines state that treatment should be temporarily discontinued in the event of malignant dysrhythmias (5), if the corrected QT interval (QTc) is >500 ms or is prolonged by >60 ms (3). General management of predisposing factors includes correcting electrolyte abnormalities, thyroid disorders, and bradycardia, in addition to avoiding other QT prolonging drugs (antiemetics, antibiotics, and antidepressants) (3,5).

Recommendations

Please refer to Table 6.5.

CONCLUSIONS

With an increasing number of cancer survivors, the focus now lies on the optimization and treatment of cardiovascular disease associated with cancer treatment. Morbidity and mortality related to cardiotoxicity can be reduced by early risk factor modification, timely identification of cardiotoxicity with imaging and/or serum biomarkers, initiation of guideline-directed cardioprotective medical therapy, prompt referral to appropriate specialists, and development of a multidisciplinary approach for individualized care. This chapter summarizes current international guidelines and position statements, which are presently still based more on consensus than level 1 evidence. Thus, more data and research involving randomized controlled trials and large prospective registries are required to optimize patient care in this complex subspecialty.

REFERENCES

1. DeSantis CE et al. Cancer treatment and survivorship statistics, 2014. *CA Cancer J Clin.* 2014;64(4):252–71.
2. Ferlay J et al. *GLOBOCAN 2012 v1.0, Cancer Incidence and Mortality Worldwide: IARC CancerBase No. 11.* Lyon, France: International Agency for Research on Cancer; 2013 [cited October 24, 2017]. Available from: http://globocan.iarc.fr

3. Zamorano JL et al. 2016 ESC Position paper on cancer treatments and cardiovascular toxicity developed under the auspices of the ESC committee for practice guidelines. *Eur Heart J*. 2016;37(36):2768–801.

4. Armenian SH et al. Prevention and monitoring of cardiac dysfunction in survivors of adult cancers: American Society of Clinical Oncology clinical practice guideline. *J Clin Oncol*. 2016;35:893–911.

5. Virani SA et al. Canadian Cardiovascular Society guidelines for evaluation and management of cardiovascular complications of cancer therapy. *Can J Cardiol*. 2016;32(7):831–41.

6. Plana JC et al. Expert consensus for multimodality imaging evaluation of adult patients during and after cancer therapy: A report from the American Society of Echocardiography and the European Association of Cardiovascular Imaging. *J Am Sc Echocardiogr*. 2014;27:911–39.

7. Curigliano G et al. Cardiovascular toxicity induced by chemotherapy, targeted agents and radiotherapy: ESMO clinical practice guidelines. *Ann Oncol*. 2012;23(7):155–66.

8. Yancy CW et al. 2013 ACCF/AHA guidelines for the management of heart failure. *Circulation*. 2013;128(16):e240–327.

9. Lang RM et al. Recommendations for chamber quantification: A report from the American Society of Echocardiography's Guidelines and Standards Committee and the Chamber Quantification Writing Group, developed in conjunction with the European Association of Echocardiography, a branch of the European Society of Cardiology. *J Am Soc Echocardiogr*. 2005;18:1440–63.

10. Mulvagh SL et al. American Society of Echocardiography consensus statement on the clinical applications of ultrasonic contrast agents in echocardiography. *J Am Soc Echocardiogr*. 2008;21:1179–201.

11. Senior R et al. Contrast echocardiography: Evidence-based recommendations by European Association of Echocardiography. *Eur J Echocardiogr*. 2009;10:194–212.

12. Badano LP et al. Current clinical applications of transthoracic three-dimensional echocardiography. *J Cardiovasc Ultrasound*. 2012;20:1–22.

13. Nagueh SF et al. Recommendations for the evaluation of left ventricular diastolic function by echocardiography. *Eur J Echocardiogr*. 2009;10:165–93.

14. Negishi K, Negishi T, Hare JL, Haluska BA, Plana JC, Marwick TH. Independent and incremental value of deformation indices for prediction of trastuzumab-induced cardiotoxicity. *J Am Soc Echocrdiogr*. 2013;26(5):493–8.

15. Hare JL, Brown JK, Leano R, Jenkins C, Woodward N, Marwick TH. Use of myocardial deformation imaging to detect preclinical myocardial dysfunction before conventional measures in patients undergoing breast cancer treatment with trastuzumab. *Am Heart J*. 2009;158:294–301.

16. Cheng S et al. Reproducibility of speckle-tracking-based strain measures of left ventricular function in a community-based study. *J Am Soc Echocardiogr*. 2013;26:1258–62.

17. Risum N et al. Variability of global left ventricular deformation analysis using vendor dependent and independent two-dimensional speckle-tracking software in adults. *J Am Soc Echocardiogr*. 2012;25:1195–203.

18. Bellenger NG et al. Comparison of left ventricular ejection fraction and volumes in heart failure by echocardiography, radionuclide ventriculography and cardiovascular magnetic resonance, are they interchangeable? *Eur Heart J*. 2000;21(16):1387–96.

19. Naik MM, Diamond GA, Pai T, Soffer A, Siegel RJ. Correspondence of left ventricular ejection fraction determinations from two-dimensional echocardiography, radionuclide angiography and contrast cineangiography. *J Am Coll Cardiol*. 1995;25:937–42.

20. Armstrong GT et al. Screening adult survivors of childhood cancer for cardiomyopathy: Comparison of echocardiography and cardiac magnetic resonance imaging. *J Clin Oncol*. 2012;30:2876–84.

21. Thavendiranathan P, Wintersperger BJ, Flamm SD, Marwick TH. Cardiac MRI in the assessment of cardiac injury and toxicity from cancer chemotherapy: A systematic review. *Circ Cardiovasc Imaging*. 2013;6:1080–91.

22. Armstrong AC, Gidding S, Gjesdal O, Wu C, Bluemke DA, Lima JA. LV mass assessed by echocardiography and CMR, cardiovascular outcomes, and medical practice. *JACC Cardiovasc Imaging*. 2012;5:837–48.

23. Reichlin T et al. Early diagnosis of myocardial infarction with sensitive cardiac troponin assays. *N Engl J Med.* 2009;361(9):858–67.

24. Cardinale D et al. Prognostic value of troponin I in cardiac risk stratification of cancer patients undergoing high-dose chemotherapy. *Circulation.* 2004;109(22):2749–54.

25. Dodos F, Halbsguth T, Erdmann E, Hoppe UC. Usefulness of myocardial performance index and biochemical markers for early detection of anthracycline-induced cardiotoxicity in adults. *Clin Res Cardiol.* 2008;97(5):318–26.

26. Knobloch K et al. Combined NT-pro-BNP and CW-Doppler ultrasound cardiac output monitoring (USCOM) in epirubicin and liposomal doxorubicin therapy. *Int J Cardiol.* 2008;128(3):316–25.

27. Tashakkor AY, Moghaddamjou A, Chen L, Cheung WY. Predicting the risk of cardiovascular comorbidities in adult cancer survivors. *Curr Oncol.* 2013;20(5):e360–70.

28. Jones AL et al. Management of cardiac health in trastuzumab-treated patients with breast cancer: Updated United Kingdom National Cancer Research Institute recommendations for monitoring. *Br J Cancer.* 2009;100(5):684–92.

29. Swain SM, Whaley FS, Ewer MS. Congestive heart failure in patients treated with doxorubicin: A retrospective analysis of three trials. *Cancer.* 2003;97:2869–79.

30. Armenian SH et al. Incidence and predictors of congestive heart failure after autologous hematopoietic cell transplantation. *Blood.* 2011;118:6023–9.

31. van Nimwegan FA et al. Cardiovascular disease after Hodgkin lymphoma treatment: 40-year disease risk. *JAMA Intern Med.* 2015;175:1007–17.

32. Tarantini L et al. Adjuvant trastuzumab cardiotoxicity in patients over 60 years of age with early breast cancer: A multicentre cohort analysis. *Ann Oncol.* 2012;23:3058–63.

33. Chavez-MacGregor M et al. Trastuzumab-related cardiotoxicity among older patients with breast cancer. *J Clin Oncol.* 2013;31:4222–8.

34. Hooning MJ et al. Long-term risk of cardiovascular disease in 10-year survivors of breast cancer. *J Natl Cancer Inst.* 2007;99:365–75.

35. Pinder MC et al. Congestive heart failure in older women treated with adjuvant anthracycline chemotherapy for breast cancer. *J Clin Oncol.* 2007;25:3808–15.

36. Rafiyath SM et al. Comparison of safety and toxicity of liposomal doxorubicin vs conventional anthracyclines: A meta-analysis. *Exp Hematol Oncol.* 2012;1:10.

37. Smith LA et al. Cardiotoxicity of anthracycline agents for the treatment of cancer: Systematic review and meta-analysis of randomised controlled trials. *BMC Cancer.* 2010;10:337.

38. Kalam K, Marwick TH. Role of cardioprotective therapy for prevention of cardiotoxicity with chemotherapy: A systematic review and meta-analysis. *Eur J Cancer.* 2013;49:2900–9.

39. van Dalen EC et al. Cardioprotective interventions for cancer patients receiving anthracyclines. *Cochrane Database Syst Rev.* 2011;6:CD003917.

40. Petersen PM et al. Prospective phase II trial of image-guided radiotherapy in Hodgkin lymphoma: Benefit of deep inspiration breath-hold. *Acta Oncol.* 2015;54:60–6.

41. Paumier A et al. Dosimetric benefits of intensity-modulated radiotherapy combined with the deep-inspiration breath-hold technique in patients with mediastinal Hodgkin's lymphoma. *Int J Radiat Oncol Biol Phys.* 2012;82:1522–7.

42. Charpentier AM et al. Active breathing control for patients receiving mediastinal radiation therapy for lymphoma: Impact on normal tissue dose. *Pract Radiat Oncol.* 2014;4:174–80.

43. Hoppe BS et al. Effective dose reduction to cardiac structures using protons compared with 3DCRT and IMRT in mediastinal Hodgkin lymphoma. *Int J Radiat Oncol Biol Phys.* 2012;84:449–55.

44. Drafts BC et al. Low to moderate dose anthracycline-based chemotherapy is associated with early noninvasive imaging evidence of subclinical cardiovascular disease. *JACC Cardiovas Imaging.* 2013;6:877–85.

45. Ky B et al. Early increases in multiple biomarkers predict subsequent cardiotoxicity in patients with breast cancer treated with doxorubicin, taxanes, and trastuzumab. *J Am Coll Cardiol.* 2014;63:809–16.

46. Thavendiranathan P, Poulin F, Lim KD, Plana JC, Woo A, Marwick TH. Use of myocardial strain

imaging by echocardiography for the early detection of cardiotoxicity in patients during and after cancer chemotherapy: A systematic review. *J Am Coll Cardiol.* 2014;63:2751–68.

47. Lancellotti P et al. Expert consensus for multimodality imaging evaluation of cardiovascular complications of radiotherapy in adults: A report from the European Association of Cardiovascular Imaging and the American Society of Echocardiography. *Eur Heart J Cardiovasc Imaging.* 2013;14(8):721–40.

48. Suter TM et al. Trastuzumab-associated cardiac adverse effects in the herceptin adjuvant trial. *J Clin Oncol.* 2007;25(25):3859–65.

49. Gianni L et al. Neoadjuvant chemotherapy with trastuzumab followed by adjuvant trastuzumab versus neoadjuvant chemotherapy alone, in patients with HER2-positive locally advanced breast cancer (the NOAH trial): A randomised controlled superiority trial with a parallel HER2-negative cohort. *Lancet.* 2010;375(9712):377–84.

50. Seidman A et al. Cardiac dysfunction in the trastuzumab clinical trials experience. *J Clin Oncol.* 2002;20(5):1215–21.

51. Romond EH et al. Seven-year follow-up assessment of cardiac function in NSABP B-31, a randomized trial comparing doxorubicin and cyclophosphamide followed by paclitaxel (ACP) with ACP plus trastuzumab as adjuvant therapy for patients with node-positive, human epidermal growth factor receptor 2-positive breast cancer. *J Clin Oncol.* 2012;30(31):3792–9.

52. Izzedine H et al. Management of hypertension in angiogenesis inhibitor-treated patients. *Ann Oncol.* 2009;20:807–15.

53. Svoboda M, Poprach A, Dobes S, Kiss I, Vyzula R. Cardiac toxicity of targeted therapies used in the treatment for solid tumors: A review. *Cardiovasc Toxicol.* 2012;12:191–207.

54. An MM et al. Incidence and risk of significantly raised blood pressure in cancer patients treated with bevacizumab: An updated meta-analysis. *Eur J Clin Pharmacol.* 2010;66:813–21.

55. Ranpura V et al. Increased risk of high-grade hypertension with bevacizumab in cancer patients: A meta-analysis. *Am J Hypertens.* 2010;23(5):460–8.

56. Daskalopoulou SS et al. The 2015 Canadian hypertension education program recommendations for blood pressure measurement, diagnosis, assessment of risk, prevention and treatment of hypertension. *Can J Cardiol.* 2015;31:549–68.

57. Polk A, Vistisen K, Vaage-Nilsen M, Nielsen DL. A systematic review of the pathophysiology of 5-fluorouracil-induced cardiotoxicity. *BMC Pharmacol Toxicol.* 2014;15:47.

58. Saif MW, Shah MM, Shah AR. Fluoropyrimidine-associated cardiotoxicity: Revisited. *Expert Opin Drug Saf.* 2009;8(2):191–202.

59. Amsterdam EA et al. 2014 AHA/American College of Cardiology/American Heart Association guideline for the management of patients with non-ST-elevation acute coronary syndromes: A report of the American College of Cardiology/American Heart Association task force on practice guidelines. *J Am Coll Cardiol.* 2014;64(24):e139–228.

60. Cianci G et al. Prophylactic options in patients with 5-fluorouracil-associated cardiotoxicity. *Br J Cancer.* 2003;88(10):1507–9.

61. Skanes AC et al. Focussed. 2012 Update of the Canadian Cardiovascular Society atrial fibrillation guidelines: Recommendations for stroke prevention and rate/rhythm control. *Can J Cardiol.* 2012;28:125–36.

62. Larsen TB, Nielsen PB, Skjoth F, Rasmussen LH, Lip GY. Non-vitamin K antagonist oral anticoagulants and the treatment of venous thromboembolism in cancer patients: A semi systematic review and meta-analysis of safety and efficacy outcomes. *PLOS ONE.* 2014;9(12):e114445.

63. Lenihan DJ, Kowey PR. Overview and management of cardiac adverse events associated with tyrosine kinase inhibitors. *Oncologist.* 2013;19:900–8.

64. Soignet SL et al. United States multicentre study of arsenic trioxide in relapsed acute promyelocytic leukemia. *J Clin Oncol.* 2001;19:3852–60.

65. Shah RR, Morganroth J, Shah DR. Cardiovascular safety of tyrosine kinase inhibitors: With a special focus on cardiac repolarisation (QT interval). *Drug Saf.* 2013;36:295–316.

7

Prevention strategies in cardio-oncology

CAROLINA MARIA PINTO DOMINGUES CARVALHO SILVA, CRISTINA
SALVADORI BITTAR, MARILIA HARUMI HIGUCHI DOS SANTOS REHDER,
AND LUDHMILA ABRAHÃO HAJJAR

INTRODUCTION

Mortality rates due to cancer have decreased over the last 30 years owing to improvements in early detection, improved surgical approaches, and advances in cancer therapeutics (1). These survival gains, however, can be offset by long-term toxicities, including cardiotoxicity. Systemic chemotherapy, targeted agents, and radiotherapy are associated with cardiac damage, including left ventricular (LV) dysfunction and heart failure, QT interval prolongation and arrhythmic disturbances, acute coronary syndromes, thromboembolism, pericardial diseases, and hypertension (1). These conditions not only have an impact on quality of life, but also increase mortality (2). Thus, measures to prevent and ameliorate cardiovascular side effects related to cancer therapy are essential.

Management of cancer patients receiving potentially cardiotoxic cancer therapy can be conceptualized into the standard framework based in general preventative medicine. Khouri et al. adapted this framework, in the setting of cancer patients receiving potential cardiotoxic cancer treatment, to include (see Figure 7.1) (3):

1. Primordial prevention: Prophylactic measures instituted before or during cancer treatment in order to prevent future cardiac damage
2. Primary prevention: Therapy given to patients with signs of subclinical damage but preserved ventricular function, in order to prevent progress of cardiac impairment
3. Secondary prevention: Therapy given after the diagnosis of cardiac damage in order to treat cardiac deterioration
4. Treatment: Therapy directed to manage symptoms related to established heart failure

While cancer patients who are exposed to a variety of cancer treatments (surgery, chemotherapy, radiation) are clearly at risk of experiencing cardiovascular toxicity, there is a paucity of high-level evidence evaluating cardioprotective strategies in this population. As a consequence, most clinical decisions at the bedside are individualized, based

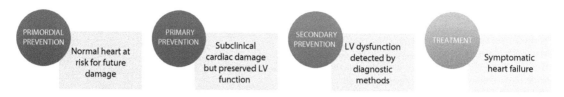

Figure 7.1 Cardiotoxicity management according to stage of cardiac damage, as proposed by Khouri et al. LV: left ventricular.

on the patients' preexisting comorbidities and planned cancer treatment. The aim of this chapter is to summarize the current available evidence on cardioprotective strategies.

INITIAL STRATEGIES

Conditions such as inappropriate diet, high alcohol intake, smoking, physical inactivity, obesity, and lack of control of blood pressure, glucose, and lipids are believed to account for 80% of the burden of cardiovascular disease (4). Risk-modifying behaviors should be encouraged prior to, during, and following cancer treatment, as per guideline-based recommendations (5,6).

For patients with previous cardiovascular disease (CVD), optimal medical treatment and clinical stabilization is mandatory before oncological treatment is started; however, ideally this should not delay the beginning of planned oncologic treatment.

According to Mitchell and Lennihan (7), patients who are exposed to cardiotoxic therapies should be considered as having Stage A heart failure (defined as being at risk for developing heart failure, but without structural heart disease or symptoms). According to the 2013 American College of Cardiology Foundation (ACCF)/American Heart Association (AHA) guidelines for the management of heart failure (8), these patients should be encouraged to adopt risk-modifying behaviors in order to control cardiovascular risk factors (class I recommendation). These recommendations have been supported by cardio-oncology statements worldwide (7).

Role of exercise in primordial and primary prevention

Physical activity plays a cardioprotective role even before cancer treatment is instituted. Cancer reduces exercise capacity even before the start of treatment, and further deterioration in functional capacity is often observed during the course of

cancer treatment (9–11). The concept of increasing cardiovascular reserve before cancer treatment is called "prehabilitation" (12), and aims to: (1) reduce the nadir drop of exercise intolerance; (2) attenuate the magnitude of reduction of cardiovascular reserve; and (3) establish an exercise routine that is likely to be continued during cancer treatment (13). For these patients, the exercise prescription follows recommendations for the general population: at least 150 minutes per week of aerobic exercise of moderate intensity associated with resistance activities (one or more sets of 8–12 repetitions for each exercise) (14,15).

Few trials have evaluated the cardioprotective effects of physical activity during chemotherapy treatment. Also, the effect of exercise on cardiac side effects of cancer treatment is unknown. Observational series and small randomized trials have demonstrated benefits of exercise on aerobic capacity, skeletal muscle strength, quality of life, and psychological outcomes (16), but there is no direct evidence regarding cancer or overall survival. However, owing to the well-established preventive role of exercise in reducing cardiovascular events and mortality (16,17), it is reasonable to recommend exercise during chemotherapy. Owing to the heterogeneity of cancer populations, oncologic treatment type, exercise routine, and outcomes assessed in exercise trials, there are no standard exercise recommendations. Thus, exercise prescription should be personalized.

Risk stratification and cardiac monitoring

Risk stratification and regular cardiac monitoring are an important part of cardiovascular surveillance, as this permits early diagnosis and prompt initiation of medications that might preserve ventricular function. Late detection of cardiotoxicity may result in irreversible cardiac damage such as end-stage heart failure. Quantifying risk of cardiotoxicity for patients starting cancer treatment is challenging, as there are few scoring systems available (18–20). Their use is limited by the lack of prospective validation in large cohorts. As a result, cardiac risk stratification in these patients is conducted on an individualized basis. In clinical practice, high-risk patients are frequently defined as those with previous cardiovascular disease or multiple cardiac risk factors (one should examine both number and severity of risk factors). Figure 7.2 outlines the main risk factors for cardiotoxicity.

It is important to emphasize that there are many different cardiac monitoring protocols available, often based on specialists' expertise; however, there is no definitive evidence that supports any timing of cardiac monitoring. Also, cost-effectiveness studies are needed to define the optimal frequency of tests. In low-risk patients (which are the majority of cases in clinical practice), frequent monitoring has limited clinical benefit, but a high cost (21). Despite some guidelines advocating specific timings of cardiac monitoring, clinical decision-making should take into account the patient's cardiovascular risk profile, risks of the planned antitumor regimen, availability of alternative regimens, and more importantly, how the results of the cardiac test proposed would affect the course of cancer treatment.

ONCOLOGIC STRATEGIES

The most effective strategy in the prevention of anthracycline-induced cardiotoxicity is to avoid this drug in cancer patients at high risk or limit the cumulative dose. The risk of heart failure is dose-dependent: at a cumulative dose of 400 mg/m², there is an approximately 5% risk of heart failure, which increases to near 26% with cumulative doses of 550 mg/m² (22). However, studies have shown cardiac damage with lower doses, leading to the concept that there is no truly safe dose of anthracyclines. Therefore, limiting the cumulative dose (whenever feasible) is an effective preventive strategy.

Administration of anthracyclines via continuous infusion, vs. intravenous bolus, is associated with lower rates of cardiotoxicity (2); nonetheless, this approach is rarely used because it requires hospitalization. Liposomal doxorubicin formulations

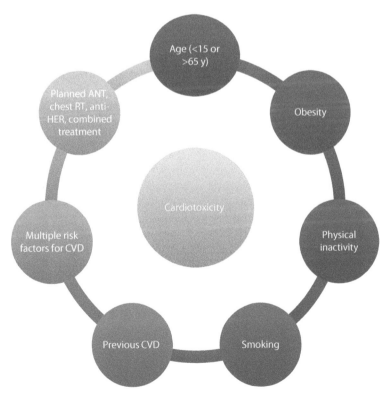

Figure 7.2 Main risk factors for cardiotoxicity. CVD: cardiovascular disease; ANT: anthracyclines; RT: radiotherapy; HER: human epidermal growth factor receptor.

Table 7.1 Summary of the initial steps for primary and primordial prevention plan

	Initial steps for primordial/primary prevention
General strategies	Healthy diet, weight management
	Low alcohol intake, smoking cessation
	Blood pressure control, glucose and lipids control
	Physical activity
	Optimal medical treatment and clinical stabilization of underlying CVD
	Risk stratification, regular monitoring
Oncologic strategies	Limit anthracycline cumulative dose
	Continuous anthracycline administration
	Use of liposomal doxorubicin formulations
	Limit thoracic radiation dose

Abbreviation: CVD: cardiovascular disease.

are manufactured by the liposomal encapsulation of doxorubicin molecules (23). These formulations have proven to reduce cardiotoxicity with similar antitumor efficacy (24). The rationale for this strategy relies on the fact that liposomes are a vehicle for delivering anticancer agents that are able to increase the concentration of the drug delivered to cancer cells while reducing its concentration on normal cells (23).

In radiation oncology, contemporary techniques have been designed to improve efficacy while reducing side effects related to the irradiation of nontumor structures. Mediastinal, thoracic, and neck radiation are associated with an increased risk of endothelial dysfunction, accelerated atherosclerosis, valvular disease, pericardial disease, and autonomic dysfunction (25). Heart-sparing techniques include 3D treatment planning, prone position radiotherapy, deep-inspiration breath holding and respiratory gating, IMRT (intensity-modulated radiation therapy), and proton therapy. The risk of radiation-related cardiotoxicity increases 7% per Gy absorbed by the heart (26). Therefore, the most effective preventive strategy is keeping radiation doses to the heart as low as possible.

Table 7.1 summarizes the initial steps (including general strategies and oncologic strategies) to conduct a primordial and primary prevention plan.

PHARMACOLOGICAL STRATEGIES IN PRIMORDIAL AND PRIMARY PREVENTION

Table 7.2 shows the cardiologic drugs evaluated for primordial and primary prevention in patients

receiving anthracycline and trastuzumab treatment, including the main characteristics of respective trials. The agents that have demonstrated cardioprotective effects in cancer patients are dexrazoxane, beta-blockers, angiotensin antagonists, statins, and aldosterone antagonists, as shown in Figure 7.3. The cardioprotective effects of pharmacologic agents administered to patients receiving chemotherapy have been studied mainly with anthracycline and trastuzumab-based regimens. Most studies evaluated surrogate endpoints (such as biomarkers, cardiac diameters, or left ventricular ejection fraction—LVEF), suggesting that modest drops in ventricular function could be attenuated with the use of beta-blockers, angiotensin-converting enzyme (ACE) inhibitors, or angiotensin-receptor blockers (ARBs) (27–30).

In primordial and primary prevention settings, the majority of trials have included low-risk patients. These studies had a lower incidence of cardiotoxicity than predicted, reducing the statistical power of analysis. In addition, there were differences in cardiac endpoints, cardiac imaging modalities (echocardiogram, cMRI), as well as frequency and timing of cardiac imaging. As a consequence, results of these studies are not robust enough to provide an evidence-based recommendation for the use of cardioprotective drugs in clinical practice.

Dexrazoxane

The cardioprotective effect of dexrazoxane (DEX) is proposed to be related to its iron chelating action. This effect results in reduction of toxic

Table 7.2 Cardiologic agents evaluated for prevention of cardiotoxicity and summary of characteristics of main trials

	Author, year	CT	Drug	Control	N	FU	Main result of experimental drug
Beta-blocker and RAAS inhibitors	Kalay et al. (2006) (27)	ANT	Carvedilol	Placebo	50	6 mo	Prevented EF drop
	Kaya et al. (2003) (28)	ANT	Nebivolol	placebo	45	6 mo	Prevented EF drop
	Bosch et al. (2013) (51) (OVERCOME trial)	Different regimens	Enalapril + carvedilol	no treatment	90	6 mo	Prevented EF drop
	Avila et al. (2018) (48) (CECCY trial)	ANT	Carvedilol	placebo	200	6 mo	No effects in EF drop
	Cardinale et al. (2018) (46) (ICOS-ONE trial)	ANT	Enalapril	enalapril only if troponin elevation	273	12 mo	No effects in troponin elevation
	Nakamae et al. (2005) (29)	ANT	Valsartan	placebo	40	7 days	Prevented LVEDD raise
	Pituskin et al. (2017) (50) (MANTICORE trial)	TZB	Perindopril or bisoprololl	placebo	94	52 weeks	No effect in LVEDi; attenuated EF decline
	Gulati et al. (2016) (49) (PRADA trial)	ANT with or without TZB	Candesartan or metoprolol	placebo	130	10–61 weeks	No change in EF
	Georgakopoulos et al. (2010) (30)	ANT	Metoprolol or enalapril	no treatment	125	variable from 12 to 36 mo	No change in EF nor clinical heart failure
	Cardinale et al. (2006) (45)	Different regimens	Enalapril	placebo	114	12 mo	Prevented EF drop
Aldosterone antagonists	Akpek et al. (2015) (47)	ANT	Spironolactone	placebo	83	24 weeks	Prevented EF drop
Statins	Acar et al. (2011) (56)	ANT	Atorvastatin	placebo	40	6 mo	Prevented EF drop

Abbreviations: ANT, anthracyclin; CT, chemotherapy; EF, ejection fraction; FU, follow-up; LVEDVi, indexed left ventricular end diastolic volume; LVEDD, left ventricular end diastolic diameter; RAAS, renin–angiotensin–aldosterone system; TZB, trastuzumab.

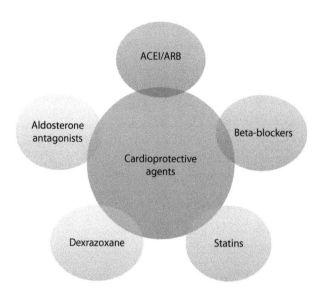

Figure 7.3 Pharmacologic agents tested against chemotherapy-related cardiotoxicity. ACEI: angiotensin-converting enzyme inhibitors; ARB: angiotensin receptor blockers.

intracellular free radicals, reducing cardiomyocyte injury (31). However, the administration of more potent iron chelating agents has not demonstrated cardioprotection, suggesting that DEX preserves myocardial cells by other pathways as well (32). Experimental study has shown that DEX can inhibit anthracycline binding by changing spatial arrangement of topoisomerase IIB. (33).

Patients receiving DEX concomitant with anthracycline regimens experience a lower incidence of heart failure (2,34,35). However, long-term follow-up in the pediatric population suggested a signal in direction of a higher incidence of secondary malignancies and higher tumor recurrence (36), leading to limitation of DEX use in adults. Recent publications, however, indicate that DEX has no effects on the antitumor activity of anthracyclines nor in progression-free or overall survival (37–40). In spite of this new data, consensus recommendations still do not advocate the routine use of DEX. Current indications for adults in the USA are restricted to metastatic breast cancer patients who achieved cumulative doxorubicin dose of 300 mg/m^2 (or equivalent) who need to continue on doxorubicin chemotherapy for tumor control (41). Although the European labeling for this drug removed its contraindication for children and adolescents, this has not been followed by other countries yet (42). As a consequence of these controversies, adult use of DEX in clinical practice is limited.

Renin-angiotensin-aldosterone blockers and beta-blockers

The observation of the effects of beta-blockers (BB) and renin-angiotensin-aldosterone system (RAAS) blockers in heart failure outcomes has raised the hypothesis that these drugs could also play a role in prevention of cardiotoxicity. These effects have been extensively demonstrated, and include neurohumoral activation control, symptoms control, and reduction of mortality (43,44). These robust data on heart failure outcomes have led researchers to start testing the role of these drugs in cardiotoxicity prevention.

RAAS BLOCKERS

Enalapril was the first cardiologic drug evaluated in a randomized trial with a cardioprotective intention (45). Cardinale et al. (45) randomized 114 patients, receiving high dose chemotherapy, who showed a troponin I increase soon after chemotherapy (with or without anthracyclines) to enalapril or placebo during treatment and continued for 1 year. This landmark trial showed a striking incidence of primary outcome (LVEF drop of 10% from baseline with a decline <50%) in the placebo group in comparison to the enalapril group (43% vs. 0%, $p < 0.001$). However, as troponin elevation does indicate subclinical cardiac damage, one can argue that this could be considered a secondary prevention trial. The same group recently published the open-label ICOS-ONE

(International Cardio-Oncology Society-One) trial (46), 12 years later. This trial randomized 273 patients scheduled to receive anthracyclines to enalapril started before chemotherapy vs. started only if there were rises in troponin. Troponin elevation was similar in both groups (23% vs. 26%, $p = 0.50$), showing that enalapril was not able to prevent cardiac injury when given prophylactically before anthracyclines. Interestingly, despite high rates of troponin elevation (near 1/4 of sample), only 1.1% of patients developed cardiotoxicity (defined as 10% point reduction of LVEF, with values lower than 50%). These findings could be attributed to lower doses of anthracyclines, enrollment of patients with a low cardiovascular risk profile, different patient populations, and insufficient power to detect differences. The role of ARBs in cardioprotection was suggested by a small randomized trial (29) of 40 patients exposed to the CHOP regimen (cyclophosphamide, doxorubicin, vincristine, and prednisolone), showing that valsartan administration prevented increase of LV end-diastolic diameter in a short 7-day follow-up period. It is important to point that none of these trials evaluated heart failure outcomes. Aldosterone antagonism was evaluated in a clinical trial with 83 breast cancer patients randomized to spironolactone or placebo during anthracycline-containing chemotherapy (47). In this study, spironolactone prevented decrease in LVEF and blunted the increase in troponin and N-terminal pro b-type natriuretic peptide (NT-proBNP), besides preserving diastolic function (47).

BETA-BLOCKERS

Carvedilol and nebivolol have been studied in small populations of anthracycline-treated patients, demonstrating a reduction in the occurrence of left ventricular dysfunction (27,28). However, no clinical outcomes (e.g., hospitalization, cardiac events, mortality) were evaluated. Recently, the CECCY (Carvedilol Effect in preventing Chemotherapy induced CardiotoxicitY) trial (48) randomized 200 breast cancer patients to receive carvedilol or placebo during chemotherapy containing doxorubicin. There were no differences between groups regarding primary outcome ($\geq$10% decline in LVEF at 6 months). LVEF remained above 60% during the follow-up period; however, the percentages of patients with positive troponin I levels were significantly different between the groups (41.6% placebo vs. 26.0% carvedilol, $p = 0.003$), suggesting a possible effect of carvedilol on reduction of

myocardial injury. The implications of these findings are unknown, as myocardial injury in this population did not correlate to any significant clinical outcome.

MULTI-DRUG TRIALS

PRADA (PRevention of cAardiac Dysfunction during Adjuvant breast cancer therapy) trial (49), in a factorial 2×2 design, evaluated the use of metoprolol succinate, candesartan, or matching placebos in 130 patients receiving chemotherapy for breast cancer containing epirubicin. No effect of metoprolol was observed in the primary end-point (decline in LVEF by cardiac MRI), but candesartan attenuated reduction of LVEF from 2.6 percentage points to 0.8 ($p = 0.026$). It's important to underline that mean EF at baseline and during the follow-up period was above 60% in all groups, indicating no functional cardiac impairment during the trial. The MANTICORE (Multidisciplinary Approach to Novel Therapies In Cardio-Oncology REsearch) 101-Breast trial (50) randomized 94 HER-2 positive breast cancer patients to receive bisoprolol, perindopril, or placebo in a 1:1:1 ratio for the duration of trastuzumab therapy. In this population, neither bisoprolol nor perindopril resulted in changes in the primary outcome, defined as changes in indexed LV end diastolic volume (LVEDVi) on cardiac MRI from baseline to completion of trastuzumab therapy. However, it was observed that mean absolute decline in LVEF was attenuated in bisoprolol-treated patients (1%) when compared to perindopril (3%) and placebo (5%) groups ($p = 0.001$). Similarly to the PRADA trial, mean LVEF values in all groups during the follow-up period did not meet cardiotoxicity criteria. Regarding combination treatment, the OVERCOME (preventiOn of left Ventricular dysfunction with Enalapril and caRvedilol in patients submitted to intensive ChemOtherapy for the treatment of Malignant hEmopathies) trial (51) randomized 90 patients with hematological malignancies to enalapril and carvedilol vs. placebo. The primary end-point for this trial was absolute change in LVEF from baseline. In the intervention group, there was no change, whereas LVEF decreased approximately 3% ($p = 0.035$) in the control group, though LVEF values were above 55% in both groups.

Notably, in the cardio-oncology setting, no trial compared different types of beta-blockers head-to-head (e.g., there is no comparison between two different beta-blockers), and similarly no comparison data exists for RAAS blockers. Hence, there is no evidence that supports the recommendation of any agent as first choice for these patients; however, it seems reasonable to extrapolate data from the heart failure literature regarding the choice of agents. Accordingly, heart failure guideline-based recommendations (52,53) should be followed.

Statins

Statins exert antioxidative, anti-inflammatory, and other pleiotropic effects in addition to reducing the low-density lipoprotein (LDL) cholesterol. The cardioprotective effects of statins were tested in animal models with positive results on reduction of cardiac inflammation (54). Retrospective data in humans showed an association between statin use and lower incidence of heart failure (55). Prospectively, a small clinical trial of 40 patients with normal LVEF before anthracycline chemotherapy showed preservation of LVEF in atorvastatin treated patients vs. 8% absolute decrease in controls (56).

SECONDARY PREVENTION

Secondary prevention in cardio-oncology setting relates to management of patients after cardiac damage is detected, in order to: (1) reduce the impact of cardiac injury; (2) avoid clinical deterioration; and (3) prevent recurrence of cardiovascular events (3). Clinical interventions in this scenario include not only treatment of detected cardiac dysfunction, but also the management of cancer survivors after treatment.

Management of cardiac damage

After the diagnosis of chemotherapy-induced cardiomyopathy, prompt initiation of heart failure (57) therapy is recommended, as decreased time to institution of heart failure treatment and New York Heart Association functional class have been identified as independent predictors of LVEF recovery (58). Cardinale et al. followed a cohort of 2625 patients receiving anthracyclines for 5 years, and was able to demonstrate that early detection and treatment with HF medications were associated with LVEF improvement (59). Importantly, it was also demonstrated that heart failure treatment started after 6 months of completion of anthracycline was associated with incomplete recovery of LVEF (58).

Similarly, treatment of trastuzumab-related cardiotoxicity with heart failure drugs is associated with recovery of LVEF (60). Maintenance of these medications during trastuzumab rechallenge resulted in stable cardiac function in asymptomatic patients (61). Therefore, heart failure drugs in maximally tolerated doses must be initiated as soon as possible after diagnosis of cardiotoxicity regardless of symptoms. In a retrospective series of ~250 patients, appropriate cardiac treatment resulted in LVEF recovery (at least partially), and continuation of planned cancer therapy in 76% of cases (54). Heart failure guideline-based recommendations such as the 2017 American College of Cardiology (ACC)/AHA/Heart Failure Society of America (HFSA) Focused Update of the 2013 ACCF/AHA Guideline for the Management of Heart Failure and the 2016 ESC Guidelines for the diagnosis and treatment of acute and chronic heart failure (52,53) should be followed.

Survivorship programs

Long-term cancer survivors are continuously increasing in number, and now they account for around 5% of the U.S. population (62). The knowledge of late cardiotoxic effects of cancer treatment gained notoriety after data from childhood cancer survivors' cohorts were published, showing striking numbers: nearly 60% of survivors have at least one chronic health condition (63); they have a 10-fold excess in overall mortality (64); and when compared to siblings, they have an incidence of cardiovascular events by 45 years of age 5-fold higher (65). The knowledge of long-term cardiovascular complication in pediatric cancer survivors has raised awareness of the risk of potential long-term cancer treatment-related cardiac dysfunction in adult cancer survivors.

Strategies to improve cardiovascular health in adult cancer survivors should include:

a. Determination of CV risk based on cancer treatment-related risk predictors (e.g., use of high-dose doxorubicin regimen, thoracic radiation >30 Gy, etc.)
b. Control of traditional CV risk factors (hypertension, diabetes, dyslipidemia, lifestyle changes, etc.)
c. Exercise promotion (discussed later in this chapter)
d. Cardiac imaging surveillance with the aim of early detection of cardiac damage.

Although several organizations have published recommendations on cardiac surveillance strategies in adult cancer survivors (see Table 7.3), it is important to note there is no robust evidence to support any specific frequency of cardiac imaging in this population. Current recommendations on cardiac surveillance strategies are based largely on groups' expertise and opinions; however, a yearly appointment for general clinical evaluation and cardiovascular assessment seems consensual.

Role of exercise in secondary prevention

Cardiorespiratory fitness declines between 5% and 26% during exposure to chemotherapy, and it may not return to initial level after completion of cancer therapy (70,71). There are multiple factors accounting for this fact, as described in Figure 7.4.

Cancer patients experience a progressive decrease in peak oxygen uptake (VO$_2$ peak), the gold standard measurement of cardiorespiratory fitness, with the deepest decline noted after chemotherapy (72). VO$_2$ peak reflects cardiovascular function and is a robust and independent predictor of cardiovascular and all-cause mortality (73).

Aerobic training is the most effective strategy to improve peak VO$_2$, and it has been demonstrated to be safe and well tolerated in cancer patients (74). Thus, exercise is thought to be an essential part of cancer patients' management. Exercise trials in this context lack data on hard endpoints such as mortality; however, they show relevant benefits in quality of life, physical functioning, mobility, cardiorespiratory fitness, fatigue, and depression (13).

The role of physical activity in secondary prevention (after diagnosis of cardiac dysfunction) is supported by the literature as part of medical treatment (75). In this setting, exercise prescription should be personalized according to each individual's functional parameters guided by cardiopulmonary test. The benefits of exercise in cancer survivors seem to be even more solid. Two large trials in breast cancer survivors (nearly 3000 patients) (76) and childhood survivors (nearly 1200 patients) (77) were able to demonstrate that physical activity reduces cardiovascular events including coronary artery disease and heart failure. Most experts support *The American College of Sports Medicine's* recommendation for cancer patients, which follow general public recommendations: at least 150 minutes per week of aerobic

Table 7.3 Summary of main recommendations of international organizations regarding long-term follow-up of cancer survivors

Organization	Population	Recommendation
ASCO (66)	Adults exposed to anthracyclines, thoracic radiation, trastuzumab	Consider echocardiogram 6–12 months after treatment completion, and after this period, according to clinical judgment
ESMO (67)	Adults exposed to anthracyclines and thoracic radiation	Echocardiogram after 6 months, then annually for 2 or 3 years; after this period, at 3–5-year intervals for life. For those exposed to thoracic radiation: screening according to clinical judgment, imaging modality based on local availability
ASE/EACI (68)	Adults exposed to thoracic radiation	Echocardiogram after 10 years (or 5 years if multiple risk factors); coronary artery disease screening after 5–10 years (reevaluations every 5 years)
COG (69)	Children exposed to anthracyclines or thoracic radiation	Consider echocardiogram 12 months after treatment completion, and after this period, each 1–5 years depending on individual risk profile

Abbreviations: ASCO: American Society of Clinical Oncology; ESMO: European Society of Medical Oncology; ASE: American Society of Echocardiography; EACI: European Association of Cardiovascular Imaging; COG: Children's Oncology Group.

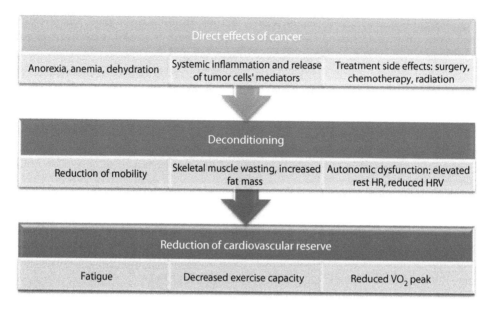

Figure 7.4 Factors related to exercise intolerance in cancer patients. HR: heart rate; HRV: heart rate variability; VO₂: oxygen uptake.

exercise of moderate intensity associated with resistance activities (one or more sets of 8–12 repetitions for each exercise) (15).

CONCLUSION

In conclusion, cardiotoxicity involves a wide range of manifestations. Cardioprotective strategies have focused mainly on prevention of LV dysfunction; however, there are a paucity of robust data in this area. Further research is needed to support evidence-based guidelines. Cardioprotective strategies should be considered on an individualized basis in order to permit the best oncological treatment. A multidisciplinary team and close collaboration between cardiologists and oncologists is essential to ameliorate the potential cardiovascular consequences of cancer treatments.

REFERENCES

1. Yeh ET et al. Cardiovascular complications of cancer therapy: Diagnosis, pathogenesis, and management. *Circulation.* 2004;109(25):3122–31.
2. Smith LA et al. Cardiotoxicity of anthracycline agents for the treatment of cancer: Systematic review and meta-analysis of randomised controlled trials. *BMC Cancer.* 2010;10:337.
3. Khouri MG et al. Cancer therapy-induced cardiac toxicity in early breast cancer: Addressing the unresolved issues. *Circulation.* 2012;126(23):2749–63.
4. Writing Group M, Mozaffarian D et al. Heart disease and stroke statistics—2016 update: A report from the American Heart Association. *Circulation.* 2016;133(4):e38–360.
5. Piepoli MF et al. 2016 European Guidelines on cardiovascular disease prevention in clinical practice: The Sixth Joint Task Force of the European Society of Cardiology and other societies on cardiovascular disease prevention in clinical practice (constituted by representatives of 10 societies and by invited experts) developed with the special contribution of the European Association for Cardiovascular Prevention & Rehabilitation (EACPR). *Eur Heart J.* 2016;37(29):2315–81.
6. Lloyd-Jones DM et al. Estimating longitudinal risks and benefits from cardiovascular preventive therapies among Medicare patients: The million hearts longitudinal ASCVD risk assessment tool: A special report from the American Heart Association and American College of Cardiology. *J Am Coll Cardiol.* 2017;69(12):1617–36.
7. Mitchell J, Lenihan DJ. *Management of Cancer-Therapy-Induced LV Dysfunction:*

Can the Guidelines Help? American College of Cardiology; 2018. Available from: https://www.acc.org/latest-in-cardiology/articles/2018/10/30/09/08/management-of-cancer-therapy-induced-lv-dysfunction

8. Writing Committee M, Yancy CW et al. 2013 ACCF/AHA guideline for the management of heart failure: A report of the American College of Cardiology Foundation/American Heart Association Task Force on practice guidelines. *Circulation.* 2013;128(16): e240–327.

9. Cramer L et al. Cardiovascular function and predictors of exercise capacity in patients with colorectal cancer. *J Am Coll Cardiol.* 2014;64(13):1310–9.

10. Scott JM, Nilsen TS, Gupta D, Jones LW. Exercise therapy and cardiovascular toxicity in cancer. *Circulation.* 2018;137(11):1176–91.

11. Lakoski SG, Eves ND, Douglas PS, Jones LW. Exercise rehabilitation in patients with cancer. *Nat Rev Clin Oncol.* 2012;9(5):288–96.

12. Silver JK, Baima J. Cancer prehabilitation: An opportunity to decrease treatment-related morbidity, increase cancer treatment options, and improve physical and psychological health outcomes. *Am J Phys Med Rehabil.* 2013;92(8):715–27.

13. Squires RW, Shultz AM, Herrmann J. Exercise training and cardiovascular health in cancer patients. *Curr Oncol Rep.* 2018;20(3):27.

14. Lobelo F et al. Routine assessment and promotion of physical activity in healthcare settings: A scientific statement from the American Heart Association. *Circulation.* 2018;137(18):e495–522.

15. Schmitz KH et al. American College of Sports Medicine roundtable on exercise guidelines for cancer survivors. *Med Sci Sports Exerc.* 2010;42(7):1409–26.

16. Jones LW, Alfano CM. Exercise-oncology research: Past, present, and future. *Acta Oncol.* 2013;52(2):195–215.

17. Kwan G, Balady GJ. Cardiac rehabilitation 2012: Advancing the field through emerging science. *Circulation.* 2012;125(7):e369–73.

18. Ezaz G, Long JB, Gross CP, Chen J. Risk prediction model for heart failure and cardiomyopathy after adjuvant trastuzumab therapy for breast cancer. *J Am Heart Assoc.* 2014;3(1):e000472.

19. Chow EJ et al. Individual prediction of heart failure among childhood cancer survivors. *J Clin Oncol.* 2015;33(5):394–402.

20. Herrmann J, Lerman A, Sandhu NP, Villarraga HR, Mulvagh SL, Kohli M. Evaluation and management of patients with heart disease and cancer: Cardio-oncology. *Mayo Clin Proc.* 2014;89(9):1287–306.

21. Nolan MT, Plana JC, Thavendiranathan P, Shaw L, Si L, Marwick TH. Cost-effectiveness of strain-targeted cardioprotection for prevention of chemotherapy-induced cardiotoxicity. *Int J Cardiol.* 2016;212:336–45.

22. Shan K, Lincoff AM, Young JB. Anthracycline-induced cardiotoxicity. *Ann Intern Med.* 1996;125(1):47–58.

23. Lao J et al. Liposomal doxorubicin in the treatment of breast cancer patients: A review. *J Drug Deliv.* 2013;2013:456409.

24. Xing M, Yan F, Yu S, Shen P. Efficacy and Cardiotoxicity of liposomal doxorubicin-based chemotherapy in advanced breast cancer: A meta-analysis of ten randomized controlled trials. *PLOS ONE.* 2015;10(7): e0133569.

25. Raghunathan D, Khilji MI, Hassan SA, Yusuf SW. Radiation-induced cardiovascular disease. *Curr Atheroscler Rep.* 2017;19(5):22.

26. Darby SC et al. Risk of ischemic heart disease in women after radiotherapy for breast cancer. *N Engl J Med.* 2013;368(11):987–98.

27. Kalay N et al. Protective effects of carvedilol against anthracycline-induced cardiomyopathy. *J Am Coll Cardiol.* 2006;48(11): 2258–62.

28. Kaya MG et al. Protective effects of nebivolol against anthracycline-induced cardiomyopathy: A randomized control study. *Int J Cardiol.* 2013;167(5):2306–10.

29. Nakamae H et al. Notable effects of angiotensin II receptor blocker, valsartan, on acute cardiotoxic changes after standard chemotherapy with cyclophosphamide, doxorubicin, vincristine, and prednisolone. *Cancer.* 2005;104(11):2492–8.

30. Georgakopoulos P et al. Cardioprotective effect of metoprolol and enalapril in doxorubicin-treated lymphoma patients: A prospective, parallel-group, randomized, controlled study with 36-month follow-up. *Am J Hematol.* 2010;85(11):894–6.

31. Hershko C, Link G, Tzahor M, Pinson A. The role of iron and iron chelators in anthracycline cardiotoxicity. *Leuk Lymphoma*. 1993;11(3–4):207–14.

32. Sterba M et al. Oxidative stress, redox signaling, and metal chelation in anthracycline cardiotoxicity and pharmacological cardioprotection. *Antioxid Redox Signal*. 2013;18(8):899–929.

33. Lyu YL et al. Topoisomerase IIbeta mediated DNA double-strand breaks: Implications in doxorubicin cardiotoxicity and prevention by dexrazoxane. *Cancer Res*. 2007;67(18):8839–46.

34. Kalam K, Marwick TH. Role of cardioprotective therapy for prevention of cardiotoxicity with chemotherapy: A systematic review and meta-analysis. *Eur J Cancer*. 2013;49(13):2900–9.

35. van Dalen EC, Caron HN, Dickinson HO, Kremer LC. Cardioprotective interventions for cancer patients receiving anthracyclines. *Cochrane Database Syst Rev*. 2011;15(6):CD003917.

36. Tebbi CK et al. Dexrazoxane-associated risk for acute myeloid leukemia/myelodysplastic syndrome and other secondary malignancies in pediatric Hodgkin's disease. *J Clin Oncol*. 2007;25(5):493–500.

37. Chow EJ et al. Late mortality after dexrazoxane treatment: A report from the Children's Oncology Group. *J Clin Oncol*. 2015;33(24):2639–45.

38. Seif AE et al. Dexrazoxane exposure and risk of secondary acute myeloid leukemia in pediatric oncology patients. *Pediatr Blood Cancer*. 2015;62(4):704–9.

39. Shaikh F, Dupuis LL, Alexander S, Gupta A, Mertens L, Nathan PC. Cardioprotection and second malignant neoplasms associated with dexrazoxane in children receiving anthracycline chemotherapy: A systematic review and meta-analysis. *J Natl Cancer Inst*. 2016;108(4).

40. Kim H, Kang HJ, Park KD, Koh KN, Im HJ, Seo JJ et al. Risk factor analysis for secondary malignancy in dexrazoxane-treated pediatric cancer patients. *Cancer Res Treat*. 2019;51(1):357–67.

41. Hensley ML et al. American Society of Clinical Oncology 2008 clinical practice guideline update: Use of chemotherapy and radiation therapy protectants. *J Clin Oncol*. 2009;27(1):127–45.

42. Reichardt P, Tabone MD, Mora J, Morland B, Jones RL. Risk-benefit of dexrazoxane for preventing anthracycline-related cardiotoxicity: Re-evaluating the European labeling. *Future Oncol*. 2018;14(25):2663–76.

43. Xie W, Zheng F, Song X, Zhong B, Yan L. Renin-angiotensin-aldosterone system blockers for heart failure with reduced ejection fraction or left ventricular dysfunction: Network meta-analysis. *Int J Cardiol*. 2016;205:65–71.

44. Cleland JGF et al. Beta-blockers for heart failure with reduced, mid-range, and preserved ejection fraction: An individual patient-level analysis of double-blind randomized trials. *Eur Heart J*. 2018;39(1):26–35.

45. Cardinale D et al. Prevention of high-dose chemotherapy-induced cardiotoxicity in high-risk patients by angiotensin-converting enzyme inhibition. *Circulation*. 2006;114(23):2474–81.

46. Cardinale D et al. Anthracycline-induced cardiotoxicity: A multicenter randomised trial comparing two strategies for guiding prevention with enalapril: The International Cardio-Oncology Society-One trial. *Eur J Cancer*. 2018;94:126–37.

47. Akpek M et al. Protective effects of spironolactone against anthracycline-induced cardiomyopathy. *Eur J Heart Fail*. 2015;17(1):81–9.

48. Avila MS et al. Carvedilol for prevention of chemotherapy related cardiotoxicity. *J Am Coll Cardiol*. 2018;71(20):2281–90.

49. Gulati G et al. Prevention of cardiac dysfunction during adjuvant breast cancer therapy (PRADA): A 2 × 2 factorial, randomized, placebo-controlled, double-blind clinical trial of candesartan and metoprolol. *Eur Heart J*. 2016;37(21):1671–80.

50. Pituskin E et al. Multidisciplinary approach to novel therapies in cardio-oncology research (MANTICORE 101-Breast): A randomized trial or the prevention of trastuzumab-associated cardiotoxicity. *J Clin Oncol*. 2017;35(8):870–7.

51. Bosch X et al. Enalapril and carvedilol for preventing chemotherapy-induced left ventricular systolic dysfunction in patients with malignant hemopathies: The OVERCOME trial (preventiOn of left Ventricular dysfunction with Enalapril and caRvedilol in patients submitted to intensive ChemOtherapy for

the treatment of Malignant hEmopathies). *J Am Coll Cardiol.* 2013;61(23):2355–62.

52. Yancy CW et al. 2017 ACC/AHA/HFSA Focused Update of the 2013 ACCF/AHA Guideline for the management of heart failure: A report of the American College of Cardiology/American Heart Association task force on clinical practice guidelines and the Heart Failure Society of America. *Circulation.* 2017;136(6):e137–e61.

53. Ponikowski P et al. 2016 ESC Guidelines for the diagnosis and treatment of acute and chronic heart failure: The task force for the diagnosis and treatment of acute and chronic heart failure of the European Society of Cardiology (ESC) developed with the special contribution of the Heart Failure Association (HFA) of the ESC. *Eur Heart J.* 2016;37(27):2129–200.

54. Riad A et al. Pretreatment with statin attenuates the cardiotoxicity of doxorubicin in mice. *Cancer Res.* 2009;69(2):695–9.

55. Seicean S, Seicean A, Plana JC, Budd GT, Marwick TH. Effect of statin therapy on the risk for incident heart failure in patients with breast cancer receiving anthracycline chemotherapy: An observational clinical cohort study. *J Am Coll Cardiol.* 2012;60(23): 2384–90.

56. Acar Z et al. Efficiency of atorvastatin in the protection of anthracycline-induced cardiomyopathy. *J Am Coll Cardiol.* 2011;58(9): 988–9.

57. Parker BL et al. Multiplexed temporal quantification of the exercise-regulated plasma peptidome. *Mol Cell Proteomics.* 2017;16(12):2055–68.

58. Cardinale D et al. Anthracycline-induced cardiomyopathy: Clinical relevance and response to pharmacologic therapy. *J Am Coll Cardiol.* 2010;55(3):213–20.

59. Cardinale D et al. Early detection of anthracycline cardiotoxicity and improvement with heart failure therapy. *Circulation.* 2015;131(22):1981–8.

60. Oliva S et al. Administration of angiotensin-converting enzyme inhibitors and beta-blockers during adjuvant trastuzumab chemotherapy for nonmetastatic breast cancer: Marker of risk or cardioprotection in the real world? *Oncologist.* 2012;17(7):917–24.

61. Ewer MS et al. Reversibility of trastuzumab-related cardiotoxicity: New insights based on clinical course and response to medical treatment. *J Clin Oncol.* 2005;23(31):7820–6.

62. Mayer DK, Nasso SF, Earp JA. Defining cancer survivors, their needs, and perspectives on survivorship health care in the USA. *Lancet Oncol.* 2017;18(1):e11–e8.

63. Oeffinger KC et al. Chronic health conditions in adult survivors of childhood cancer. *N Engl J Med.* 2006;355(15):1572–82.

64. Mertens AC et al. Late mortality experience in five-year survivors of childhood and adolescent cancer: The childhood cancer survivor study. *J Clin Oncol.* 2001;19(13):3163–72.

65. Armstrong GT et al. Modifiable risk factors and major cardiac events among adult survivors of childhood cancer. *J Clin Oncol.* 2013;31(29):3673–80.

66. Armenian SH et al. Prevention and monitoring of cardiac dysfunction in survivors of adult cancers: American Society of Clinical Oncology Clinical Practice Guideline. *J Clin Oncol.* 2017;35(8):893–911.

67. Curigliano G et al. Cardiovascular toxicity induced by chemotherapy, targeted agents and radiotherapy: ESMO clinical practice guidelines. *Ann Oncol.* 2012;23(Suppl 7): vii155–66.

68. Kwa MC, Silverberg JI. association between inflammatory skin disease and cardiovascular and cerebrovascular co-morbidities in US Adults: Analysis of nationwide inpatient sample data. *Am J Clin Dermatol.* 2017;18(6):813–23.

69. Landier W et al. Development of risk-based guidelines for pediatric cancer survivors: The Children's Oncology Group long-term follow-up guidelines from The Children's Oncology Group Late Effects Committee and Nursing Discipline. *J Clin Oncol.* 2004;22(24):4979–90.

70. Hurria A, Jones L, Muss HB. Cancer treatment as an accelerated aging process: Assessment, biomarkers, and interventions. *Am Soc Clin Oncol Educ Book.* 2016;35:e516–22.

71. Jarden M, Hovgaard D, Boesen E, Quist M, Adamsen L. Pilot study of a multimodal intervention: Mixed-type exercise and psychoeducation in patients undergoing allogeneic stem cell transplantation. *Bone Marrow Transplant.* 2007;40(8):793–800.

72. Klassen O et al. Cardiorespiratory fitness in breast cancer patients undergoing adjuvant therapy. *Acta Oncol.* 2014;53(10):1356–65.

73. Kavanagh T et al. Prediction of long-term prognosis in 12169 men referred for cardiac rehabilitation. *Circulation.* 2002;106(6):666–71.

74. Jones LW et al. Effect of exercise training on peak oxygen consumption in patients with cancer: A meta-analysis. *Oncologist.* 2011;16(1):112–20.

75. Cattadori G. Exercise and heart failure: An update. *ESC Heart Fail.* 2018;5(2):222–32.

76. Jones LW et al. Exercise and risk of cardiovascular events in women with non-metastatic breast cancer. *J Clin Oncol.* 2016;34(23):2743–9.

77. Jones LW et al. Exercise and risk of major cardiovascular events in adult survivors of childhood Hodgkin lymphoma: A report from the childhood cancer survivor study. *J Clin Oncol.* 2014;32(32):3643–50.

8

Cancer survivorship and cardiovascular disease

MICHAEL CHETRIT, SABIN FILIMON, NINA GHOSH, AND NEGAR MOUSAVI

NATURAL CARDIOVASCULAR HISTORY OF CANCER SURVIVORS

Introduction

Five-year survival rates for common cancers such as breast cancer have improved significantly over the past three decades; the number of cancer survivors in the USA is estimated to reach 20.3 million by 2026 (1,2). Commensurate with this improved survival, however, is the long-term cardiovascular morbidity and mortality risk associated with anticancer therapies, as well as baseline cardiovascular risk factors including increasing age. There is also interaction between anticancer treatments and traditional risk factors. Indeed, cardiovascular disease exceeded cancer related deaths in one cohort of survivors of breast cancer patients over the age of 65 (3).

Much of the focus in the field of cardio-oncology has been geared toward the care of patients experiencing cardiovascular problems *during* cancer treatment, when tertiary-quaternary-based oncologists/cardio-oncologists are actively engaged in the patient's care. Cardiovascular morbidity and mortality related to cancer treatment may not develop for months to years after the cancer patient has been discharged into community-based practice settings. This chapter focuses on cancer survivorship care and the specific challenges related to the management of patients who have completed cancer treatment and been discharged from specialized care. In order to develop strategies to mitigate long-term cancer treatment–related cardiovascular toxicity, a thorough understanding of the natural history of cardiovascular disease (CVD) in cancer survivors is important.

Long-term cardiovascular side effects

CARDIOMYOPATHY

Cardiomyopathy and heart failure are potential devastating consequences of cancer treatment with evidence suggesting that early detection and treatment can improve outcomes (4). In oncology, a number of treatments are associated with cardiomyopathy including anthracyclines, anti-HER2 agents, anti-angiogenesis agents, and radiation.

The mechanism of anthracycline-induced cardiac injury includes structural cardiomyocyte alterations and cell death induced by reactive oxygen species (ROS) and disturbances in DNA topoisomerase 2-β (Top2β) metabolism (5). Although symptomatic heart failure is thought to develop in only 5% of patients exposed to anthracycline-based chemotherapy, this additional risk factor for heart failure is significant when superimposed on a high baseline risk of developing heart failure, particularly in the elderly population. In a surveillance, epidemiology, and end results (SEER) database review of elderly breast cancer patients, the cumulative incidence of heart failure at 10 years was 38% after anthracyclines, 32.5% with nonanthracycline chemotherapy regimens, and 29% with no chemotherapy (6). Other predictors of heart failure in this cohort included peripheral and coronary atherosclerotic disease, diabetes, hypertension, and emphysema.

Targeted agents have variable effects on the myocardium, with the best studied agents being trastuzumab. Although trastuzumab exposure can result in left ventricular (LV) dysfunction and heart failure, the effect is generally reversible and studies have shown no substantial increase in cardiovascular (CV) events over 8 to 10 years (7). There is a paucity of data on the long-term trajectory of patients who develop cardiomyopathy during treatment with antiangiogenic-based cancer treatment such as sunitinib. Data to date suggest that LV dysfunction seems to occur early in treatment and improve with adequate treatment (8).

Generally, mediastinal radiation–related myocardial toxicity results in the restrictive phenotype of cardiomyopathy (e.g., heart failure with preserved ejection fraction), although radiation may sensitize the myocardium to the toxic effects of anthracyclines (9).

ATHEROSCLEROSIS

Several factors may contribute to an increased risk of atherosclerotic heart disease in cancer survivors. Survivors tend to be older than the general population and may be more likely to develop atherosclerotic disease due to modifiable risk factors common to both cancer and atherosclerotic heart disease such as smoking and physical inactivity (10,11). These factors interact with the effects of certain cancer therapies including radiation treatment, and possibly androgen deprivation therapy, to increase risk of atherosclerotic events such as myocardial infarction and stroke (12).

A history of mediastinal radiation exposure is associated with an increased risk for the development of both coronary and carotid artery disease. The pathophysiology includes oxidative stress and endothelial dysfunction at both the macro- and microvascular level, leading to accelerated atherosclerosis. Although there have been increasing efforts to minimize the involvement of coronary arteries from the radiation field over time, data suggest that patients treated with mediastinal radiation in more contemporary cohorts are still at risk. In a cohort of breast cancer patients treated from 2005 to 2008, there was a 3.3% incidence of an acute coronary event over a median of 7.6 years (13).

Androgen deprivation therapy (ADT), widely used for the treatment of prostate cancer, has been shown to be associated with several adverse metabolic effects including dyslipidemia, increased visceral adiposity, and increased insulin resistance (14). Studies examining the link between ADT and cardiovascular death have conflicting outcomes. A joint statement by the American Heart Association, the American Cancer Society, the American Urological Association, and the American Society for Radiation Oncology suggests a possible relationship between ADT and cardiovascular events and death (15). The mode of ADT may also play a role. In an analysis of men from the SEER-Medicare database, ADT exposure but not orchiectomy was associated with an increased 10-year risk of coronary artery disease, acute myocardial infarction, and sudden cardiac death (16). Similarly, in an analysis of men comparing gonadotropin releasing hormone (GnRH) antagonists versus GnRH agonists, men with pre-existing CVD experienced fewer cardiac events with GnRH antagonists than with GnRH agonist (17).

VALVULAR DISEASE

Valvular stenosis and/or regurgitation are established long-term consequences of mediastinal radiation (18). The most common valvular abnormality has been shown to be aortic stenosis, followed by mitral valve disease, including mitral regurgitation and stenosis (18). As expected, higher doses of mediastinal radiation are associated with increased risk of valvular heart disease (19). Clinically significant valvular disease generally occurs years to decades following exposure to mediastinal radiation. Large observational studies of Hodgkin's lymphoma survivors suggest that clinically significant radiation-induced valvular disease develops a median of 15 years following radiation therapy (19).

Future directions

Although patients may experience cardiovascular toxicity during cancer treatment, many of the cardiovascular manifestations of cancer therapy occur months to years following treatment. Furthermore, traditional cardiovascular risk factors may interact with the cancer treatment to modify risk for cardiovascular events. Therefore, for cancer survivors, addressing traditional risk factors and monitoring for and identifying cardiovascular toxicity related to cancer treatment may fall primarily into the hands of community-based providers. The following sections will review preventative measures, modes of surveillance, and care models for the cardiovascular care of cancer survivors.

PREVENTATIVE CARDIOVASCULAR CARE OF CANCER SURVIVORS

Introduction

In the last decades, cancer mortality has decreased considerably and it will continue to decrease in the face of novel therapies; however, this improved survival may be tempered by the adverse effects of cancer treatment modalities on cardiovascular health. Cardiovascular disease (CVD) is the second most common cause of death in cancer survivors (20,21) and, according to some studies, exceeds that of tumor recurrence (3,21,23). The field of cardio-oncology is growing at a fast pace, with the emergence of guidelines for prevention, diagnosis, and treatment of cardiovascular toxicity (24–32). Despite this, many aspects of cancer therapy–related cardiac dysfunction still need to be elucidated—especially prevention. In this section, we will summarize the existing expert consensus on preventative cardiovascular care in cancer survivors.

The high-risk patient

Development of cancer therapy related cardiac dysfunction (CTRCD) can be insidious and often asymptomatic. Screening and preventative measures are of utmost importance since cardiac dysfunction if detected early, can be treated effectively, resulting in good functional recovery, without having to stop cancer therapy (25). However, not all cancer patients develop CTRCD. Preventative measures with careful monitoring could be applied to all, though the incurred costs would be unsustainable. Furthermore, access to cardio-oncology services is limited at this point. Identifying patients at risk of cardiotoxicity based on patient-related and therapy-related risk factors might be a better strategy (See Chapter 3).

Cardio-preventative measures in cancer survivors

With new achievements in cancer therapy, an increasing number of survivors live longer after diagnosis (33). Cardiac complications posttreatment represent major contributors to morbidity and mortality in these patients (34). Because these complications may occur years later, clinical suspicion should remain high (31). In patients on long-term trastuzumab and high-dose (cumulative dose of 500 mg/m^2 doxorubicin) anthracyclines, heart failure can appear even 10+ years post-treatment (35). Valvular heart disease and coronary artery disease (CAD) usually start after 5 years post-radiotherapy (RT); however, the risk continues until the third decade (28).

At each follow-up visit, the oncologist and primary care providers should continue to take a thorough history and perform a physical examination. Counseling patients to maintain a healthy lifestyle based on appropriate diet, minimal alcohol intake, no smoking, and regular exercise remains one of the best preventative methods against CVD (25). Conventional therapies against existing CVD should be continued with good compliance.

For symptomatic patients new tests should be ordered and the results should be compared to the baseline pretreatment. Echocardiography (cardiac magnetic resonance imaging [CMR]) or multigated acquisition scan (MUGA) according to the test initially used) and cardiac enzymes are strongly indicated before referral to a cardiologist (31). For patients that demonstrated LV dysfunction during treatment with recovery, discontinuation of cardioprotective heart failure therapy is contraindicated (25). As per European Society of Cardiology (ESC) 2016 guidelines (24), this therapy should be indefinitely used even if LV function remains stable; however, clinical data on this subject are still lacking.

The recommendations for asymptomatic patients are still based on administrative databases since there are no studies that have compared the efficacy of different cardiac surveillance strategies. The true incidence and natural history of cardiac dysfunction after completion of cancer treatment remains a subject for future studies. To date, the American Society of Clinical Oncology (ASCO) and ESC guidelines recommend an echocardiogram (or the initial imaging modality used) to be performed between 6 and 12 months after completion of treatment. Patients identified as having asymptomatic cardiac dysfunction are to be referred to cardio-oncology for further management (24,31). No recommendation can be made for further surveillance past the 1-year mark owing to lack of data. Nonetheless, the European Association of Cardiovascular Imaging and American Society of Echocardiography (ASE) recommend screening for valvular disease in patients treated with chest RT 10 years postradiation and every 5 years thereafter (31).

Finally, the reality of a cancer survivor includes the risk of relapse and secondary cancers. The doses of anthracyclines that increase the risk of cardiac dysfunction are calculated as a cumulative lifetime dose. The effects of these drugs occur either early, within the first year of treatment, or late with a median presentation of 7 years posttreatment (36). When possible, selecting a nonanthracycline regimen, or treating with cumulative doses below the high-risk threshold, with avoidance of chest RT, will lower the risk of cardiotoxicity.

Future directions

Various recommendations for cardiopreventative strategies during cancer treatment have been established and should be followed as per current guidelines (24–26,31). Cardioprotective strategies postcancer treatment (Table 8.1) in cancer survivors are based on principles of primary prevention in the general population and theoretical risk of long-term cardiotoxicity. More data are needed to support screening strategies for CVD following specific cancer treatment with potential long-term cardiotoxicity such as anthracycline chemotherapy and thoracic radiation. Therefore, clinicians should endeavour to adopt novel cardioprotective strategies as clinical data emerges.

CARDIAC SURVEILLANCE IN SURVIVORS OF CANCER

Introduction

Current therapies in oncology have resulted in marked improvement in childhood cancer survival with an estimated 5-year survival upwards of 80% (36). As a result, the number of patients surviving for long periods of time after having received cancer treatment has increased significantly (37,38). With a 15-fold increased risk of developing congestive heart failure and 7-fold risk

Table 8.1 Summary of preventative strategies to reduce cardiotoxicity after cancer treatment

Prevention posttreatment	• Order echocardiography ± serum biomarkers guided by symptoms and duration posttreatment
	• Screening for valvular disease in patients with chest RT by echocardiography 10 years posttreatment and 5 years thereafter
	• Avoid use of high cumulative doses of anthracyclines for future cancer treatments
	• Continuous management of CV risk factors and screening for cardiotoxicity
	• Balanced diet, regular physical exercise, quit smoking, and minimal alcohol intake

of sudden death, cardiovascular complications have emerged as a leading cause of morbidity and mortality in this demographic (36). This is the result of cardiotoxic effects of some chemotherapeutic agents, as well as chest radiotherapy, both of which can have long latency periods (>10 years) (39). Although the magnitude of the risk of chemotherapy-related cardiac dysfunction (CRCD) and radiation-induced heart failure (RIHD) with modern radiotherapy techniques are not yet well defined, screening and follow-up examinations are clearly warranted (40).

Echocardiography remains the mainstay in initiation and follow-up for monitoring survivors of cancer. The American Society of Clinical Oncology (ASCO), the American College of Cardiology (ACC), and the Canadian Cardiovascular Society, among other societies, have all offered general guidance; however, owing to lack of data, recommendations regarding initiation and frequency of surveillance are largely based on consensus. This chapter will outline the various available imaging modalities and the parameters that are recommended for surveillance, and summarize the current recommendations from the various societies.

Initial imaging modality for patient surveillance

Echocardiography (2D) with Doppler is a radiation-free, reproducible, readily available, and noninvasive modality that has become the cornerstone of cardiac imaging in preparation for, and follow-up after chemotherapy, and is recommended by all societies (41–44). Echocardiography is recommended to detect and/or follow radiation-induced valvulopathy, evaluate and follow LV systolic function, and assess for structural heart disease (40). The American Society of Echocardiography (ASE) recommends a 3D echocardiogram as the primary imaging modality if available, owing to its superiority in test-retest variability (45). It is important to remain consistent with imaging techniques for comparability of serial studies (46). Radionuclide angiography or CMR are suggested in individuals for whom echocardiography is not technically feasible or image quality is suboptimal. Preference is given to CMR due to its lack of ionizing radiation and potential for additional information regarding cardiac structure, function, and myocardial characterization.

Recommended parameters

The European Society of Cardiology (ESC) consensus for the multimodality imaging evaluation of cardiovascular complications after cancer therapy currently recommends a detailed evaluation of the LV systolic function and right ventricle, assessment of diastolic function, and assessment of the valves and pericardium (24).

LEFT VENTRICULAR EJECTION FRACTION

Left ventricular ejection fraction (LVEF) is currently the most widely studied measure of cardiac function in cancer patients and is recommended prior to cancer treatment and continuing throughout survivorship. The American and European Societies/Association of Echocardiography and the European Association of Cardiovascular Imaging currently endorse a 2D echocardiographic measurement using Simpson's biplane method of discs for the assessment of ejection fraction (44). Moreover, the wall motion index score based on the 16−segment model has been demonstrated to be a sensitive marker for anthracycline-induced cardiomyopathy when coupled with LVEF and is also recommended when assessing the LV function (44,47). Other adjunctive measurements such as the mitral annular plane systolic excursion (MAPSE) by M-mode echocardiography and peak systolic velocity (s') of the mitral annulus by pulsed-wave doppler tissue imaging (DTI) could help in the assessment of LV function, however the data is less robust (48).

LVEF should be assessed using the best available and least variable technique. Follow-up echocardiograms should be compared directly to minimize inter-observer variability. LVEF measurements have been criticized due to the lack of sensitivity when detecting small changes in LV function namely because of the use of geometric assumptions, inadequate visualization of all the segments of the left ventricle, and the inability to detect subtle wall motion abnormalities (49). Otterstad et al. demonstrated that sequential measurements of the LVEF by 2D echocardiography were only able to detect a change of 10%, causing many to question its ability to detect subclinical LV dysfunction given that the definition of cardiotoxicity is currently a 10% decrease in LVEF or a 5% decrease in the presence of heart failure symptoms (50). Detecting a decrease in LVEF after anthracyclines may in fact be too late, suggesting that there is a need for more sensitive markers in the detection of subclinical cardiotoxicity, during and after cancer therapy (51). More recent studies have compared the various echocardiographic techniques to assess LV function serially by 2D Simpson's biplane, 2D tri-plane, 3D echocardiography and contrast ultrasonography, and have determined that 3D echo has the lowest test-retest variability over 1 year of follow up. 3D echocardiography is also devoid of geometric assumptions and foreshortening and more importantly is able to detect changes in LV function in the 1%–10% range (45). 3D echocardiography, when available, can alleviate some of the limitations of 2D echocardiography, but societies have looked elsewhere to find markers of increased sensitivity.

MYOCARDIAL DEFORMATION INDICES, STRAIN, AND STRAIN RATE

Myocardial deformation may be a more sensitive tool to identify subclinical left ventricular systolic dysfunction. Many studies have demonstrated the predictive value of myocardial strain imaging. Studies also demonstrated that chemotherapy does not appear to preferentially impair one particular layer of the muscle (either the subendocardium, midmyocardium or subepicardial layers), rendering the measure of global longitudinal strain (GLS) to be the most predictive (44). More specifically, a 10%–15% reduction in GLS predicted subsequent LV systolic dysfunction in a systematic review, supporting the ASE's recommendations to include GLS in patients' protocols before and during treatment with anthracyclines and/or trastuzumab (44). Interestingly, decreases in global longitudinal strain appeared to persist at least partially throughout the treatment, but its persistence and predictive value throughout the years of survivorship is not well defined.

Two studies have evaluated deformation parameters in long-term cancer survivors ranging from 2 to 30 years after treatment. Tsai et al. and Cheung et al. were able to show that those having received higher doses of anthracyclines were at higher risk for CRCD and had both an abnormal LVEF and strain. In addition, both studies detected a decrease in strain parameters when compared to age-matched control patients, reinforcing this technique as a sensitive tool to detect subclinical LV dysfunction (52,53). The value of myocardial strain imaging in follow-up of patients outside of detecting subclinical LV dysfunction remains to be elucidated as there are no studies that have evaluated this. What is suggested is that if a baseline GLS has been measured, serial imaging should be compared to the baseline to detect changes over 15%, which has been deemed to be abnormal (54). It is important to note that GLS, while an automated technique, is dependent on many factors such as the vendor and the version of the analysis software, as well as the preload status. Serial evaluations of GLS should be performed using the same vendor's machine and software given variability in normal GLS ranges between vendors (44).

DIASTOLIC FUNCTION

The European Society of Cardiology consensus for multimodality imaging evaluation of cardiovascular complications after cancer therapy currently endorses a comprehensive assessment of LV diastolic function including mitral valve inflow early diastolic filling velocity (E) to lated diastolic filling velocity (A) ratio (E/A ratio) and isovolumic relaxation time (IVRT), grading the diastolic function and estimating the LV filling pressures in accordance with ASE and European Association of Echocardiography (EAE) recommendations. While Stoddard et al. were able to demonstrate an association between prolongation of IVRT and a 10% decrease in LVEF, this was not reproduced by larger studies. Currently, the diagnostic and therapeutic utility of diastolic function is not established in the serial assessment of survivors of cancer therapy (55).

RIGHT VENTRICULAR FUNCTION

The European Society of Cardiology consensus for multimodality imaging evaluation of cardiovascular complications after cancer therapy currently recommends a complete quantitative and qualitative assessment of the right ventricle (RV) and right atrium as well as assessment of RV systolic function using M-mode derived tricuspid annular plane systolic excursion (TAPSE), pulsed DTI systolic peak annular velocity (s'), and RV fractional area shortening. When feasible, it is also recommended to sample the tricuspid regurgitation jet and get an estimate of RV systolic pressure. The latter is particularly important with chemotherapeutic agents that induce pulmonary hypertension such as tyrosine kinase inhibitors (e.g., dasatinib) (56). That being said, the prognostic value of RV function as well as its value in longitudinal follow-up in patients having survived cancer has not been established (44).

VALVULAR HEART DISEASE

Chemotherapeutic agents do not appear to directly induce clinically relevant valvulopathy; however, progressive annular dilatation or leaflet tethering secondary to LV dysfunction and remodeling may occur as a result of these agents. There is a higher incidence of left- and right-sided valvular regurgitation in the years following mediastinal radiation therapy (more than 10 years) with a slow progression to severe valvulopathy (18). Transthoracic echocardiography is the recommended modality to assess for valvulopathy. It is currently recommended that a full assessment for valvular heart disease be included in studies in accordance with the current ASE and EAE guidelines.

PERICARDIAL DISEASES

Chemotherapeutic agents and radiation may cause pericardial disease including pericarditis, pericardial effusions and cardiac tamponade (57). Many agents spanning various classes have been shown to cause pericardial disease, including anthracyclines and cyclophosphamide to name a few (58–60). As it pertains to survivorship, reoccurrence of disease may manifest with metastases to the pericardium, endomyocardial fibrosis, and constrictive pericarditis (more commonly associated with radiation injury) occurring in the years following treatment (61,62). Transthoracic echocardiography is the recommended modality to assess the pericardium. Evaluation of the pericardium should be undertaken when there is suspicion of pericardial disease as per the current ASE and EAE guidelines.

Contrast echocardiography

There is consensus amongst the various societies that the use of contrast echocardiography should be limited to the studies in which two continuous LV segments from any apical view are not well seen. Although the addition of contrast to 2D echocardiography is believed to increase the interobserver variability, it is not recommended in routine follow-up unless otherwise indicated. Studies have looked at the incremental value of contrast to 3D echocardiography for the measurement of LV volumes and function and have not found any additional benefit (54,63,64).

Stress echocardiography

There are two major applications of stress echocardiography in the surveillance of patients with a history of radiation therapy and chemotherapy. The first application is evaluation for the presence of coronary artery disease and the second is to evaluate for sub-clinical LV dysfunction. The indication for stress echocardiography is to unveil significant CAD in patients having been treated with thoracic radiation or treatments with chemotherapeutic agents that may cause ischemia including: fluorouracil, bevacizumab, sorafenib, and sunitinib. The role of stress echocardiography in survivorship is limited to patients presenting with clinical symptoms suggesting coronary artery disease or in asymptomatic patients having been treated with left chest radiation (lymphoma and breast) (65).

Detection of subclinical LV dysfunction using contractile reserve has been investigated in the last several years. Civelli et al. found a 5-unit fall in LV contractile reserve to be predictive of a subsequent drop in LVEF below 50% (66). Grosu et al. demonstrated that the transient recovery of LV function during stress echocardiography may be associated with a better prognosis (67). While stress echocardiography may allow for the early identification of LV compromise, there is currently insufficient evidence for its routine use and hence it should be limited to screening of CAD in intermediate-/high-risk survivors (43).

Other imaging modalities

While echocardiography is currently the recommended initial modality for surveillance of survivors of chemotherapy and radiation therapy, other cardiac modalities have emerged as alternatives to evaluate the effects of these therapies on the heart. These modalities include CMR imaging and radionucleotide angiography. The current recommendation is to utilize these modalities when echocardiography is suboptimal or not feasible. If both modalities are available, CMR is given preference due to the lack of ionizing radiation and ability to evaluate structure along with function (36,40).

Cardiac magnetic resonance

CMR has become the gold standard for the non-invasive assessment of the heart due to its safety, interobserver consistency, quantitative accuracy, and ability to characterize the myocardial tissue. It has also been deemed a sensitive and reproducible alternative to echocardiography in cancer survivors (68). In a cross-sectional study of 114 adult survivors of childhood cancer, 12 individuals had an LVEF quoted to be greater than 50% by Simpson's biplane on 2D echocardiography, amongst which 14% were found to have an EF less than 50% by CMR (69,70).

CMR, in addition to having high spatial resolution, and providing quantitative measurements, can characterize the myocardial tissue. Tham et al. followed 30 pediatric patients with a normal LV function at baseline (71). After just 2 years of anthracycline therapy, an increase in extracellular volume and fibrosis was noted in the myocardium. These findings correlated with the cumulative dose of anthracycline as well as endpoints such as decreased LV mass and wall thickness. Neilan et al. showed an association between impaired diastolic function and increased extracellular volume in 42 adult survivors who had completed anthracycline-based chemotherapies (71,72).

Although CMR is not the first-line modality for assessing cardiotoxicity due to high cost and limited access, major societies favor it as an alternative to first-line modalities because there is minimal exposure to ionizing radiation. Much like other modalities, however, access and costs are too prohibitive for it to be the primary imaging modality. Moreover, not enough evidence is currently available to recommend CMR imaging as the first line in surveillance during survivorship.

Multigated acquisition scan

MUGA scan by myocardial perfusion is a well-established alternative to echocardiograms when the latter is not feasible or available. MUGA scan has been proven to provide accurate and reproducible measurement of the LV cavity size and function, all of which have been prognostically validated. The major limitation of the MUGA scan outside of the technical aspects of image acquisition (i.e., limited in presence of arrhythmia) is the exposure to ionizing radiation. This technique does not allow for evaluation of diastolic function, valvular disease, or the pericardium. When echocardiogram and/or CMR are not available it is reasonable to check EF using MUGA; however, if CMR is available it is prioritized due to the lack of ionizing radiation (40,43).

Risk for chemotherapy-related cardiac dysfunction and radiation-induced heart disease

The various societies (Children's Oncology Group [COG], Dutch Childhood Oncology Group [DCOG], Canadian Cardiovascular Society [CCS], ACC, ESC) have agreed that a history of anthracycline treatment, chest radiation, and pre-existing cardiovascular risk factors warrants cardiomyopathy surveillance. When following these cancer survivors it is important to have a well-documented history of their cancer therapy to understand their risk category.

The highest risk groups for developing heart failure after receiving chemotherapy include (36,40,43):

- Having been treated with $\geq$250–300 mg/m^2 of doxorubicin, $\geq$600 mg/m^2 of epirubicin
- Combination of anthracycline and chest radiation (even at the lower doses, i.e., $\geq$100 mg/m^2 anthracyclines and $\geq$15 Gy of chest radiation)
- A history of transient cardiomyopathy during treatment
- Pregnancy during survivorship given the increased cardiometabolic demand on the heart
- Treatment with anthracyclines (even at lower doses) or trastuzumab with at least one cardiovascular risk factor including:
  - Older age ($\geq$60)
  - Abnormal cardiac function (including borderline EF of 50%–55%)
  - History of myocardial infarction
  - $\geq$ Moderate valvular dysfunction
  - $\geq$2 Traditional cardiac risk factors
- Treatment with low-dose anthracyclines followed by trastuzumab in sequential fashion

Moderate risk groups include those having received 100 mg/m^2 to <250 mg/m^2 of anthracyclines. Low risk is defined as individuals who have been treated with <100 mg/m^2 of anthracyclines.

The highest risk group of developing heart failure after receiving radiation therapy include (36,40):

- Having received high doses of chest radiation $\geq$30–35 Gy, specifically the left chest as is done in Hodgkin's and left sided chest radiation.
- Received chest radiation with one or more CV risk factors as defined by:

- Young patients (less than 50 years of age)
- High dose of radiation fractions (>2 Gy/day)
- Proximity and extent of tumor in or near the heart
- Lack of shielding during therapy
- CV risk factors
- Previous CV disease

Individuals having been treated with moderate doses of chest radiation (15 Gy –<35 Gy) are considered at high risk of developing heart failure according to a more recent harmonized set of guidelines set forth by Armenian et al. (36)

There is a paucity of data on the cardiotoxic risks of lower doses of chest radiation (2 Gy to <15 Gy) and therefore the exact risk remains unknown. Nonetheless there seems to be a lifelong risk (36,44).

Echocardiographic follow-up in survivors having completed cancer therapy with cardiotoxic agents (chemotherapy and radiation therapy)

The American Society of Clinical Oncology (ASCO), the American College of Cardiology (ACC), and the Canadian Cardiovascular Society all recognize the need for follow-up with an imaging modality, but due to lack of data, recommendations regarding initiation and frequency vary. No studies compare the efficacy of one cardiac surveillance strategy to another with regard to frequency and efficacy in cancer survivors. Most societies have agreed on lifelong surveillance performed at a minimum of every 5 years, except for surveillance after undergoing treatment with trastuzumab (unless there is persistent LV dysfunction after cessation of therapy).

ECHOCARDIOGRAPHIC FOLLOW-UP IN SURVIVORS HAVING HAD CHEMOTHERAPY: ACC/ASCO/ESC GUIDELINES

The American College of Cardiology (ACC) recommends to the American Society of Clinical Oncology guidelines recommend an echocardiogram in everyone who is symptomatic (43). For asymptomatic survivors, they recommend a single echocardiogram at 6–12 months in individuals after completion of anthracycline-based chemotherapy. If the echocardiogram demonstrates systolic dysfunction, the recommendation is for the survivor to be referred to a cardio-oncologist. There is no recommendation or additional guidance for further management. There is no recommendation made if the echocardiogram shows normal systolic function during the 6–12 month study.

The American College of Cardiology agrees with the consensus statement issued by the European Society of Cardiology Task Force (24) and the joint European Association of Cardiovascular Imaging and American Society of Echocardiography (EACVI/ASE) position statement for guidance on follow-up (31). The position paper suggests an echocardiogram at completion of cancer treatment, then at 6 months, 12 months and 5 years. There are no recommendations for survivorship in patients having been treated with other chemotherapeutic agents other than anthracyclines and trastuzumab. As for the Task Force, they recognize the need for long-term periodic surveillance with imaging in survivors having been treated with anthracyclines, but they do not specify the timing of initiation or frequency. They also recommend immediate assessment if a survivor becomes symptomatic.

ECHOCARDIOGRAPHIC FOLLOW-UP AFTER RADIATION: JOINT ASE/EACVI STATEMENT

Although the long-term effects of RIHD are well established, the optimal methods and frequency for surveillance are unclear. The joint ASE/EAVCI statement recommends that new symptoms suggestive of LV systolic dysfunction should prompt an imaging follow-up. Those who remain asymptomatic should have an imaging study 10 years after treatment and every 5 years thereafter. In those with high-risk cardiovascular disease, the surveillance could begin as early as 5 years post-treatment with 5-year follow-ups and periodic stress imaging.

Screening for valvular heart disease and CAD

Chemotherapy has not been shown to cause primary valvular disease, and most of the risk attributed to CAD and valvulopathy is from chest radiotherapy during the years of survivorship.

The highest risk groups of developing heart failure/valvulopathy after receiving radiation therapy include those (36,40):

- Having received high doses of chest radiation $\geq$30–35 Gy, specifically the left chest as is done in Hodgkin's and left-sided more than right-sided breast cancer).
- Having received chest radiation with one or more CV risk factors as defined by:
  - Younger patients (less than 50 years of age)
  - High dose of radiation fractions (>2 Gy/day)
  - Presence and extent of tumor in or near the heart
  - Lack of shielding during therapy
  - CV risk factors
  - Previous CV disease.

The EACVI/ASE recommend an echocardiographic exam in symptomatic patients. For asymptomatic patients, the EACVI/ASE recommend a screening stress echocardiogram at 5–10 years postradiation followed by serial exams every 5 years thereafter irrespective of their risk profile (31). The Task Force for cancer treatments and cardiovascular toxicity of the European Society of Cardiology suggests starting screening earlier (5 years posttreatment) and then at least every 5 years thereafter, again devoid of risk profile (24).

The Canadian Cardiovascular Society endorses the Children's Oncology Group's long-term follow-up guidelines. They recommend a cardiology consultation 5–10 years post–chest radiation therapy to evaluate the risk for CAD in patients having received $\geq$40 Gy of therapy or $\geq$30 Gy if there was concomitant anthracycline therapy (42).

Special circumstances

PREGNANCY

Current congenital cardiology data and the limited experience in childhood cancer survivors suggest that women having had abnormal LV systolic function (less than 40%) prior to pregnancy, all etiologies included, have an increased risk of further deterioration in LV systolic function postpartum, and in the case of chemotherapy this is irrespective of the cumulative lifetime dose of anthracyclines.

The current recommendation by The International Late Effects of Childhood Cancer Guideline Harmonization Group, the only society to address this demographic, is to screen women with an imaging modality prior to pregnancy and/or in the first trimester in any survivor having been treated with anthracyclines and/or chest radiation. While those with abnormal systolic function should be followed closely, no recommendations could be formulated for women found to have normal LV systolic function prior to or during the first trimester of pregnancy (73,74).

Conclusion

The number of cancer survivors living after treatment with chemotherapy and radiation is increasing and the toxic effects of treatment may only manifest years after treatment. High dose anthracyclines and left-sided chest radiation are just a couple of therapies that are deemed high risk. While there is lack of data about surveillance during survivorship, it has been recognized as a lifelong necessity. Various societies have put forth recommendations for monitoring but more studies are needed to determine the most cost-effective follow-up strategy.

THE OTTAWA MODEL: A COMMUNITY-BASED MODEL FOR LONGITUDINAL CARDIOVASCULAR CARE OF CANCER SURVIVORS

Introduction

In the transition of patients from oncology and tertiary care cardio-oncology to community-based settings, care should be taken to make providers aware of possible long-term consequences of cancer treatment. For instance, in a study surveying a large group of oncologists and primary care physicians, 95% of oncologists but only 55% of primary care physicians reported awareness of cardiac dysfunction as a late effect of doxorubicin (75).

Traditional cardiovascular risk factors are also important modifiers of short and long-term cardiovascular toxicity. Therefore, the most impactful approach to risk reduction in cancer survivors is likely related to adherence to primary prevention guidelines for the general population. However, recent data show that cardiovascular risk factors are not being adequately addressed or are being under-treated in this patient population compared to their noncancer survivor counterparts (76,77). In a large survey of cancer survivors, a substantial proportion of survivors at risk for CVD reported lack of health promotion discussions with their providers (78). Several factors may contribute to inadequate CVD preventative interventions. First, providers caring for cancer survivors may need additional education regarding how to screen and provide referrals or interventions for this patient population. Furthermore, risk factor counseling may be challenging in the context of brief oncology visits after cancer treatment and busy primary care encounters.

Community-based cancer survivorship and cardiovascular care programs: The Ottawa model

Given that the anticipated number of cancer survivors at risk of long-term CVD related to cancer treatments outweighs the capacity of most cancer centers and cardio-oncology programs to follow them in the long term, rational strategies to optimize the longitudinal cardiovascular care of these patients in the community are needed. Once discharged into the community, providers need not only be aware of a patient's cancer diagnosis, but also the treatments given and implications of these treatments on long-term risk of cardiovascular morbidity and morality. At minimum, survivorship care plans provided to primary care providers, should be include information regarding potential long-term cardiotoxicities of cancer treatment and strategies for risk factor modification (79).

However, a more targeted strategy for surveillance of high-risk patients, or of those who developed cardiovascular complications during cancer treatments may allow for more timely intervention and mitigation of cardiovascular morbidity and mortality.

One such model is currently being championed as a pilot strategy in breast cancer survivors by a tertiary cardio-oncology program in collaboration with a community-based cardiovascular center in Ottawa, Canada (80). Patients at high risk of cardiovascular complications after cancer therapy (Figure 8.1) or those with cardiovascular diagnoses identified during cancer treatment (Figure 8.2) are referred for long-term follow-up to a community-based "Cancer Survivorship and Cardiovascular Care" program. The goal of this program is

two-fold: to provide optimal care and surveillance of cancer survivors at risk of cardiovascular complications or who have established CV disease; and to track the characteristics and outcomes of this population. Importantly, information acquired by tracking these patients over the long term could facilitate the development of more evidence-based surveillance strategies.

The objectives of a community-based cancer survivorship and cardiovascular care program are:

1. To provide a common portal for longitudinal follow-up of cancer survivors at increased risk of developing long-term cardiovascular complications of cancer and cancer therapy.
   a. Rationale:
      i. Referral to clinicians with expertise and a vested interest in this field would facilitate evidence-based and timely institution of primary preventative measures and identification and treatment of cancer treatment–related cardiovascular complications.
      ii. Clinicians would seek to remain current with emerging evidence in the field and in turn to implement evidence-based interventions as the field evolves.
2. To develop a registry to track interventions and outcomes in this patient population.
   a. Data collected would be analyzed to better understand the natural history of this patient population. A registry would facilitate scholarly activity to contribute to the broader field of cardio-oncology at the national and international levels.
   b. Data from such a registry would serve as a vehicle to continually evaluate and improve quality of care to this patient population.
3. To provide educational resources to clinicians and the public about cancer- and cancer treatment–related cardiovascular effects (Figures 8.1 and 8.2).

In summary, given that most cardio-oncology programs have finite resources, longitudinal follow-up of cancer survivors at high risk of long-term cardiotoxicity needs to be shared with community providers. The "Ottawa Model" provides a framework by which such patients can be followed in the community with the objectives of prevention, detection, documentation and treatment of long-term cancer-related cardiotoxicity.

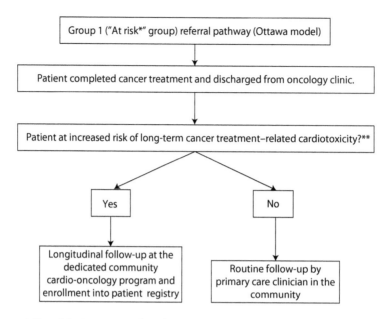

Figure 8.1 Group 1 ("at risk*" group) referral pathway (Ottawa model). *Patients at increased risk of long-term cancer treatment–related cardiotoxicity; **risk assessment would be based on established treatment- and patient-related risk factors for cardiotoxicity based on cancer site.

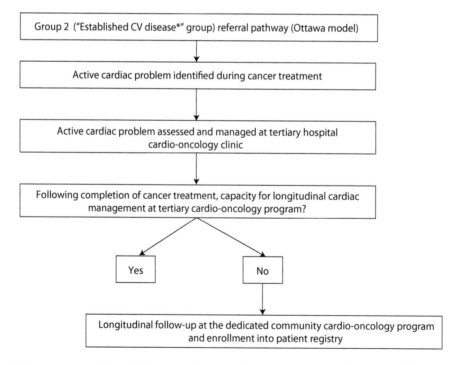

Figure 8.2 Group 2 ("established CV disease" group) referral pathway (Ottawa model). *Patients with an established diagnosis of cardiovascular disease identified prior to or during cancer treatment.

REFERENCES

1. www.cancer.gov/about-cancer/understanding/statistics.

2. Force T, Kolaja KL. Cardiotoxicity of kinase inhibitors: The prediction and translation of preclinical models to clinical outcomes. *Nat Rev Drug Discov.* 2011;10:111–26.

3. Patnaik JL, Byers T, DiGuiseppi C, Dabelea D, Denberg TD. Cardiovascular disease competes with breast cancer as the leading cause of death for older females diagnosed with breast cancer: A retrospective cohort study. *Breast Cancer Res.* June 20, 2011;13(3):R64.

4. Hamo CE, Bloom MW, Cardinale D, Ky B, Nohria A, Baer L, Skopicki H, Lenihan DJ, Gheorghiade M, Lyon AR, Butler J. Cancer therapy-related cardiac dysfunction and heart failure: Part 2: Prevention, treatment, guidelines, and future directions. *Circ Heart Fail.* February 2016;9(2):e002843.

5. Zhang S et al. Identification of the molecular basis of doxorubicin-induced cardiotoxicity. *Nat Med.* 2012;18:1639–42.

6. Pinder MC, Duan Z, Goodwin JS, Hortobagyi GN, Giordano SH. Congestive heart failure in older women treated with adjuvant anthracycline chemotherapy for breast cancer. *J Clin Oncol.* 2007;25:3808–15.

7. Procter M et al. Longer-term assessment of trastuzumab-related cardiac adverse events in the Herceptin Adjuvant (HERA) trial. *J Clin Oncol.* 2010;28(21):3422.

8. Narayan V et al. Prospective evaluation of sunitinib-induced cardiotoxicity in patients with metastatic renal cell carcinoma. *Clin Cancer Res.* 2017;23(14):3601.

9. Myrehaug S, Pintilie M, Tsang R, Mackenzie R, Crump M, Chen Z, Sun A, Hodgson DC. Cardiac morbidity following modern treatment for Hodgkin lymphoma: Supra-additive cardiotoxicity of doxorubicin and radiation therapy. *Leuk Lymphoma.* 2008;49(8):1486.

10. Felicetti F et al. Prevalence of cardiovascular risk factors in long-term survivors of childhood cancer: 16 years follow up from a prospective registry. *Eur J Prev Cardiol.* 2015;22:762–70.

11. Meacham LR et al. Cardiovascular risk factors in adult survivors of pediatric cancer—a report from the childhood cancer survivor study. *Cancer Epidemiol Biomarkers Prev.* 2010;19:170–81.

12. Bhatia N, Santos M, Jones LW, Beckman JA, Penson DF, Morgans AK, Moslehi J. Cardiovascular effects of androgen deprivation therapy for the treatment of prostate cancer: ABCDE steps to reduce cardiovascular disease in patients with prostate cancer. *Circulation.* February 2, 2016;133(5):537–41.

13. van den Bogaard VA et al. Validation and modification of a prediction model for acute cardiac events in patients with breast cancer treated with radiotherapy based on three-dimensional dose distributions to cardiac substructures. *J Clin Oncol.* 2017;35(11):1171.

14. Collier A, Ghosh S, McGlynn B, Hollins G. Prostate cancer, androgen deprivation therapy, obesity, the metabolic syndrome, type 2 diabetes, and cardiovascular disease: A review. *Am J Clin Oncol.* October 2012;35(5):504–9.

15. Levine GN et al. American Heart Association Council on Clinical Cardiology and Council on Epidemiology and Prevention, the American Cancer Society, and the American Urological Association. Androgen-deprivation therapy in prostate cancer and cardiovascular risk: A science advisory from the American Heart Association, American Cancer Society, and American Urological Association: Endorsed by the American Society for Radiation Oncology. *Circulation.* 2010;121:833–40.

16. Keating NL, O'Malley AJ, Smith MR. Diabetes and cardiovascular disease during androgen deprivation therapy for prostate cancer. *J Clin Oncol.* September 20, 2006;24(27):4448–56.

17. Albertsen PC, Klotz L, Tombal B, Grady J, Olesen TK, Nilsson J. Cardiovascular morbidity associated with gonadotropin releasing hormone agonists and an antagonist. *Eur Urol.* 2014;65:565–73.

18. Hull MC, Morris CG, Pepine CJ, Mendenhall NP. Valvular dysfunction and carotid, subclavian, and coronary artery disease in survivors of Hodgkin lymphoma treated with radiation therapy. *JAMA.* 2003;290(21):2831–7.

19. Galper SL, Yu JB, Mauch PM, Strasser JF, Silver B, Lacasce A, Marcus KJ, Stevenson MA, Chen MH, Ng AK. Clinically significant

cardiac disease in patients with Hodgkin lymphoma treated with mediastinal irradiation. *Blood*. 2011;117(2):412.

20. Curigliano G, Cardinale D, Dent S, Criscitiello C, Aseyev O, Lenihan D, Cipolla CM. Cardiotoxicity of anticancer treatments: Epidemiology, detection, and management. *CA Cancer J Clin*. July 2016;66(4):309–25.

21. Carver JR, Shapiro CL, Ng A, Jacobs L, Schwartz C, Virgo KS, Hagerty KL, Somerfield MR, Vaughn DJ, ASCO Cancer Survivorship Expert Panel. American Society of Clinical Oncology clinical evidence review on the ongoing care of adult cancer survivors: Cardiac and pulmonary late effects. *J Clin Oncol*. September 1, 2007;25(25):3991–4008.

22. Silber JH et al. Enalapril to prevent cardiac function decline in long-term survivors of pediatric cancer exposed to anthracyclines. *J Clin Oncol*. March 1, 2004;22(5):820–8.

23. Plana JC et al. Expert consensus for multimodality imaging evaluation of adult patients during and after cancer therapy: A report from the American Society of Echocardiography and the European Association of Cardiovascular Imaging. *Eur Heart J Cardiovasc Imaging*. October 2014;15(10):1063–93.

24. Zamorano JL et al. 2016 ESC Position Paper on cancer treatments and cardiovascular toxicity developed under the auspices of the ESC Committee for Practice Guidelines: The task force for cancer treatments and cardiovascular toxicity of the European Society of Cardiology (ESC). *Eur Heart J*. September 21, 2016;37(36):2768–801.

25. Curigliano G, Cardinale D, Suter T, Plataniotis G, de Azambuja E, Sandri MT, Criscitiello C, Goldhirsch A, Cipolla C, Roila F, ESMO Guidelines Working Group. Cardiovascular toxicity induced by chemotherapy, targeted agents and radiotherapy: ESMO Clinical Practice Guidelines. *Ann Oncol*. October 2012;23(Suppl 7):vii155–66.

26. Chang HM, Moudgil R, Scarabelli T, Okwuosa TM, Yeh ETH. Cardiovascular complications of cancer therapy: Best practices in diagnosis, prevention, and management: Part 1. *J Am Coll Cardiol*. November 14, 2017;70(20):2536–51.

27. Chang HM, Okwuosa TM, Scarabelli T, Moudgil R, Yeh ETH. Cardiovascular complications of cancer therapy: Best practices in diagnosis, prevention, and management: Part 2. *J Am Coll Cardiol*. November 14, 2017;70(20):2552–65.

28. Hamo CE et al. Cancer therapy-related cardiac dysfunction and heart failure: Part 2: Prevention, treatment, guidelines, and future directions. *Circ Heart Fail*. February 2016;9(2):e002843.

29. Bloom MW et al. Cancer therapy-related cardiac dysfunction and heart failure: Part 1: Definitions, pathophysiology, risk factors, and imaging. *Circ Heart Fail*. January 2016;9(1):e002661.

30. Armenian SH, Lacchetti C, Lenihan D. Prevention and monitoring of cardiac dysfunction in survivors of adult cancers: American Society of Clinical Oncology Clinical Practice Guideline Summary. *J Oncol Pract*. April 2017;13(4):270–5.

31. Lancellotti P et al. Expert consensus for multimodality imaging evaluation of cardiovascular complications of radiotherapy in adults: A report from the European Association of Cardiovascular Imaging and the American Society of Echocardiography. *J Am Soc Echocardiogr*. September 2013;26(9):1013–32.

32. McCabe MS, Bhatia S, Oeffinger KC, Reaman GH, Tyne C, Wollins DS, Hudson MM. American Society of Clinical Oncology statement: Achieving high-quality cancer survivorship care. *J Clin Oncol*. February 10, 2013;31(5):631–40.

33. Lenihan DJ, Oliva S, Chow EJ, Cardinale D. Cardiac toxicity in cancer survivors. *Cancer*. January 1, 2013;119(Suppl 11):2131–42.

34. de Azambuja E et al. Cardiac assessment of early breast cancer patients 18 years after treatment with cyclophosphamide-, methotrexate-, fluorouracil- or epirubicin-based chemotherapy. *Eur J Cancer*. November 2015;51(17):2517–24.

35. Steinherz LJ, Steinherz PG, Tan CT, Heller G, Murphy ML. Cardiac toxicity 4 to 20 years after completing anthracycline therapy. *JAMA*. September 25, 1991;266(12):1672–7.

36. Armenian SH et al. Recommendations for cardiomyopathy surveillance for survivors of childhood cancer: A report from the

International Late Effects of Childhood Cancer Guideline Harmonization Group. *Lancet Oncol.* 2015;16(3):e123–36.

37. Lenihan DJ, Oliva S, Chow EJ, Cardinale D. Cardiac toxicity in cancer survivors. *Cancer.* 2013;119(Suppl:2131–2142).

38. Hequet O et al. Subclinical late cardiomyopathy after doxorubicin therapy for lymphoma in adults. *J Clin Oncol.* 2004;22(10):1864–71.

39. de Azambuja E et al. Cardiac assessment of early breast cancer patients 18 years after treatment with cyclophosphamide-, methotrexate-, fluorouracil- or epirubicin-based chemotherapy. *Eur J Cancer.* 2015;51(17):2517–24.

40. Lancellotti P et al. Expert consensus for multimodality imaging evaluation of cardiovascular complications of radiotherapy in adults: A report from the European Association of Cardiovascular Imaging and the American Society of Echocardiography. *Eur Heart J Cardiovasc Imaging.* 2013;14(8):721–40.

41. Kenigsberg B, Wellstein A, Barac A. Left ventricular dysfunction in cancer treatment: Is it relevant? *JACC Heart Fail.* 2018;6(2):87–95.

42. Virani SA et al. Canadian Cardiovascular Society guidelines for evaluation and management of cardiovascular complications of cancer therapy. *Can J Cardiol.* 2016;32(7):831–41.

43. Armenian SH et al. Prevention and monitoring of cardiac dysfunction in survivors of adult cancers: American Society of Clinical Oncology Clinical Practice Guideline. *J Clin Oncol.* 2017;35(8):893–911.

44. Plana JC et al. Expert consensus for multimodality imaging evaluation of adult patients during and after cancer therapy: A report from the American Society of Echocardiography and the European Association of Cardiovascular Imaging. *J Am Soc Echocardiogr.* 2014;27(9):911–39.

45. Mor-Avi V, Lang RM. Is echocardiography reliable for monitoring the adverse cardiac effects of chemotherapy? *J Am Coll Cardiol.* 2013;61(1):85–7.

46. Tan TC, Scherrer-Crosbie M. Assessing the cardiac toxicity of chemotherapeutic agents: Role of echocardiography. *Curr Cardiovasc Imaging Rep.* 2012;5(6):403–9.

47. Lang RM et al. Recommendations for cardiac chamber quantification by echocardiography in adults: An update from the American Society of Echocardiography and the European Association of Cardiovascular Imaging. *J Am Soc Echocardiogr.* 2015; 28(1):1–39.e14.

48. Tassan-Mangina S et al. Tissue Doppler imaging and conventional echocardiography after anthracycline treatment in adults: Early and late alterations of left ventricular function during a prospective study. *Eur J Echocardiogr.* 2006;7(2):141–6.

49. Jacobs LD et al. Rapid online quantification of left ventricular volume from real-time three-dimensional echocardiographic data. *Eur Heart J.* 2006;27(4):460–8.

50. Otterstad JE, Froeland G, St John Sutton M, Holme I. Accuracy and reproducibility of biplane two-dimensional echocardiographic measurements of left ventricular dimensions and function. *Eur Heart J.* 1997;18(3):507–13.

51. Cardinale D et al. Anthracycline-induced cardiomyopathy: Clinical relevance and response to pharmacologic therapy. *J Am Coll Cardiol.* 2010;55(3):213–20.

52. Tsai H-R et al. Left ventricular function assessed by two-dimensional speckle tracking echocardiography in long-term survivors of Hodgkin's lymphoma treated by mediastinal radiotherapy with or without anthracycline therapy. *Am J Cardiol.* 2011;107(3):472–7.

53. Cheung Y, Hong W, Chan GCF, Wong SJ, Ha S. Left ventricular myocardial deformation and mechanical dyssynchrony in children with normal ventricular shortening fraction after anthracycline therapy. *Heart.* 2010;96(14):1137–41.

54. Thavendiranathan P, Poulin F, Lim K-D, Plana JC, Woo A, Marwick TH. Use of myocardial strain imaging by echocardiography for the early detection of cardiotoxicity in patients during and after cancer chemotherapy: A systematic review. *J Am Coll Cardiol.* 2014;63(25 Pt A):2751–68.

55. Stoddard MF, Seeger J, Liddell NE, Hadley TJ, Sullivan DM, Kupersmith J. Prolongation of isovolumetric relaxation time as assessed by Doppler echocardiography predicts doxorubicin-induced systolic dysfunction in humans. *J Am Coll Cardiol.* 1992;20(1):62–9.

56. Montani D et al. Pulmonary arterial hypertension in patients treated by dasatinib. *Circulation.* 2012;125(17):2128–37.

57. Gaya AM, Ashford RFU. Cardiac complications of radiation therapy. *Clin Oncol (R Coll Radiol).* 2005;17(3):153–9.

58. Yamamoto R et al. Myopericarditis caused by cyclophosphamide used to mobilize peripheral blood stem cells in a myeloma patient with renal failure. *Bone Marrow Transplant.* 2000;26(6):685–8.

59. Tohda S et al. Acute pericarditis caused by daunorubicin in acute myelocytic leukemia. *Rinsho Ketsueki.* 1988;29(6):874–8.

60. Hermans C, Straetmans N, Michaux JL, Ferrant A. Pericarditis induced by high-dose cytosine arabinoside chemotherapy. *Ann Hematol.* 1997;75(1–2):55–7.

61. Kane GC, Edie RN, Mannion JD. Delayed appearance of effusive-constrictive pericarditis after radiation for Hodgkin lymphoma. *Ann Intern Med.* 1996;124(5):534–5.

62. Tulleken JE, Kooiman C, van der Werf TS, Zijlstra JG, de Vries EGE. Constrictive pericarditis after high-dose chemotherapy. *Lancet.* 1997;350(9091):1601.

63. Mulvagh SL et al. American Society of Echocardiography consensus statement on the clinical applications of ultrasonic contrast agents in echocardiography. *J Am Soc Echocardiogr.* 2008;21(11):1179–201; quiz 1281.

64. Senior R et al. Contrast echocardiography: Evidence-based recommendations by European Association of Echocardiography. *Eur J Echocardiogr.* 2009;10(2):194–212.

65. Douglas PS et al. Developing an action plan for patient radiation safety in adult cardiovascular medicine: Proceedings from the Duke University Clinical Research Institute/American College of Cardiology Foundation/American Heart Association Think Tank held on February 28. *J Am Coll Cardiol.* 2012;59(20):1833–47.

66. Civelli M et al. Early reduction in left ventricular contractile reserve detected by dobutamine stress echo predicts high-dose chemotherapy-induced cardiac toxicity. *Int J Cardiol.* 2006;111(1):120–6.

67. Grosu A, Bombardini T, Senni M, Duino V, Gori M, Picano E. End-systolic pressure/volume relationship during dobutamine stress echo: A prognostically useful non-invasive index of left ventricular contractility. *Eur Heart J.* 2005;26(22):2404–12.

68. Krawczuk-Rybak M, Dakowicz L, Hryniewicz A, Maksymiuk A, Zelazowska-Rutkowska B, Wysocka J. Cardiac function in survivors of acute lymphoblastic leukaemia and Hodgkin's lymphoma. *J Paediatr Child Health.* 2011;47(7):455–9.

69. Armstrong AC, Gidding S, Gjesdal O, Wu C, Bluemke DA, Lima JAC. LV mass assessed by echocardiography and CMR, Cardiovascular outcomes, and medical practice. *JACC Cardiovasc Imaging.* 2012;5(8):837–48.

70. Wassmuth R et al. Subclinical cardiotoxic effects of anthracyclines as assessed by magnetic resonance imaging-a pilot study. *Am Heart J.* 2001;141(6):1007–13.

71. Tham EB et al. Diffuse myocardial fibrosis by T1-mapping in children with subclinical anthracycline cardiotoxicity: Relationship to exercise capacity, cumulative dose and remodeling. *J Cardiovasc Magn Reson.* 2013;15:48.

72. Neilan TG et al. Myocardial extracellular volume by cardiac magnetic resonance imaging in patients treated with anthracycline-based chemotherapy. *Am J Cardiol.* 2013;111(5):717–22.

73. Thompson KA. Pregnancy and cardiomyopathy after anthracyclines in childhood. *Front Cardiovasc Med.* 2018;5:14.

74. van Dalen EC, van der Pal HJH, van den Bos C, Kok WEM, Caron HN, Kremer LCM. Clinical heart failure during pregnancy and delivery in a cohort of female childhood cancer survivors treated with anthracyclines. *Eur J Cancer.* 2006;42(15):2549–53.

75. Nekhlyudov L, Aziz NM, Lerro C, Virgo KS. Oncologists' and primary care physicians' awareness of late and long-term effects of chemotherapy: Implications for care of the growing population of survivors. *J Oncol Pract.* March 2014;10(2):e29–36.

76. Ammon M et al. Cardiovascular management of cancer patients with chemotherapy-associated left ventricular systolic dysfunction in real-world clinical practice. *J Card Fail.* 2013;19:629–34.

77. Yoon GJ et al. Left ventricular dysfunction in patients receiving cardiotoxic cancer

therapies: Are clinicians responding optimally? *J Am Coll Cardiol.* 2010;56:1644–50.

78. Weaver KE, Foraker RE, Alfano CM, Rowland JH, Arora NK, Bellizzi KM, Hamilton AS, Oakley-Girvan I, Keel G, Aziz NM. Cardiovascular risk factors among long-term survivors of breast, prostate, colorectal, and gynecologic cancers: A gap in survivorship care? *J Cancer Surviv.* June 2013;7(2):253–61.

79. Lawrence RA, McLoone JK, Wakefield CE, Cohn RJ. Primary care physicians' perspectives of their role in cancer care: A systematic review. *J Gen Intern Med.* October, 2016;31(10):1222–36.

80. Dent S, Law A, Ghosh N, Johnson C. Coordinating cardio-oncology care. Gottlieb RA and Mehta PK (eds) *Cardio-Oncology: Principles, Prevention and Management.* Elselvier, 2017.

9

Survivorship: Pediatric cancer survivors

SHAHNAWAZ AMDANI, NEHA BANSAL, EMMA RACHEL LIPSHULTZ,
MICHAEL JACOB ADAMS, AND STEVEN E. LIPSHULTZ

BACKGROUND

Major and rapid advancements in managing childhood cancers have remarkably improved the survival of these patients. More than 80% of children diagnosed with cancer in the USA now survive at least 5 years (1). The mortality rate of survivors has declined from 6.3 per 100,000 population in 1970 to 2.1 in 2011 (2). This reduction is largely attributed to improved treatments and high rates of participation in clinical trials.

Unfortunately, the same treatments that cure cancer often cause adverse effects in other organ systems, especially the cardiovascular system (3). Cancer therapies, aimed at stopping rapidly dividing neoplastic cells, also potentially interfere with normal tissue growth, as evidenced clearly by long-term cancer survivors who never attain normal height (4). In the 2017 St. Jude Lifetime Cohort Study, 99.9% of 5054 survivors had a chronic health condition by age 50 years. Utilizing the St. Jude Children's Research Hospital-modified version of the National Cancer Institute's Common Terminology Criteria for Adverse Events (CTCAE) (version 4.03), the authors found that 96% had a chronic health condition that was severe or disabling (grade 3), life-threatening (grade 4), or fatal (grade 5) by age 50 years (5).

Cardiovascular-related disease is the leading cause of morbidity and mortality in survivors after cancer itself (6–10). Among 1853 adult survivors of childhood cancer, cardiomyopathy was present in 7.4%, coronary artery disease in 3.8%, valvular regurgitation or stenosis in 28.0%, and conduction or rhythm abnormalities in 4.4% (11). Treatment-related cardiotoxicity is not limited to acute complications; long-term survivors of childhood cancer are at increased risk for cardiovascular complications for the rest of their lives (Table 9.1) (6,12–16). Anthracycline-containing regimens and radiation treatment especially have been associated with increased risk of these cardiovascular complications (7,8,10,17–19). A large proportion of survivors exposed to cardiotoxic treatments have subclinical

Table 9.1 Characteristics of the different types of anthracycline-associated cardiotoxicity

Characteristic	Acute cardiotoxicity	Early onset, chronic progressive cardiotoxicity	Late onset, chronic progressive cardiotoxicity
Onset	Within the first week of anthracycline treatment	<1 year after the completion of anthracycline therapy	>1 year after the completion of anthracycline therapy
Risk factor dependence	Unknown	Yes	Yes
Clinical features in adults	Transient depression of myocardial contractility; myocardial necrosis (cardiac troponin T [cTnT] elevation); arrhythmia	Dilated cardiomyopathy; arrhythmia	Dilated cardiomyopathy; arrhythmia
Clinical features in children	Transient depression of myocardial contractility; myocardial necrosis (cTnT elevation); arrhythmia	Restrictive cardiomyopathy and/or dilated cardiomyopathy; arrhythmia	Restrictive cardiomyopathy and/or dilated cardiomyopathy; arrhythmia
Course	Usually reversible on discontinuation of anthracycline	Can be progressive	Can be progressive

Source: From Lipshultz SE et al. *Heart* 2008;94:525–33. Adams MJ, Lipshultz SE: Pathophysiology of anthracycline- and radiation-associated cardiomyopathies: Implications for screening and prevention. *Pediatr Blood Cancer.* 2005.44.600–6. Copyright Wiley-VCH Verlag GmbH & Co. KGaA. Reproduced with permission.

cardiotoxicity (13–16,20) that ranges from pericardial or valvular damage associated with cardiac radiation exposure to decreased left ventricular (LV) systolic and diastolic function associated with anthracycline chemotherapy (13–16). This cardiotoxicity appears to be progressive and can lead to clinical cardiovascular disease (CVD) (15).

Currently, most survivors of childhood cancer will live for at least a decade after successful treatment of their original cancer (21). Thus, small, subclinical changes can become more severe over a lifetime and can cause marked cardiovascular morbidity that adult survivors do not experience. In addition, the adverse effects of cancer treatment may be especially problematic in children, because developmental immaturity does not allow them to compensate for therapy-related insults (22). Thus, heart failure (HF) rates are higher in children than in adults treated with the same anthracycline dose when adjusted for body size (23).

A recent preclinical study confirms the relative sensitivity of younger cells to chemotherapy (24). Whereas the mitochondria from the heart and brain tissues of adult mice and humans become "apoptosis refractory," the mitochondria in children are still subject to cell death in response to genotoxic damage (24). Thus, children with cancer are subject to severe side effects of radiation and chemotherapy from which older adults are relatively spared.

In this chapter, we review the treatment-related cardiovascular complications associated with treating childhood cancers and discuss methods for preventing, screening, and treating them. Providers caring for childhood cancer survivors need to understand these complications to improve the care for these patients.

MECHANISMS OF CARDIOTOXICITY FROM ANTHRACYCLINES

For several decades, anthracyclines, such as doxorubicin, daunorubicin, epirubicin, and idarubicin, have been instrumental in treating a variety of hematologic and solid tumors in children. More than 50% of childhood cancer survivors are estimated to have received anthracycline therapy (25). That anthracyclines are associated with clinically important cardiotoxicity is well established, and awareness of this fact among providers is critical, both during and after treatment of these patients (18).

The mechanisms of anthracycline-induced cardiotoxicity are complex, but one of the most broadly acknowledged mechanisms is the "oxidative stress hypothesis" (26–29). Anthracyclines readily enter cells through passive diffusion and reach intracellular concentrations several hundred times greater than those in extracellular compartments. Intracellularly, anthracyclines can undergo a series of redox reactions that result in a self-perpetuating cycle in which reactive oxygen radicals are produced. Intracellular anthracyclines may also form complexes with intracellular iron, which can produce free radicals. Reactive oxygen species and free radicals can then damage DNA and lipid peroxidation. Glutathione peroxidase, a cardiac antioxidant, is depleted in the presence of anthracyclines (30). Thus, the damaged cell mitochondria are unable to adjust to the increased oxidative stress, resulting in more damage and ultimately cell death.

Cardiolipins, which are abundant on the inner cell membrane of mitochondria, have an affinity for anthracyclines that allows anthracyclines to enter the cells more easily (31,32). This affinity can lead to anthracycline accumulation in the mitochondria, which may damage the stability of the mitochondrial membrane or the mitochondrial DNA through intercalation. Such damage may impair the cell's ability to produce energy, as well as its ability to handle added oxidative stress (26,33–35).

Several other mechanisms for anthracycline-related cardiotoxicity have been proposed, including the induction of apoptosis, the production of vasoactive amines, the formation of toxic metabolites, the upregulation of nitric oxide synthetase, and the inhibition of transcription and translation (36–38).

Cardiomyocytes exposed to anthracyclines show other changes, which may or may not depend on the oxidative pathway. These changes include depleted cardiac stem cells, impaired DNA synthesis, impaired cell signaling that triggers cell death, altered gene expression, inhibited calcium release from the sarcoplasmic reticulum, impaired formation of the protein titin in sarcomeres, and impaired mitochondrial creatine kinase activity and function (39–45). By impairing mitochondrial calcium regulation, they also destabilize the mitochondrial membrane, decrease ATP synthesis, and ultimately may cause cell death. Many of these subcellular sequelae progress for weeks after exposure to anthracyclines, which provides insight into mechanisms of chronic cardiomyopathy (46).

Over the past several years, topoisomerase-II β (Top2β) alterations have been considered as a possible mechanism of doxorubicin-mediated cardiotoxicity (47,48). As the only Top2 gene in heart tissue, Top2β is well established as the molecular target of anthracyclines' anticancer activity (49). The Top2β-doxorubicin-DNA ternary cleavage complex induces DNA double-strand breaks, killing cells (50). In mice, cardiomyocyte-specific deletion of Top2β protects cardiomyocytes from doxorubicin-induced DNA double-strand breaks and transcriptome changes, which would otherwise result in defective mitochondria and generate reactive oxygen species (47). Furthermore, the expression of Top2β on peripheral blood leukocytes was higher in anthracycline-sensitive patients than it was in anthracycline-resistant patients, which suggests that Top2β is a potential surrogate marker for susceptibility to anthracycline-induced cardiotoxicity. Here, anthracycline-sensitive patients were defined as those with a LV ejection fraction (LVEF) of 10% or greater below baseline values and an LVEF of less than 50%, despite receiving a cumulative doxorubicin dose no greater than 250 mg/m^2, and anthracycline-resistant patients were defined as those receiving a cumulative doxorubicin dose of at least 450 mg/m^2 with an LVEF of 50% or more (51). Furthermore, again in mice, deleting Top2β from cardiomyocytes prevented anthracycline-induced cardiotoxicity. These insights into molecular changes may lead to new strategies for preventing anthracycline-induced cardiotoxicity by targeting Top2β (52).

EFFECTS OF ANTHRACYCLINE CARDIOTOXICITY

Anthracycline cardiotoxicity can be categorized at the time of presentation as either acute or chronic, with chronic cases further categorized as early- or late-onset (Table 9.1) (53). In each category, HF may develop secondary to LV dysfunction and decreased exercise capacity (54). Acute toxicity, which presents during treatment, occurs in less than 1% of patients and often manifests as arrhythmias, electrocardiogram (EKG) abnormalities, HF, or as a myocarditis-pericarditis syndrome (25,53,55,56). Although some patients may present with potentially fatal HF, especially at higher cumulative doses of anthracyclines, some abnormalities may be transient, disappearing after cancer treatment (25,56); however, some abnormalities are persistent and progress for years after treatment. In fact, severe cardiotoxicity detected during or shortly after treatment, even with an intervening asymptomatic period, is strongly associated with eventual HF. In a follow-up study of childhood cancer survivors treated with anthracyclines and with acute HF, all recovered temporarily, although nearly half of the survivors later had recurrent HF (13). Lowering the dose of anthracyclines substantially reduced the incidence of acute cardiac complications, to less than 1%; however, chronic LV dysfunction remains a major clinical concern (55). The greatest risk of cardiac dysfunction is to those patients in whom abnormal cardiac function is diagnosed during or immediately after therapy (15).

Early-onset cardiomyopathy may present with LV dysfunction, EKG changes, and potentially fatal HF (25,53–55,57,58). The cumulative incidence of HF in 115 long-term survivors was 2.8% at a mean follow-up of 6.3 years after a mean cumulative dose of 301 mg/m² of anthracyclines (doxorubicin, daunorubicin, idarubicin, epirubicin, alone or in combination) (59). However, a 2005 study reported that this dilated cardiomyopathy progresses toward a restrictive pattern during extended follow-up (15).

Late-onset cardiomyopathy is caused by changes occurring during therapy that do not cause immediate symptoms. Ventricular function deteriorates and often shows a loss of cardiomyocytes (13–15). This loss results in progressive LV dilation, LV wall thinning, and decreases in LV contractility (60).

Echocardiographic findings include decreases in left ventricular fractional shortening (LVFS), LV mass, LV contractility, and LV end-diastolic posterior wall thickness (25). With marked LV dilation, the heart is unable to compensate further to meet increased metabolic demands from events such as acute viral illness, growth-hormone-induced growth spurts, weightlifting, pregnancy-induced hypervolemia, or vaginal birth (15,61–63). Although the estimated incidence of chronic HF in survivors treated with anthracyclines ranges from 1% to 16%, the true rate may be even higher with more extended follow-up (15,64).

In 115 survivors of acute lymphoblastic leukemia (ALL) or osteogenic sarcoma treated with the anthracycline doxorubicin, 6 years after treatment, LV wall thickness was decreased relative to body surface area (13–15). LVFS was reduced in one-fourth of the survivors studied. A follow-up study of these survivors 8 years after treatment found that younger age at diagnosis and longer follow-up were associated with decreased LV wall thickness (Figure 9.1) (14). Increased individual anthracycline dose was associated with LV dilation. Female sex and higher cumulative anthracycline dose were also associated with reduced LV contractility. Another follow-up study of these patients 12-years after treatment found that the anthracycline-related abnormalities of LV structure (LV mass) and function (LV contractility) had progressed (Figure 9.2), indicating worsening health of cardiac muscle cells

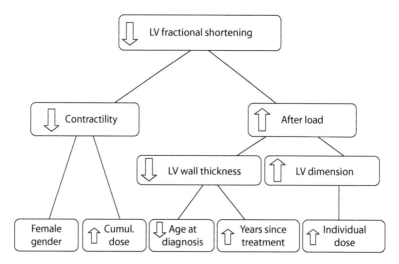

Figure 9.1 Factors associated with cardiac abnormalities and progression to left ventricular dysfunction in childhood cancer survivors treated with anthracyclines. LV, left ventricular. (Reproduced from Wouters KA et al. *Br J Haematol.* 2005;131:561–78. With permission.)

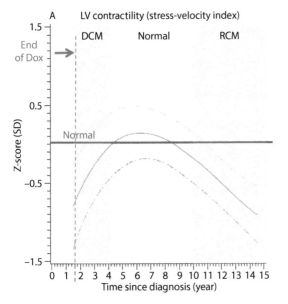

Figure 9.2 Changes in left ventricular structure and function over time, reported as Z-scores, from a study of 115 survivors of childhood acute lymphoblastic leukemia. Solid line, overall group means; dashed lines, upper and lower bounds of the 95% confidence interval for left ventricular contractility (LV stress-velocity index). Dox, doxorubicin; DCM, dilated cardiomyopathy; RCM, restrictive cardiomyopathy. (Modified from Lipshultz SE et al. *J Clin Oncol.* 2005;23:2629–63.)

in the LV over time. This study also reported that even survivors who received low cumulative doses of anthracyclines were still at risk for chronic cardiotoxicity years after therapy, indicating that there is no safe dose of anthracyclines (15).

At a mean of 17-years after treatment, in 115 survivors, LV dimension-to-body-surface area had decreased and LV thickness-to-body-surface area subsequently increased, resulting in a normal LV thickness-to-dimension ratio, indicating ventricular remodeling (Figure 9.3). This shrinking myocardial cavity for body surface area, which we have called "Grinch Syndrome," indicating a heart too small for body size, is a chronic cardiomyopathy, which may lead to HF, heart transplantation, or premature death in long-term survivors (65).

The restrictive-like nature of anthracycline cardiotoxicity may be important because it suggests that theories and treatments based on studies of dilated cardiomyopathy may not help understand anthracycline cardiotoxicity over a lifetime (66). Abnormal LV structure and function, as well as a restrictive-like cardiomyopathy, are also found in other long-term follow-up studies of other anthracycline-treated survivors (67–69). Endomyocardial biopsies from survivors with chronic anthracycline cardiotoxicity show both individual cardiomyocyte hypertrophy and cytoplasmic and nuclear enlargement (12,13). These biopsies have also revealed varying degrees of interstitial fibrosis, which may partially explain the restrictive-like cardiomyopathy seen in survivors.

CARDIOTOXICITY FROM RADIOTHERAPY

In survivors of childhood and adolescent cancer, radiotherapy (RT) that exposes the heart to radiation can increase the incidence of several cardiac abnormalities, as well as death (70,71). Such therapy includes mediastinal irradiation for Hodgkin's lymphoma (HL), cranial-spinal irradiation for

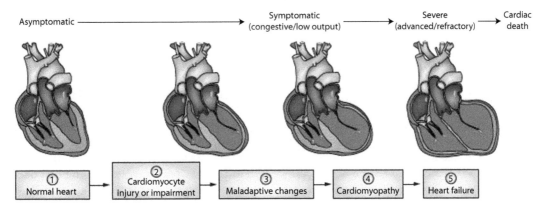

Figure 9.3 Stages in the development of pediatric ventricular dysfunction. (Permission from Nature Publishing Group, Lipshultz SE et al. *Nat Rev Clin Oncol.* 2013;10:697–710.)

high-risk acute lymphoblastic lymphoma and brain cancer, and abdominal irradiation for Wilms' tumor (72,73). Although this review focuses primarily on cardiac complications, RT that exposes the carotid arteries can increase the risk of stroke in survivors of childhood cancer, which must also be remembered when caring for survivors of brain cancer and HL (74,75). Additionally, survivors treated with high doses of cranial radiation are more likely to have hormonal abnormalities that can increase the incidence of elevated CVD risk factors, such as hypothyroidism, obesity, and hypertension (76–79).

The direct effects of therapeutic doses of radiation to the heart can cause several cardiac complications, including myocardial infarction (MI), cardiomyopathy and HF, valvular defects, arrhythmia, and pericarditis (Table 9.2). The common pathological mechanism of cardiac radiation injury appears to be the destruction of the cardiac microcirculation, which leads to further cell death through ischemia and finally, fibrosis (80,81); however, the pathological mechanism for valvular defects remains unclear because they are avascular.

Historically, RT was not focused, thereby affecting multiple structures in the mediastinum (heart, lungs, thyroid, skeletal muscle). This approach increased the risk of cardiac complications (Table 9.3). Although less likely to be a problem with the more focused methods of delivering RT used in the past two decades, these effects should be considered, especially in those survivors treated with older RT techniques.

Generally, the time between treatment and a marked increase in the risk of cardiovascular complications is 5–15 years, but this period depends on the particular side effect, the cumulative dose of radiation, other cardiotoxic therapies received, and baseline cardiovascular risk factors (Table 9.4) (10,17). Cumulative dose to the heart is by far the most important risk factor of radiotherapy. The overall risk of CVD caused by radiation is apparent amongst the 4,122 childhood cancer survivors in Great Britain and France, diagnosed before 1986, in whom the CVD death rate was 5 times as high as that in the age-matched general population. The risk of CVD death is statistically significantly higher than that in non-irradiated survivors at a mean cardiac dose of 5Gy or higher (10).

MI causes more than two-thirds of the cardiac deaths among patients with HL treated with radiation (82,83). With older RT techniques, including cumulative doses greater than 40Gy, the risk of fatal MI was 41.5 times as high among survivors of childhood HL than among the age-matched general population (72). Among children with a variety of childhood malignancies treated with RT in the Childhood Cancer Survivors Study, the risk of MI was dose-dependent and was significantly greater only among those receiving 15Gy or more compared to those treated without cardiac radiation (17). Myocardial infarction presents in this population as it does in the general population, with two exceptions. Survivors are less likely to feel cardiac pain caused by radiation-induced nerve fibrosis, and their baseline b-type natriuretic peptide (BNP) concentrations and possibly troponin concentrations are elevated (6,70,84).

Cardiomyopathy

Cardiac dysfunction caused by radiation differs from that caused by anthracyclines. Radiation causes myocardial fibrosis, which leads to a restrictive cardiomyopathy characterized by diastolic dysfunction. In survivors treated only with anthracyclines, systolic dysfunction is usually the primary abnormality, although those treated as children have important aspects of diastolic dysfunction with increasing follow-up as well (19). Nevertheless, given high enough doses and longer lengths of time in follow-up mediastinal RT has been shown to lead to systolic dysfunction (70).

Many studies have documented the fact that the impact of mediastinal radiation is greater on LV diastolic dysfunction than on LV systolic dysfunction (16,85–87). Diastolic dysfunction ranges from 12% to 83% at a mean of 15–17 years after diagnosis, whereas the prevalence of LV systolic dysfunction ranges from 9% to 36%. Cardiac event-free survival is substantially worse, as is quality of life, in survivors of HL with LV diastolic dysfunction than in those without it (6,82). For example, among 48 survivors of HL treated with mediastinal RT between 15 and 25 years old, mostly without anthracyclines, 54% had an abnormal E/A ratio (a sign of possible diastolic dysfunction), 30% had abnormally low peak oxygen consumption during exercise, and less than 10% had abnormally low LVEFs (16). Further, peak oxygen consumption was correlated with worse quality of life at the time of screening and at follow-up about 5 years later

Table 9.2 Spectrum of radiation-induced cardiovascular disease

Manifestation	Comments	References
Pericarditis	1. During therapy—Associated with mediastinal tumor and some chemotherapeutic agents such as cyclophosphamide 2. Posttherapy—Acute effusion, chronic effusion, pericarditis, constrictive pericarditis	(80)
Myocarditis	1. Fibrosis secondary to microvasculature changes 2. Frequently with normal LV dimensions, LVEF, and LVFS as measured by radionuclide scan or echocardiogram 3. Can have progressive, restrictive cardiomyopathy with fibrosis. Can cause pulmonary vascular disease and pulmonary hypertension 4. Diastolic dysfunction often occurs alone as well as with systolic dysfunction	(80,190)
Coronary artery disease	1. Premature fibrosis and also probably accelerates atherosclerosis 2. Distribution of arteries affected tend to be anterior with anterior weighted therapy 3. Lesions tend to be proximal and even ostial 4. ↑ Rates of silent ischemia, acute MI and possibly the proportion of clinically unsuspected MIs (see autonomic effects)	(80,81,191,192)
Valvular disease	1. Left-sided valve damage predominates 2. ↑ Regurgitation and stenosis with ↑ time since therapy 3. May progress to significant disease 10–20 years later, even in those with normal valves at the completion of therapy	(16,85,92)
Conduction system/ arrhythmia	1. High rate of complete or incomplete right bundle branch block is suggestive of right bundle branch fibrosis 2. Can progress to complete heart block and cause HF, requiring a pacemaker 3. Complete heart block rarely occurs without other radiation-induced abnormalities to the heart 4. ↑ Left ventricular fibrosis associated with ↑ high grade ventricular ectopic activity 5. ↑ Right atrial pressure associated with ↑ risk of atrial arrhythmia	(193)
Autonomic dysfunction	1. Frequent cardiac dysfunction with tachycardia, loss of circadian rhythm and respiratory phasic heart rate variability 2. This is similar to a denervated heart, suggesting autonomic nervous system damage 3. ↓ Perception of anginal pain	(16)
Vascular changes	1. May cause significant pulmonary artery stenosis and hypoplasia, especially in those treated in early childhood	(190)

Source: Adams MJ et al. Radiation. In: Crawford MH, DiMarco JP, eds. *Cardiology*. London: Mosby International Ltd; 2001; pp. 8.15.1–8. With permission.

(16,88). The prevalence of LV dysfunction increases with higher radiation dose volumes, higher anthracycline doses, and longer follow-up. Prevalence also depends on the screening modality.

Radiation increases the cardiotoxicity of anthracyclines. In long-term survivors of childhood cancer, LV function is lower in those who received anthracyclines and chest radiation than it is in those who received chest radiation alone and lower than that seen in those who received anthracyclines alone at a substantially higher mean total dose (89). In a Dutch cohort of survivors of HL

Table 9.3 Indirect effects of mediastinal radiation on the cardiovascular system

Manifestation	Comments	References
Mediastinal fibrosis	↓ Success of cardiovascular surgery	(194,5)
Lung fibrosis	Chronic, restrictive and can be progressive	(66)
Scoliosis and ↓ skeletal muscle	↓ Cardiovascular and lung function	(66)
Thyroid	Usually hypothyroid	(71)
	Affects cardiovascular function and lipid profile	

Source: Modified from Adams MJ et al. Radiation. In: Crawford MH, DiMarco JP, eds. Cardiology. London: Mosby International Ltd; 2001. pp. 8.15.1–8. With permission.
Note: Indirect effects based on survivors treated with older RT techniques so may be delayed or less frequent with modern RT techniques.

diagnosed before age 41 between 1965 and 1995, anthracyclines greatly increased the risks of HF and valvular disorders over those from mediastinal RT alone, which was already two to seven times higher for MI, angina, HF, and valvular disorders (90). The 25 year cumulative incidence of HF was 10.7% after combined RT and anthracycline therapy but just 7.5% after RT alone.

Valvular disease

Several studies have documented increased valvular abnormalities after RT. The pathologic mechanism is unclear. The fact that changes to valves on the left side of the heart are more common and severe than changes to those on the right side, regardless of dose distribution, suggests that the higher pressures of the systemic circulation are important in pathogenesis (81,91). Among the 48 survivors of HL treated between the ages of 15 and 25, in which only four received anthracyclines, 20 (42%) had rates of mitral and/or aortic regurgitation higher than expected in the general population (16). Another study of HL survivors treated with RT at any age reported higher than expected rates of valve surgeries and coronary revascularization procedures 10–20 years after therapy (92). Both the 1986 British-French study and the Childhood Cancer Survivor Study previously cited confirmed that the risk of valvular disease increases with radiation dose and that the incidence increases with time since diagnosis (10,17).

Other cardiovascular effects

Pericarditis, with or without effusion, may have been one of the most severe effects from very high dose RT. Pericarditis can occur during therapy, in which it is associated with tumors near the heart, but it occurs more often as soon as 4 months or up to years after RT. However, with the longstanding limitation of daily fraction size, changes in techniques, and efforts to limit cumulative doses, the incidence of radiation-associated, delayed acute and chronic pericarditis has fallen substantially (93). Nevertheless, the RT-related potential for increased fibrosis in the pericardial sac and damage to the lymphatic vessels draining it should be considered when planning cardiac surgeries, even in survivors treated with more modern RT techniques. In survivors, pericarditis can remain clinically silent or present with the sudden onset of typical signs and symptoms: pleuritic chest pain, dyspnea, fever, friction rub, ST segment and T-wave changes, and decreased QRS voltage.

Arrhythmias related to RT range from severe, life-threatening heart block to subtle changes in heart rate variability, each of which can occur years after therapy. They both result from fibrosis of the myocardial cells involved with conduction or damage to the nerves innervating the heart (e.g., the vagal nerve), and are a late consequence of cardiomyopathy. Serious abnormalities reported after RT include atrioventricular nodal bradycardia and all levels of heart block, including complete heart block and sick sinus syndrome (70). A more recent case series at one institution suggests that, in survivors, the length of the QTc interval and radiation dose are associated with later new-onset LV dysfunction, as detected by echocardiography (94).

CARDIOTOXICITY FROM OTHER CHEMOTHERAPIES COMMONLY USED IN CHILDREN

Chemotherapeutic agents commonly used to treat childhood cancers, other than anthracyclines and RT, can also be cardiotoxic. The most rapidly

Table 9.4 Risk factors for the different manifestations of radiation-induced heart diseases

Risk factor	Pericarditis	CM	CAD	Arrhythmia	Valvular disease	All causes CD	References
Total dose; (≥15 Gy) (>35 Gy)	X	X	X	X	X	X	(17,69,80,85)
Fractionated dose; (≥2.0 Gy a day)	X	X	X	Likely	Likely	X	(80)
Volume of heart exposed	X	X	X	Likely	Likely	X	(80)
Relative weighting of radiation portals and thus how much radiation is delivered to different parts of the heart and not using subcarinal blocking	X	X	X	Likely	Likely		(72,80,82)
The presence of tumor next to the heart	X	–	–	–	–	–	(80)
Younger age at exposure	–	X	X	Likely	Likely	X	(80,82)
Increased time since exposure	–	X	X	X	X	X	(17,91,193)
Type of radiation source	X	X	X	Likely	Likely	X	(80)
Use of adjuvant cardiotoxic chemotherapy	–	X	–	X	X	X	(80)
The presence of other known risk factors in each individual such as current age, weight, lipid profile, and habits such as smoking	–	–	X	–	–	X	(80)

Source: Updated from Adams MJ et al. Radiation. In: Crawford MH, DiMarco JP, eds. *Cardiology.* London: Mosby International Ltd; 2001·pp. 8.15.1–8. With permission.
Abbreviations: – = no known association; likely = unknown but likely association; X = associations of specific risk factors with specific presentation. CAD = coronary artery disease, CD = cardiac death, CM = cardiomyopathy.

growing class of chemotherapeutic drugs used in childhood cancers are tyrosine kinase inhibitors (TKIs) (95,96). These drugs are primarily used to treat cancer in adults; however, they are of interest in treating cancer in children because their ubiquitous nature creates viability in many types of cancer development. TKIs are not solely selective for cancer cells, so they can cause adverse cardiac effects, including arrhythmias, myocardial injury, and HF in adults (97,98). Because their use in treating childhood cancer is limited, the cardiac effects of TKIs in children are unknown, but worthy of attention.

Most of what is known about the cardiotoxicity caused by TKIs comes from the commonly used TKI such as imatinib (99,100). Trastuzumab inhibits the HER2 receptor, which is overexpressed in 20%–30% of women with breast cancer and is associated with more aggressive disease (100). Although effective, trastuzumab is associated with an increased incidence of HF, both when used as monotherapy and when used with other cardiotoxic treatments, such as anthracyclines and alkylating agents (101). Although trastuzumab is likely to remain limited to treating breast cancer, other TKIs are increasingly used to treat a variety of childhood cancers (102,103). Short- and long-term monitoring of the cardiac status of children exposed to TKIs will be important in evaluating these drugs.

Imatinib is highly effective in treating several types of cancer, most notably chronic myelogenous leukemia. Imatinib has been associated with cardiac injury, but only rarely (104). Despite a lack of evidence-based guidelines, patients with cardiac disease or those at risk of LV dysfunction should be carefully monitored during treatment with imatinib because many patients with imatinib-related HF also appear to have had other risk factors before treatment, such as HF, coronary disease, or high arterial blood pressure. Cardiac troponin T (cTnT) concentrations are a good indicator of cardiac damage after imatinib treatment (105,106).

In a retrospective study of 219 patients with sarcoma treated with imatinib, cardiac complications were rare (107). Less severe cardiotoxic effects, such as edema or effusions, occurred in 8.2% of these patients. A recent prospective study of 59 patients with chronic myeloid leukemia treated with imatinib for 3.4 years found no evidence of myocardial deterioration (108). Although similar reports show that imatinib is less cardiotoxic than other chemotherapies, such as the anthracyclines, its long-term consequences are largely unknown, especially when it is administered with other cardiotoxic agents and to children or adolescents.

MONITORING CARDIOTOXICITY

Anthracycline-induced cardiomyopathy

Given the long-term effects of chemotherapy on the cardiovascular system, cancer survivor clinician groups have recommended regular surveillance for patients receiving cardiotoxic treatments (71,109,110). Surveillance should include a physical examination, diagnostic testing (EKG, echocardiography), and assessing and managing other factors that can increase the risk of CVD (obesity, hypertension, smoking, and diabetes).

ASSESSMENT DURING CHEMOTHERAPY

Early monitoring is important to identify subtle abnormalities that might potentially be reversible (109,111). Moreover, early monitoring would provide data that could be monitored over time to identify any abnormalities. Although several groups have recommended monitoring guidelines, none are evidence-based.

Among monitoring guidelines published between 1966 and 2006 (112), only one by Steinherz et al., proposed guidelines for monitoring children during and after anthracycline chemotherapy (113). This guideline proposed changing cancer chemotherapy, given abnormal cardiac findings. Unfortunately, none of the studies cited in these guidelines prospectively evaluated the effects of changing an anthracycline dose on cardiac function, oncologic efficacy, and overall mortality (114). Adjusting doses based primarily on changes in LVFS and LVEF could harm patients without the purported benefit.

The modalities often used to monitor these patients include EKG, echocardiography, cardiac magnetic resonance imaging (MRI), radionuclide angiography, and serum biomarker concentrations (115).

Electrocardiograms are mainly used to monitor QTc intervals because many chemotherapeutic agents, such as amsacrine, arsenic trioxide, TKIs, and anthracyclines, can prolong QTc intervals (116–121).

Echocardiography continues to be the most commonly used modality to assess cancer patients during chemotherapy because it is widely available, easy to use, and noninvasive (112). However, traditional measures of evaluating function (LVFS and LVEF) are load-dependent measures and may not detect early abnormalities in cardiac function (122). These traditional measures include strain imaging, myocardial performance index, LV end-systolic wall stress, and the velocity of circumferential fiber shortening. Although most of the newer modalities have not been used during treatment, their utility has been evaluated in long-term follow-up. Among 14 asymptomatic patients with normal LVEFs treated with anthracyclines, 2D-strain imaging found regional wall motion abnormalities (123). Dobutamine stress-testing echocardiography and measuring LV end-systolic wall stress have also been suggested for identifying subtle cardiac dysfunction (124,125). Magnetic resonance imaging provides better assessments of cardiac function, especially in children with poor acoustic windows. Also, fibrosis and perfusion abnormalities can also be assessed; however, MRI can be more time-consuming and can require sedating young children. In anthracycline-treated children, MRI can detect acute and chronic subclinical cardiotoxicity (126). In 10 women with breast cancer and trastuzumab-induced cardiomyopathy, MRI revealed late gadolinium enhancement along the subepicardial lateral wall in all 10 (127).

ASSESSMENT AFTER CHEMOTHERAPY

The most common measures used in serial follow-up of patients with anthracycline-related cardiomyopathy are LVFS and LVEF (113). However, as mentioned previously, these measures may not detect subclinical cardiotoxicity, which may occur in up to 60% of treated patients (128). Moreover, LVFS and LVEF are load-dependent measures. Recently, strain and strain-rate imaging measured by speckle tracking echocardiography has been used. Among 56 asymptomatic patients evaluated 2–15 years after anthracycline treatment (doses <300 mg/m^2), although traditional measures of ventricular function (LVFS and LVEF) did not differ, systolic myocardial deformation decreased, as did radial and longitudinal peak systolic strain (69). However, long-term evaluations of pediatric cancer survivors exposed to cancer chemotherapeutics using strain imaging have not been validated.

FREQUENCY OF MONITORING

The goal of routine monitoring is to identify children at highest risk of developing cardiovascular dysfunction. The hope is that identifying at-risk children early can allow interventions to stop further cardiovascular deterioration. Unfortunately, many recommendations for guiding clinicians are not evidence-based. The 2004 Children's Oncology Group guidelines provide recommendations for the long-term follow-up of cancer survivors (128) (Table 9.5). These guidelines provide a framework for identifying what needs to be assessed (history, physical exam, EKG, and echocardiographic measures) in patients at highest risk for cardiovascular dysfunction. European guidelines on evaluating patients with treated HL suggest that EKG should be performed at every visit, whereas screening for coronary artery disease and valvular disease should start 10 years after RT (129). Such tests should be repeated every 5 years or when new symptoms of CVD arise.

CARDIAC BIOMARKERS FOR FOLLOWING PATIENTS WITH CHEMOTHERAPY-INDUCED CARDIOTOXICITY

Biomarkers of cardiac toxicity (cTnT, cardiac troponin I [cTnI], and N-terminal pro-brain natriuretic peptide [NT-proBNP]) are being used to monitor cancer survivors. In 201 survivors, some exposed to both anthracyclines and radiation and some unexposed, concentrations of NT-proBNP and markers of cardiometabolic dysfunction (non-high-density lipoprotein cholesterol, insulin, and C-reactive protein concentrations) were higher in survivors than in their sibling controls during a median follow-up of 11 years (6). These data suggest that cancer survivors, either with or without exposure to anthracyclines and radiation, are at increased risk for cardiovascular dysfunction. Another study in patients with high-risk ALL showed that both cTnT and NT-proBNP concentrations increased during the first 90 days of therapy with doxorubicin (130). The rise in cTnT concentrations was associated with reduced LV mass and LV end-diastolic posterior wall thickness 4 years later. Moreover, a rise in NT-proBNP concentrations was also related to an abnormal LV thickness-to-dimension ratio 4 years later. These data suggest that cTnT and NT-proBNP may be used to detect cardiotoxicity in these patients.

Table 9.5 Monitoring cardiovascular disease in cancer survivors

Therapeutic agent	Potential late effect	Highest risk factor	Recommendation	Guideline score
Anthracyclines	Cardiomyopathy	<5 years old at time of treatment	Annual history and physical examination	1
	Arrhythmias	Female gender	Baseline echocardiography or multiple gated acquisition scan, then periodically, with frequency based on age at treatment, radiation dose, and cumulative anthracycline dose	
			Baseline electrocardiogram for evaluation of QTc	
	Subclinical left	Black or of African descent		
	Ventricular dysfunction	*Cumulative dose:* 300 mg/m^2 (<18 years of age at time of treatment), 550 mg/m^2 (age ≥18 years at time of treatment), any dose in infants; chest radiation: ≥30 Gy longer time elapsed since treatment		
Mediastinal radiation	Congestive heart failure	Female gender	Annual history and physical examination	1
	Cardiomyopathy	Black or of African descent	Baseline echocardiography, then periodically, with frequency based on age at treatment, radiation dose, and cumulative anthracycline dose	
	Pericarditis	<5 years old at time of treatment		
	Pericardial fibrosis	Anteriorly weighted radiation fields		
	Valvular disease	Lack of subcarinal shielding		
	Myocardial infarction	Doses of ≥30 Gy in patients who have received anthracyclines	Baseline electrocardiogram for evaluation of QTc	
	Arrhythmia			
	Atherosclerotic heart disease	Doses of ≥40 Gy in patients who have not received anthracyclines Longer time since treatment	Fasting glucose and lipid profile every 3–5 years	
Neck radiation of ≥40 Gy	Carotid and subclavian artery disease	NA	Annual history and physical examination; Doppler ultrasound as clinically indicated	2A

Source: From Shankar SM et al. *Pediatrics.* 2008;121(2):e387–96.
NA, not applicable.

Radiation-induced cardiotoxicity

Consensus guidelines and statements by the pediatric cardiology and pediatric oncology communities provide reasonable minimum standards and suggestions for screening, although no screening regimens have been rigorously tested (71,109,131). As in survivors treated with cardiotoxic chemotherapies, screening should be long-term and guided by the frequency and intensity of risk factors (Table 9.4). On the other hand, all survivors treated with thoracic RT should be monitored continually for traditional CVD risk factors, such as obesity, hypertension, dyslipidemias, and diabetes, because of survivors' known increased risk, the large public health burden of CVD, and the availability of effective preventive measures. Screening should begin soon after therapy, regardless of the patient's age, given that fatal MIs have occurred in survivors during adolescence. Radiation exposure should be considered a risk factor when using general population guidelines to determine the need for and goal of therapy (132).

Serial echocardiographic examinations are important for assessing cardiac anatomy, such as the pericardium, ventricular walls, and valves in patients treated with RT. Particular attention must be paid to diastolic function because diastolic dysfunction is more likely to occur than systolic dysfunction in survivors treated with thoracic RT.

Exercise or pharmacologic stress testing augments the diagnosis of ischemic heart disease and cardiac dysfunction compared to rest-only studies. Radionuclide myocardial perfusion imaging during exercise is 90% sensitive and specific for ischemic heart disease in the general population; however, its sensitivity and specificity in irradiated patients has not been well studied. Myocardial perfusion imaging appears to detect radiation-induced microvascular damage in the myocardium, but the ability of perfusion scanning to distinguish microvascular abnormalities from coronary heart disease in this population is unclear (133). Detecting microvascular damage, however, may identify survivors at highest risk for HF and death from cardiac causes, although this relationship requires further study (134,135).

Peak oxygen consumption, which can be measured during exercise stress tests, can be prognostic in patients with cardiomyopathy (136,137). Peak oxygen consumption is surprisingly low in many patients with a history of mediastinal irradiation, including those who do not have symptoms of cardiac dysfunction (16,138). Of all the measures of cardiac status analyzed, maximal oxygen consumption was the only one highly correlated with the physical component of quality of life on the 36-Item Short Form Health Survey (the SF36) (16). The extent to which pulmonary dysfunction, which correlates with quality of life in HL survivors treated with mediastinal RT, decreases maximal oxygen consumption is unclear (139).

Although screening for electrical conduction abnormalities and arrhythmias may be reasonable in theory because they may remain silent until fatal, these abnormalities may not occur frequently enough to warrant screening all survivors who received mediastinal RT. The prognostic value of the various nonspecific conduction abnormalities observed in this population also remain unknown.

MANAGING CARDIOMYOPATHY

Preventing cardiotoxicity

Preventing anthracycline-induced cardiotoxicity has long been a priority. Proposed methods include concomitant use of dexrazoxane and changing anthracycline dosing and formulations (e.g., liposomal anthracyclines and anthracycline analogs).

DEXRAZOXANE

In the 1980s, a study in dogs revealed that dexrazoxane was superior to *n*-acetyl cysteine in preventing doxorubicin-induced chronic cardiotoxicity (140). This finding was confirmed in a randomized trial of 92 women with advanced breast cancer, in which dexrazoxane did not reduce the efficacy of chemotherapy (141). A subsequent trial revealed that the incidence of cardiac events (HF, decline in LVEF $\geq$20% points, decline from baseline $\geq$10%, and decline to below the institutional lower limit of normal or to $\geq$5% below institutional lower limit of normal) was 3.5 times lower in women with metastatic breast cancer receiving dexrazoxane than in those receiving the placebo during chemotherapy with fluorouracil, doxorubicin, and cyclophosphamide (142).

Dexrazoxane acts by chelating iron, thus preventing myocardial damage secondary to reactive oxygen species (71,112,143,144). Dexrazoxane also reduces doxorubicin-induced DNA damage,

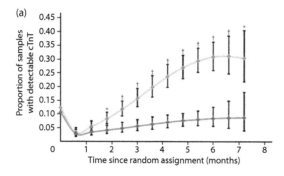

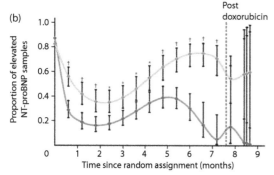

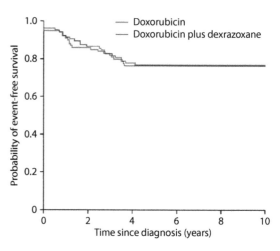

Figure 9.5 Event-free survival. All patients randomly assigned to treatment (n = 205) were eligible for assessment of event-free survival, but by convention, events of induction failure and induction death have been recorded at 0 years. (From Lipshultz SE et al. *Lancet Oncol.* 2010;11:950–61.)

Figure 9.4 A model-based estimated probability of having an increased cardiac troponin T (cTnT) concentration at each depicted time point in patients treated with doxorubicin with or without dexrazoxane. (From Lipshultz SE et al. *J Clin Oncol.* 2012;30:1042–9.)

perhaps by the formation of Top2-DNA covalent complexes (145).

Children with high-risk ALL treated with dexrazoxane and doxorubicin had better LVFS and LV end-systolic dimension Z-scores 5 years after completing treatment than children who did not receive dexrazoxane (143). This study also showed that the effect was greater in girls treated with dexrazoxane. Moreover, another study on the same cohort suggested that the dexrazoxane-treated group had lower concentrations of cTnT (a marker of cardiac injury) and NT-proBNP (a maker of cardiac stress) at the end of chemotherapy (Figure 9.4) (130).

An apparent increased risk of secondary malignancies in patients treated with dexrazoxane raised concern, but the conclusions from this study have been questioned (146–148). Subsequent studies have found that dexrazoxane does not increase the incidence of malignancies (Figure 9.5) (143,149,150).

ANTHRACYCLINE DOSING

That higher cumulative doses of anthracyclines lead to progressive declines in cardiac function years later is well documented (13,15,151). In 189 children with ALL, cardiac dysfunction was unlikely when the total anthracycline dose was less than 300 mg/m^2 (152); although, lowering the total dose to prevent cardiotoxicity may be appealing, it may also reduce efficacy (153). Moreover, there is no absolute safe lower limit for anthracyclines at which cardiotoxicity will not occur (15).

LIPOSOMAL ANTHRACYCLINE

Encapsulating an anthracycline in a liposome allows it to accumulate in the tumor, which reduces its concentration in plasma and cardiomyocytes and thus reduces cardiotoxicity (154,155). This formulation reduces cardiotoxicity without reducing efficacy (156,157).

ANTHRACYCLINE ANALOGS

No extensive clinical trials in children have compared the efficacy of analogs to conventional anthracyclines in preventing cardiotoxicity, but a few studies have shown promise. Epirubicin, an epimer of doxorubicin, reduced cardiotoxicity in 172 children with soft tissue sarcoma (158). Idarubicin is a structural analog of daunorubicin.

In children less than 14 years old with acute myelogenous leukemia, idarubicin was more effective than daunorubicin in achieving complete remission (71% vs. 58%, respectively; $p = 0.03$) (159); however, the incidence of HF did not differ significantly between groups (25% vs. 31%).

Mitoxantrone, an anthracenedione derivative, is believed to reduce cardiotoxicity. However, a meta-analysis of 16 studies evaluating its cardiotoxic profile found that the true incidence of mitoxantrone-induced cardiotoxicity could not be evaluated because the studies had serious methodological limitations (160). The authors suggested it might be premature to conclude that mitoxantrone is less-cardiotoxic than conventional anthracyclines.

CONTINUOUS ANTHRACYCLINE INFUSION

Some studies have suggested that giving anthracycline over 6 hours or as 48–96 hour continuous infusions may reduce cardiotoxicity. However, one randomized trial found that the cardiotoxicity profiles of children with high-risk ALL receiving doxorubicin infusion over 48 hours did not differ significantly from those receiving bolus doses (161–163). In another study of children receiving daunorubicin over 6 hours, cardiotoxicity profiles again did not differ from those receiving bolus doses after a mean follow-up of 5 years (164).

Treating cardiomyopathy

Beta-blockers and angiotensin converting enzyme (ACE) inhibitors are the standard of care in managing patients with depressed ventricular function (165). Patients with chemotherapy-induced cardiotoxicity may present later with features of dilated cardiomyopathy or restrictive cardiomyopathy. Hence, management should be based on the presenting phenotype.

ANGIOTENSIN CONVERTING ENZYME INHIBITORS

The ability of ACE inhibitors to treat anthracycline-induced cardiomyopathy has generated interest (66). A review evaluating the efficacy of enalapril in 18 long-term survivors treated with doxorubicin revealed that, although LV dimension, LV afterload, LVFS, and LV mass improved during the first 6 years of therapy, LV dysfunction subsequently progressed between 6 and 10 years

(166). A randomized, double-blind controlled clinical trial comparing enalapril to placebo in 135 long-term survivors of childhood cancer revealed that enalapril lowered LV end-systolic wall stress but did not significantly improve maximal cardiac index, LVFS, or LVEF (167). These results could have been related to the small sample size or to an inadequate follow-up period (median time 3 years) (66). In both studies, LV wall stress declined without ventricular remodeling, which is often seen in patients with dilated cardiomyopathy treated with ACE inhibitors. In fact, patients treated with anthracyclines often have a restrictive phenotype, which does not respond well to ACE inhibitors. Unfortunately, given the lack of robust data on the long-term efficacy of ACE inhibitors in treating anthracycline-induced cardiomyopathy, its use in this condition remains debated (66,167). In the After Anthracycline (AAA) Study, the incidence of hypotension and fatigue was significantly higher in patients receiving enalapril than in those receiving placebo (22% vs. 3%; $p < 0.001\%$, 10% vs. 0%, $p = 0.01$), respectively (167). Some data suggest an increased risk of malignancy in adults on prolonged ACE inhibitor therapy (168). More importantly, ACE inhibitors can have teratogenic effects (169). In addition, because no study has clearly shown that ACE inhibitors improve health-related quality of life or prevent HF or death, the wisdom of using them in the absence of proven efficacy is uncertain (170).

BETA-BLOCKERS

Beta-blockers decrease progression of myocardial dysfunction and can even reverse remodeling when used in patients with dilated cardiomyopathy (171). In a small case series of children with anthracycline-induced cardiomyopathy already taking other HF medications, beta-blockers improved New York Heart Association class and LVFS (172). Another study of adults compared the effects of beta-blockers in patients with doxorubicin-induced cardiomyopathy to those in patients with idiopathic-dilated cardiomyopathy. Left ventricular ejection fraction improved to the same extent in both groups, suggesting that its efficacy in patients with anthracycline-related cardiomyopathy is similar to that in cardiomyopathies with other causes (173).

Carvedilol is a combination of a nonselective beta-blocker and an α-1 blocker. In rats, its antioxidant activity protected against doxoru-bicin-induced mitochondrial damage (174). In children with ALL, pretreatment with carvedilol before Adriamycin administration reduced tro-ponin I and lactate dehydrogenase concentra-tions after treatment more than concentrations in patients not pretreated with carvedilol. Also, pretreated patients had significantly higher LVFS and global peak systolic strain than did nontreated patients (175). In a more recent randomized trial in women with breast cancer about to receive anthra-cyclines, prophylactic carvedilol preserved LVEF and significantly lowered cTnI concentrations 30 days after treatment (176).

MECHANICAL CIRCULATORY SUPPORT DEVICES AND TRANSPLANTATION

Cancer survivors who are refractory to stan-dard medical management for HF may require advanced therapies, including mechanical circula-tory support devices and/or heart transplantation. Patients with active malignancy can be palliated using mechanical support devices as destination therapy when they are not transplant candidates (177). However, in patients with no active malig-nancy, heart transplant has been performed with success (178). A multi-institutional study of pedi-atric heart transplant centers revealed that patients with anthracycline cardiomyopathy can be trans-planted successfully with 1-, 2-, and 5-year surviv-als of 100%, 92%, and 60% respectively (179).

CARDIOMETABOLIC MORBIDITIES IN CHILDHOOD CANCER SURVIVORS

The burden of chronic health conditions in survi-vors of childhood cancer is substantial and vari-able. The St. Jude Lifetime Cohort Study collected data on all chronic conditions in patients treated for childhood cancer at the St. Jude Children's Research Hospital who survived 10 years or lon-ger after their initial diagnosis. The mean number of chronic CVD (grades 1 through 5) per survivor nearly quadrupled, from 1.2 at age 30 years to 4.4 by age 50 years. In contrast, the burden of chronic health conditions for other organ systems started high and only slowly increased with age (5).

Cardiovascular disease is the leading noncan-cer contributor to early morbidity and mortal-ity in survivors of childhood cancer in the USA

(7,11,71,180–182). Survivors of childhood cancer also have a risk of ischemic heart disease and stroke that is more than 10 times higher than that of their siblings. Variations in cancer treat-ment exposures, such as dose-dependent, chest-directed RT and anthracycline chemotherapy, genetic predisposition, and conventional cardio-vascular risk factors, such as hypertension, dyslip-idemia, and diabetes, contribute to this increased risk among childhood cancer survivors (183). Participants in the Childhood Cancer Survivor Study ($n = 13,060$) were observed through age 50 years for the development of ischemic heart disease and stroke. The cumulative incidences of heart disease and stroke at age 50 years were less than 5% among the low-risk groups but about 20% for high-risk groups ($p < 0.001$). The cumula-tive incidence of CVD was only 1% for siblings ($p < 0.001$) (184). Much of the information avail-able immediately after children and adolescents complete cancer treatment accurately predicts subsequent heart disease and stroke and thus should be considered when planning screening and intervention strategies.

Increasing evidence indicates that children who survive cancer are at a greater risk for metabolic syndrome, which puts them at greater risk for CVD. Among 165 child survivors of ALL treated with contemporary therapy, 17% were overweight, 21.2% were obese, and 15.3% had blood pressures meeting stage 1+ hypertension thresholds. The highest category of corticosteroid exposure, com-pared to the lowest, was associated with both obe-sity and stage 1+ hypertension (185).

In another report from the St. Jude Lifetime Cohort Study of adult survivors of childhood can-cer, with a median age of 33 years, metabolic syn-drome was present in 32.5% of men and 31.0% of women, with high blood pressure and low HDL concentrations being the most prevalent compo-nents of metabolic syndrome in men and women, respectively (186). Furthermore, of the 1598 sur-vivors examined, 33% had abnormal fasting glu-cose concentrations and 47% had hypertension (186). Although these numbers are similar to those reported for large cohorts, such as the National Health and Nutrition Survey (NHANES) in the general population that link the incidence of meta-bolic syndrome to poor dietary and lifestyle hab-its, the high prevalence among a younger cohort of childhood cancer survivors indicates that this population is particularly vulnerable to risk factors for cardiac disease, such as the components of metabolic syndrome. Moreover, young survivors with these acquired modifiable cardiovascular risk factors, particularly hypertension, are at increased risk for severe, life-threatening, and fatal (grades 3–5) cardiac events (183). Thus, early diagnosis and appropriate management of hypertension, diabetes, dyslipidemia, and obesity in at-risk, aging survivors may substantially reduce their risk of premature cardiac disease.

HEALTH-RELATED QUALITY OF LIFE IN SURVIVORS OF PEDIATRIC CANCER

As the number of childhood cancer survivors has increased to nearly 80%, investigating health-related quality of life is imperative. The late effects of cancer treatment on survivors are present even a short time after treatment. Contemporary studies indicate that a substantial number of survivors present different long-term side effects that influence their quality of life. In a Polish study of 1761 childhood cancer survivors, 1557 (88.25%) had one or more symptoms or reports suggesting organ dysfunction. These symptoms suggested problems with circulation, the urinary tract, skin, teeth, and the musculoskeletal system. Of the entire cohort, 21% were obese or had short-stature syndrome (187). Health-related abnormalities can have direct effects on both mental and physical quality of life summaries.

Among 75 long-term survivors of ALL diagnosed in childhood and adolescence and diagnosed more than 10 years before the study, 12% of women and 18% of men were frankly obese by World Health Organization criteria, which is associated with an adverse impact on overall health-related quality of life (188).

In a retrospective study, 91 cancer survivors and 223 healthy controls completed the Pediatric Quality of Life Inventory 4.0 and the Hopkins Symptom Checklist-10 as a measure of health-related quality of life and distress. Survivors reported lower physical functioning health-related quality of life than did healthy controls. This result likely reflects a greater vulnerability to treatment-related toxicities (189).

Health-related quality of life in pediatric cancer survivors is tied to late effects of cancer treatment.

Minimizing these late effects will improve their health-related quality of life.

CONCLUSION

Over the last four decades, there has been a lot of advances in managing children with various malignancies. Cancer survivors exposed to anthracyclines and RT experience cardiotoxic effects. Early recognition of such cardiovascular comorbidities is beneficial. Therapies should be aimed to reduce cardiotoxicity while maintaining oncologic efficacy. Such survivors will benefit from long-term follow-up with cardiologists, however the optimal screening for these patients still needs to be determined.

REFERENCES

1. Howlader NNA et al. SEER Cancer statistics review. 1975–2014. Available from: https://seer.cancer.gov/csr/1975_2014/. Last accessed June 11, 2018.
2. Siegel RL, Miller KD, Jemal A. Cancer statistics, 2015. *Cancer J Clin.* 2015;65(1):5–29.
3. Scully RE, Lipshultz SE. Anthracycline cardiotoxicity in long-term survivors of childhood cancer. *Cardiovasc Toxicol.* 2007;7(2):122–8.
4. Didcock E et al. Pubertal growth in young adult survivors of childhood leukemia. *J Clin Oncol.* 1995;13(10):2503–7.
5. Bhakta N et al. The cumulative burden of surviving childhood cancer: An initial report from the St Jude lifetime cohort study (SJLIFE). *Lancet Oncol.* 2017;390(10112):2569–82.
6. Lipshultz SE et al. Cardiovascular status of childhood cancer survivors exposed and unexposed to cardiotoxic therapy. *J Clin Oncol.* 2012;30(10):1050–7.
7. Oeffinger KC et al. Chronic health conditions in adult survivors of childhood cancer. *N Engl J Med.* 2006;355(15):1572–82.
8. Mertens AC et al. Cause-specific late mortality among 5-year survivors of childhood cancer: The Childhood Cancer Survivor Study. *J Natl Cancer Inst.* 2008;100(19):1368–79.
9. Garwicz S et al. Late and very late mortality in 5-year survivors of childhood cancer: Changing pattern over four decades—experience from the Nordic countries. *Int J Cancer.* 2012;131(7):1659–66.

10. Tukenova M et al. Role of cancer treatment in long-term overall and cardiovascular mortality after childhood cancer. *J Clin Oncol.* 2010;28(8):1308–15.

11. Mulrooney DA et al. Cardiac outcomes in adult survivors of childhood cancer exposed to cardiotoxic therapy: A cross-sectional study. *Ann Intern Med.* 2016;164(2):93–101.

12. Goorin AM et al. Initial congestive heart failure, six to ten years after doxorubicin chemotherapy for childhood cancer. *J Pediatr.* 1990;116(1):144–7.

13. Lipshultz SE et al. Late cardiac effects of doxorubicin therapy for acute lymphoblastic leukemia in childhood. *N Engl J Med.* 1991;324(12):808–15.

14. Lipshultz SE et al. Female sex and drug dose as risk factors for late cardiotoxic effects of doxorubicin therapy for childhood cancer. *N Engl J Med.* 1995;332(26):1738–43.

15. Lipshultz SE et al. Chronic progressive cardiac dysfunction years after doxorubicin therapy for childhood acute lymphoblastic leukemia. *J Clin Oncol.* 2005;23(12):2629–36.

16. Adams MJ et al. Cardiovascular status in long-term survivors of Hodgkin's disease treated with chest radiotherapy. *J Clin Oncol.* 2004;22(15):3139–48.

17. Mulrooney DA et al. Cardiac outcomes in a cohort of adult survivors of childhood and adolescent cancer: Retrospective analysis of the Childhood Cancer Survivor Study cohort. *BMJ.* 2009;339:b4606.

18. Levitt G et al. Cardiac or cardiopulmonary transplantation in childhood cancer survivors: An increasing need? *Eur J Cancer.* 2009;45(17):3027–34.

19. Lipshultz SE, Adams MJ. Cardiotoxicity after childhood cancer: Beginning with the end in mind. *J Clin Oncol.* 2010;28(8):1276–81.

20. Leger K et al. Subclinical cardiotoxicity in childhood cancer survivors exposed to very low dose anthracycline therapy. *Pediatr Blood Cancer.* 2015;62(1):123–7.

21. Silverman LB et al. Long-term results of Dana-Farber Cancer Institute ALL Consortium protocols for children with newly diagnosed acute lymphoblastic leukemia (1985–2000). *Leukemia.* 2010;24(2):320–34.

22. Alvarez JA et al. Long-term effects of treatments for childhood cancers. *Curr Opin Pediatr.* 2007;19(1):23–31.

23. Von Hoff DD et al. Daunomycin-induced cardiotoxicity in children and adults: A review of 110 cases. *Am J Med.* 1977;62(2):200–8.

24. Sarosiek KA et al. Developmental regulation of mitochondrial apoptosis by c-Myc governs age- and tissue-specific sensitivity to cancer therapeutics. *Cancer Cell.* 2017;31(1):142–56.

25. Lipshultz SE, Alvarez JA, Scully RE. Anthracycline associated cardiotoxicity in survivors of childhood cancer. *Heart.* 2008; 94(4):525–33.

26. Lebrecht D et al. Time-dependent and tissue-specific accumulation of mtDNA and respiratory chain defects in chronic doxorubicin cardiomyopathy. *Circ J.* 2003;108(19):2423–9.

27. Minotti G et al. Anthracyclines: Molecular advances and pharmacologic developments in antitumor activity and cardiotoxicity. *Pharmacol Rev.* 2004;56(2):185–229.

28. Horenstein MS, Vander Heide RS, L'Ecuyer TJ. Molecular basis of anthracycline-induced cardiotoxicity and its prevention. *Mol Genet Metab.* 2000;71(1–2):436–44.

29. Gianni L et al. Anthracycline cardiotoxicity: From bench to bedside. *J Clin Oncol.* 2008;26(22):3777–84.

30. Doroshow JH, Locker GY, Myers CE. Enzymatic defenses of the mouse heart against reactive oxygen metabolites: Alterations produced by doxorubicin. *J Clin Invest.* 1980;65(1):128–35.

31. Nicolay K et al. Effects of adriamycin on lipid polymorphism in cardiolipin-containing model and mitochondrial membranes. *Biochim Biophys Acta.* 1985;819(1):55–65.

32. Leonard RC et al. Improving the therapeutic index of anthracycline chemotherapy: Focus on liposomal doxorubicin (Myocet). *Breast.* 2009;18(4):218–24.

33. Ashley N, Poulton J. Mitochondrial DNA is a direct target of anti-cancer anthracycline drugs. *Biochem Biophys Res Commun.* 2009;378(3):450–5.

34. Wallace KB. Doxorubicin-induced cardiac mitochondrionopathy. *Pharmacol Toxicol.* 2003;93(3):105–15.

35. Thompson KL et al. Early alterations in heart gene expression profiles associated with doxorubicin cardiotoxicity in rats. *Cancer Chemother Pharamcol.* 2010;66(2):303–14.

36. Chen B et al. Molecular and cellular mechanisms of anthracycline cardiotoxicity. *Cardiovasc Toxicol.* 2007;7(2):114–21.

37. Ito H et al. Doxorubicin selectively inhibits muscle gene expression in cardiac muscle cells in vivo and in vitro. *Proc Natl Acad Sci USA.* 1990;87(11):4275–9.

38. Peng X, Chen B, Lim CC, Sawyer DB. The cardiotoxicology of anthracycline chemotherapeutics: Translating molecular mechanism into preventative medicine. *Mol Interv.* 2005;5(3):163–71.

39. De Angelis A et al. Anthracycline cardiomyopathy is mediated by depletion of the cardiac stem cell pool and is rescued by restoration of progenitor cell function. *Circulation.* 2010;121(2):276–92.

40. Kalyanaraman B et al. Doxorubicin-induced apoptosis: Implications in cardiotoxicity. *Mol Cell Biochem.* 2002;234–235(1–2):119–24.

41. Jurcut R et al. Detection and monitoring of cardiotoxicity-what does modern cardiology offer? *Support Care Cancer.* 2008;16(5):437–45.

42. Rusconi P et al. Carvedilol in children with cardiomyopathy: 3-year experience at a single institution. *J Heart Lung Transplant.* 2004;23(7):832–8.

43. Lowis S et al. A phase I study of intravenous liposomal daunorubicin (DaunoXome) in paediatric patients with relapsed or resistant solid tumours. *Br J Cancer.* 2006;95(5):571–80.

44. Lebrecht D et al. Tissue-specific mtDNA lesions and radical-associated mitochondrial dysfunction in human hearts exposed to doxorubicin. *J Pathol.* 2005;207(4):436–44.

45. Ryberg M et al. New insight into epirubicin cardiac toxicity: Competing risks analysis of 1097 breast cancer patients. *J Natl Cancer Inst.* 2008;100(15):1058–67.

46. Tokarska-Schlattner M, Zaugg M, Zuppinger C, Wallimann T, Schlattner U. New insights into doxorubicin-induced cardiotoxicity: The critical role of cellular energetics. *J Mol Cell Cardiol.* 2006;41(3):389–405.

47. Zhang S et al. Identification of the molecular basis of doxorubicin-induced cardiotoxicity. *Nat Med.* 2012;18(11):1639–42.

48. Khiati S et al. Mitochondrial topoisomerase I (top1 mt) is a novel limiting factor of doxorubicin cardiotoxicity. *Clin Cancer Res.* 2014;20(18):4873–81.

49. Tewey KM et al. Adriamycin-induced DNA damage mediated by mammalian DNA topoisomerase II. *Science.* 1984;226(4673):466–8.

50. Lyu YL et al. Topoisomerase IIbeta mediated DNA double-strand breaks: Implications in doxorubicin cardiotoxicity and prevention by dexrazoxane. *Cancer Res.* 2007;67(18):8839–46.

51. Ong DS et al. Radiation-associated valvular heart disease. *J Heart Valve Dis.* 2013;22(6):883–92.

52. Vejpongsa P, Yeh ET. Topoisomerase 2beta: A promising molecular target for primary prevention of anthracycline-induced cardiotoxicity. *Clin Pharmacol Ther.* 2014;95(1):45–52.

53. Giantris A et al. Anthracycline-induced cardiotoxicity in children and young adults. *Crit Rev Oncol Hematol.* 1998;27(1):53–68.

54. Adams MJ, Lipshultz SE. Pathophysiology of anthracycline- and radiation-associated cardiomyopathies: Implications for screening and prevention. *Pediatric Blood Cancer.* 2005;44(7):600–6.

55. Krischer JP et al. Clinical cardiotoxicity following anthracycline treatment for childhood cancer: The pediatric oncology group experience. *J Clin Oncol.* 1997;15(4):1544–52.

56. Bristow MR et al. Doxorubicin cardiomyopathy: Evaluation by phonocardiography, endomyocardial biopsy, and cardiac catheterization. *Ann Intern Med.* 1978;88(2):168–75.

57. Barry E et al. Anthracycline-induced cardiotoxicity: Course, pathophysiology, prevention and management. *Expert Opin Pharmacother.* 2007;8(8):1039–58.

58. Grenier MA, Lipshultz SE. Epidemiology of anthracycline cardiotoxicity in children and adults. *Semin Oncol.* 1998;25(4 Suppl 10):72–85.

59. Kremer LC et al. Anthracycline-induced clinical heart failure in a cohort of 607 children: Long-term follow-up study. *J Clin Oncol.* 2001;19(1):191–6.

60. Kim DH et al. Doxorubicin-induced calcium release from cardiac sarcoplasmic reticulum vesicles. *J Molec Cell Biol.* 1989;21(5):433–6.

61. Ali MK et al. Late doxorubicin-associated cardiotoxicity in children. The possible role of intercurrent viral infection. *Cancer.* 1994;74(1):182–8.

62. Steinherz LJ, Steinherz PG, Tan C. Cardiac failure and dysrhythmias 6–19 years after anthracycline therapy: A series of 15 patients. *Med Pediatr Oncol.* 1995;24(6):352–61.

63. Steinherz LJ et al. Cardiac toxicity 4 to 20 years after completing anthracycline therapy. *JAMA.* 1991;266(12):1672–7.

64. Kremer LC et al. Frequency and risk factors of anthracycline-induced clinical heart failure in children: A systematic review. *Annal Oncol.* 2002;13(4):503–12.

65. Lipshultz SE et al. Hearts too small for body size after doxorubicin for childhood leukemia: Grinch syndrome. *J Clin Oncol.* 2014;32:10021.

66. Lipshultz SE, Colan SD. Cardiovascular trials in long-term survivors of childhood cancer. *J Clin Oncol.* 2004;22(5):769–73.

67. Armenian SH et al. Screening for cardiac dysfunction in anthracycline-exposed childhood cancer survivors. *Clin Cancer Res.* 2014;20(24):6314–23.

68. Sorensen K et al. Late anthracycline cardiotoxicity after childhood cancer: A prospective longitudinal study. *Cancer.* 2003;97(8):1991–8.

69. Ganame J et al. Myocardial dysfunction late after low-dose anthracycline treatment in asymptomatic pediatric patients. *J Am Soc Echocardiogr.* 2007;20(12):1351–8.

70. Adams MJ et al. Radiation-associated cardiovascular disease. *Crit Rev Oncol Hematol.* 2003;45(1):55–75.

71. Lipshultz SE et al. Long-term cardiovascular toxicity in children, adolescents, and young adults who receive cancer therapy: Pathophysiology, course, monitoring, management, prevention, and research directions: A scientific statement from the American Heart Association. *Circulation.* 2013;128(17):1927–95.

72. Hancock SL, Donaldson SS, Hoppe RT. Cardiac disease following treatment of Hodgkin's disease in children and adolescents. *J Clin Oncol.* 1993;11:1208–15.

73. Wright KD, Green DM, Daw NC. Late effects of treatment for Wilms tumor. *Pediatr Hematol Oncol.* 2009;26:407–13.

74. Bowers DC et al. Stroke as a late treatment effect of Hodgkin's disease: A report from the childhood cancer survivor study. *J Clin Oncol.* 2005;23(27):6508–15.

75. Bowers DC et al. Late-occurring stroke among long-term survivors of childhood leukemia and brain tumors: A report from the childhood cancer survivor study. *J Clin Oncol.* 2006;24(33):5277–82.

76. Oeffinger KC et al. Obesity in adult survivors of childhood acute lymphoblastic leukemia: A report from the childhood cancer survivor study. *J Clin Oncol.* 2003;21(7):1359–65.

77. Miller TL et al. Characteristics and determinants of adiposity in pediatric cancer survivors. *Cancer Epidemiol.* 2010;19(8):2013–22.

78. Constine LS et al. Hypothalamic-pituitary dysfunction after radiation for brain tumors. *N Engl J Med.* 1993;328(2):87–94.

79. Duffner PK. Long-term effects of radiation therapy on cognitive and endocrine function in children with leukemia and brain tumors. *Neurologist.* 2004;10(6):293–310.

80. Stewart JR et al. Radiation injury to the heart. *Int J Radiat Oncol Biol Phys.* 1995;31(5):1205–11.

81. Veinot JP, Edwards WD. Pathology of radiation-induced heart disease: A surgical and autopsy study of 27 cases. *Human Path.* 1996;27(8):766–73.

82. Mauch PM et al. Long-term survival in Hodgkin's disease: Relative impact of mortality, second tumors, infection and cardiovascular disease. *Cancer J Sci Am.* 1995;1:33–42.

83. Hoppe RT. Hodgkin's disease: Complications of therapy and excess mortality. *Ann Oncol.* 1997;8(Suppl 1):115–8.

84. Mavinkurve-Groothuis AM et al. Abnormal NT-pro-BNP levels in asymptomatic long-term survivors of childhood cancer treated with anthracyclines. *Acta Pediatri.* 2009;52:631–6.

85. Heidenreich PA et al. Asymptomatic cardiac disease following mediastinal irradiation. *J Am Coll Cardiol*. 2003;42(4):743–9.

86. Heidenreich PA et al. Diastolic dysfunction after mediastinal irradiation. *Am Heart J*. 2005;150(5):977–82.

87. Iarussi D et al. Evaluation of left ventricular function in long-term survivors of childhood Hodgkin disease. *Pediatr Blood Cancer*. 2005;45(5):700–5.

88. Adams MJ et al. Peak oxygen consumption in Hodgkin's lymphoma survivors treated with mediastinal radiotherapy as a predictor of quality of life 5 years later. *Prog Pediatr Cardiol*. 2015;39(2A):93–8.

89. Pihkala J et al. Myocardial function in children and adolescents after therapy with anthracyclines and chest irradiation. *Eur J Cancer*. 1996;32A(1):97–103.

90. Aleman BM et al. Late cardiotoxicity after treatment for Hodgkin lymphoma. *Blood*. 2007;109(5):1878–86.

91. Carlson RG et al. Radiation-associated valvular disease. *Chest*. 1991;99(3):538–45.

92. Hull MC et al. Valvular dysfunction and carotid, subclavian, and coronary artery disease in survivors of Hodgkin lymphoma treated with radiation therapy. *JAMA*. 2003;290(21):2831–7.

93. Carmel RJ, Kaplan HS. Mantle irradiation in Hodgkin's disease. *Cancer*. 1976;37:2813–5.

94. Markman TM et al. Electrophysiological effects of anthracyclines in adult survivors of pediatric malignancy. *Pediatr Blood Cancer*. 2017;64(11).

95. Krause DS, Van Etten RA. Tyrosine kinases as targets for cancer therapy. *N Engl J Med*. 2005;353(2):172–87.

96. Drake JM, Lee JK, Witte ON. Clinical targeting of mutated and wild-type protein tyrosine kinases in cancer. *Molec Cell Biol*. 2014;34(10):1722–32.

97. Guglin M, Cutro R, Mishkin JD. Trastuzumab-induced cardiomyopathy. *J Card Fail*. 2008;14(5):437–44.

98. Baron KB et al. Trastuzumab-induced cardiomyopathy: Incidence and associated risk factors in an inner-city population. *J Card Fail*. 2014;20(8):555–9.

99. Tan-Chiu E et al. Assessment of cardiac dysfunction in a randomized trial comparing doxorubicin and cyclophosphamide followed by paclitaxel, with or without trastuzumab as adjuvant therapy in node-positive, human epidermal growth factor receptor 2–overexpressing breast cancer: NSABP B-31. *J Clin Oncol*. 2005;23(31):7811–9.

100. Toikkanen S et al. Prognostic significance of HER-2 oncoprotein expression in breast cancer: A 30-year follow-up. *J Clin Oncol*. 1992;10(7):1044–8.

101. Sivagnanam K, Rahman ZU, Paul T. Cardiomyopathy associated with targeted therapy for breast cancer. *Am J Med Sci*. 2016;351(2):194–9.

102. Lee-Sherick AB et al. Efficacy of a Mer and Flt3 tyrosine kinase small molecule inhibitor, UNC1666, in acute myeloid leukemia. *Oncotarget*. 2015;6(9):6722.

103. Furman WL et al. Tyrosine kinase inhibitor enhances the bioavailability of oral irinotecan in pediatric patients with refractory solid tumors. *J Clin Oncol*. 2009;27(27):4599–604.

104. Kerkelä R et al. Cardiotoxicity of the cancer therapeutic agent imatinib mesylate. *Nature Med*. 2006;12(8):908–16.

105. Herman EH et al. A multifaceted evaluation of imatinib-induced cardiotoxicity in the rat. *Toxicol Pathol*. 2011;39(7):1091–106.

106. Atallah E et al. Congestive heart failure is a rare event in patients receiving imatinib therapy. *Blood*. 2007;110(4):1233–7.

107. Trent JC et al. Rare incidence of congestive heart failure in gastrointestinal stromal tumor and other sarcoma patients receiving imatinib mesylate. *Cancer*. 2010;116(1):184–92.

108. Estabragh ZR et al. A prospective evaluation of cardiac function in patients with chronic myeloid leukaemia treated with imatinib. *Leuk Res*. 2011;35(1):49–51.

109. Shankar SM et al. Monitoring for cardiovascular disease in survivors of childhood cancer: Report from the Cardiovascular Disease Task Force of the Children's Oncology Group. *Pediatrics*. 2008;121(2):e387–96.

110. Armenian SH et al. Recommendations for cardiomyopathy surveillance for survivors of childhood cancer: A report from the International Late Effects of Childhood Cancer Guideline Harmonization Group. *Lancet Oncol*. 2015;16(3):e123–36.

111. Fulbright JM. Review of cardiotoxicity in pediatric cancer patients: During and after therapy. *Cardiol Res Pract.* 2011;2011.

112. van Dalen EC et al. Anthracycline-induced cardiotoxicity: Comparison of recommendations for monitoring cardiac function during therapy in paediatric oncology trials. *Eur J Cancer.* 2006;42(18):3199–205.

113. Steinherz LJ et al. Guidelines for cardiac monitoring of children during and after anthracycline therapy: Report of the Cardiology Committee of the Children's Cancer Study Group. *Pediatrics.* 1992;89(5):942–9.

114. Lipshultz SE et al. Monitoring for anthracycline cardiotoxicity. *Pediatrics.* 1994;93(3):433–7.

115. Altena R et al. Cardiovascular toxicity caused by cancer treatment: Strategies for early detection. *Lancet Oncol.* 2009;10(4):391–9.

116. Louie AC, Issell B. Amsacrine (AMSA)–a clinical review. *J Clin Oncol.* 1985;3(4):562–92.

117. Weiss RB et al. Amsacrine-associated cardiotoxicity: An analysis of 82 cases. *J Clin Oncol.* 1986;4(6):918–28.

118. Huang SY et al. Acute and chronic arsenic poisoning associated with treatment of acute promyelocytic leukaemia. *Br J Haematol.* 1998;103(4):1092–5.

119. DuBois SG et al. Phase I and pharmacokinetic study of sunitinib in pediatric patients with refractory solid tumors: A children's oncology group study. *Clin Cancer Res.* 2011;17(15):5113–22.

120. Bagnes C, Panchuk PN, Recondo G. Antineoplastic chemotherapy induced QTc prolongation. *Curr Drug Saf.* 2010;5(1):93–6.

121. Albini A et al. Cardiotoxicity of anticancer drugs: The need for cardio-oncology and cardio-oncological prevention. *J Nat Cancer Instit.* 2010;102(1):14–25.

122. Colan SD, Borow KM, Neumann A. Left ventricular end-systolic wall stress-velocity of fiber shortening relation: A load-independent index of myocardial contractility. *J Am Coll Cardiol.* 1984;4(4):715–24.

123. Park JH et al. Cardiac functional evaluation using vector velocity imaging after chemotherapy including anthracyclines in children with cancer. *Korean Circ J.* 2009;39(9):352–8.

124. Yıldırım A et al. Early diagnosis of anthracycline toxicity in asymptomatic long-term survivors: Dobutamine stress echocardiography and tissue Doppler velocities in normal and abnormal myocardial wall motion. *Euro J of Echocardio.* 2010;11(10):814–22.

125. Iarussi D et al. Left ventricular systolic and diastolic function after anthracycline chemotherapy in childhood. *Clin Cardiol.* 2001;24(10):663–9.

126. Oberholzer K et al. Anthracycline-induced cardiotoxicity: Cardiac MRI after treatment for childhood cancer. *Rofo.* 2004;176(9):1245–50.

127. Fallah-Rad N et al. Delayed contrast enhancement cardiac magnetic resonance imaging in trastuzumab induced cardiomyopathy. *J Cardiovas Magn Reson.* 2008;10(1):5.

128. Landier W et al. Development of risk-based guidelines for pediatric cancer survivors: The Children's Oncology Group Long-term Follow-up Guidelines from the Children's Oncology Group Late Effects Committee and Nursing Discipline. *J Clin Oncol.* 2004;22(24):4979–90.

129. van Leeuwen-Segarceanu EM et al. Screening Hodgkin lymphoma survivors for radiotherapy induced cardiovascular disease. *Cancer Treat Rev.* 2011;37(5):391–403.

130. Lipshultz SE et al. Changes in cardiac biomarkers during doxorubicin treatment of pediatric patients with high-risk acute lymphoblastic leukemia: Associations with long-term echocardiographic outcomes. *J Clin Oncol.* 2012;30(10):1042–9.

131. Sieswerda E et al. The Dutch Childhood Oncology Group guideline for follow-up of asymptomatic cardiac dysfunction in childhood cancer survivors. *Ann Oncol.* 2012;23(8):2191–8.

132. Stone NJ et al. 2013 ACC/AHA guideline on the treatment of blood cholesterol to reduce atherosclerotic cardiovascular risk in adults. *Cardiology.* 2014;129:S1–45.

133. Pierga JY et al. Follow-up thallium-201 scintigraphy after mantle field radiotherapy for Hodgkin's disease. *Int J Radiat Oncol Biol Phys.* 1993;25(5):871–6.

134. Yu X et al. Symptomatic cardiac events following radiation therapy for left-sided breast cancer: Possible association with radiation therapy-induced changes in regional perfusion. *Clin Breast Cancer.* 2003;4(3):193–7.

135. Marks LB et al. Functional consequences of radiation (RT)-induced perfusion changes in patients with left-sided breast cancer. *Int J Radiat Oncol Biol Phys*. 2002;54.

136. Aaronson KD, Mancini DM. Is percentage of predicted maximal exercise oxygen consumption a better predictor of survival than peak exercise oxygen consumption for patients with severe heart failure? *J Heart Lung Transplant*. 1995;14(5):981–9.

137. Mancini DM et al. Value of peak exercise oxygen consumption for the optimal timing of cardiac transplantation in ambulatory patients with heart failure. *Circulation*. 1991;83:778–86.

138. Pihkala J et al. Cardiopulmonary evaluation of exercise tolerance after chest irradiation and anticancer chemotherapy in children and adolescents. *Pediatrics*. 1995;95:722–26.

139. Knobel H et al. Late medical complications and fatigue in Hodgkin's disease survivors. *J Clin Oncol*. 2001;19(13):3226–33.

140. Herman E et al. Comparison of the effectiveness of (±)-1, 2-bis (3, 5-dioxopiperazinyl-1-yl) propane (ICRF-187) and N-acetylcysteine in preventing chronic doxorubicin cardiotoxicity in beagles. *Cancer Res*. 1985;45(1):276–81.

141. Speyer JL et al. Protective effect of the bispiperazinedione ICRF-187 against doxorubicin-induced cardiac toxicity in women with advanced breast cancer. *N Engl J Med*. 1988;319(12):745–52.

142. Swain SM et al. Delayed administration of dexrazoxane provides cardioprotection for patients with advanced breast cancer treated with doxorubicin-containing therapy. *J Clin Oncol*. 1997;15(4):1333–40.

143. Lipshultz SE et al. Assessment of dexrazoxane as a cardioprotectant in doxorubicin-treated children with high-risk acute lymphoblastic leukaemia: Long-term follow-up of a prospective, randomised, multicentre trial. *Lancet Oncol*. 2010;11(10):950–61.

144. Lipinczyk T, Lipshultz S. Cardioprotective effects of dexrazoxane in children with acute lymphoblastic leukemia treated with doxorubicin: An overview. *Am J Oncol Rev*. 2005;4:103–16.

145. Lyu YL et al. Topoisomerase IIβ–mediated DNA double-strand breaks: Implications in doxorubicin cardiotoxicity and prevention by dexrazoxane. *Cancer Res*. 2007;67(18):8839–46.

146. Tebbi CK et al. Dexrazoxane-associated risk for acute myeloid leukemia/myelodysplastic syndrome and other secondary malignancies in pediatric Hodgkin's disease. *J Clin Oncol*. 2007;25(5):493–500.

147. Lipshultz SE, Lipsitz SR, Orav EJ. Dexrazoxane-associated risk for secondary malignancies in pediatric Hodgkin's disease: A claim without compelling evidence. *J Clin Oncol*. 2007;25(21):3179.

148. Hellmann K. Dexrazoxane-associated risk for secondary malignancies in pediatric Hodgkin's disease: A claim without evidence. *J Clin Oncol*. 2007;25(29):4689–90.

149. Barry EV et al. Absence of secondary malignant neoplasms in children with high-risk acute lymphoblastic leukemia treated with dexrazoxane. *J Clin Oncol*. 2008;26(7):1106–11.

150. Vrooman LM et al. The low incidence of secondary acute myelogenous leukaemia in children and adolescents treated with dexrazoxane for acute lymphoblastic leukaemia: A report from the Dana-Farber cancer institute ALL consortium. *Eur J Cancer*. 2011;47(9):1373–9.

151. Lipshultz SE et al. Female sex and higher drug dose as risk factors for late cardiotoxic effects of doxorubicin therapy for childhood cancer. *N Engl J Med*. 1995;332(26):1738–43.

152. Nysom K et al. Relationship between cumulative anthracycline dose and late cardiotoxicity in childhood acute lymphoblastic leukemia. *J Clin Oncol*. 1998;16(2):545–50.

153. Trachtenberg BH et al. Anthracycline-associated cardiotoxicity in survivors of childhood cancer. *Pediatr Cardiol*. 2011;32(3):342–53.

154. Fulbright JM et al. Can anthracycline therapy for pediatric malignancies be less cardiotoxic? *Curr Oncol Rep*. 2010;12(6):411–9.

155. Safra T. Cardiac safety of liposomal anthracyclines. *Oncologist*. 2003;8(Suppl 2):17–24.

156. Batist G et al. Reduced cardiotoxicity and preserved antitumor efficacy of liposome-encapsulated doxorubicin and cyclophosphamide compared with conventional doxorubicin and cyclophosphamide in a randomized, multicenter trial of metastatic breast cancer. *J Clin Oncol*. 2001;19(5):1444–54.

157. Harris L et al. Liposome-encapsulated doxorubicin compared with conventional doxorubicin in a randomized multicenter trial as first-line therapy of metastatic breast carcinoma. *Cancer.* 2002;94(1):25–36.

158. Stohr W et al. Comparison of epirubicin and doxorubicin cardiotoxicity in children and adolescents treated within the German Cooperative Soft Tissue Sarcoma Study (CWS). *J Cancer Res Clin Oncol.* 2006;132(1):35–40.

159. Vogler WR et al. A phase III trial comparing idarubicin and daunorubicin in combination with cytarabine in acute myelogenous leukemia: A Southeastern Cancer Study Group Study. *J Clin Oncol.* 1992;10(7):1103–11.

160. Van Dalen E et al. Cumulative incidence and risk factors of mitoxantrone-induced cardiotoxicity in children: A systematic review. *Eur J Cancer.* 2004;40(5):643–52.

161. Shapira J et al. Reduced cardiotoxicity of doxorubicin by a 6-hour infusion regimen. A prospective randomized evaluation. *Cancer.* 1990;65(4):870–3.

162. Hortobagyi GN et al. Decreased cardiac toxicity of doxorubicin administered by continuous intravenous infusion in combination chemotherapy for metastatic breast carcinoma. *Cancer.* 1989;63(1):37–45.

163. Lipshultz SE et al. Doxorubicin administration by continuous infusion is not cardioprotective: The Dana-Farber 91–01 Acute Lymphoblastic Leukemia protocol. *J Clin Oncol.* 2002;20(6):1677–82.

164. Levitt G et al. Does anthracycline administration by infusion in children affect late cardiotoxicity? *Brit J Haematol.* 2004;124(4):463–8.

165. Yancy CW et al. 2017 ACC/AHA/HFSA focused update of the 2013 ACCF/AHA guideline for the management of heart failure. *J Cardiac Fail.* 2017;23(8):628–51.

166. Lipshultz SE et al. Long-term enalapril therapy for left ventricular dysfunction in doxorubicin-treated survivors of childhood cancer. *J Clin Oncol.* 2002;20(23):4517–22.

167. Silber JH et al. Enalapril to prevent cardiac function decline in long-term survivors of pediatric cancer exposed to anthracyclines. *J Clin Oncol.* 2004;22(5):820–8.

168. Hallas J et al. Long term use of drugs affecting the renin-angiotensin system and the risk of cancer: A population-based case-control study. *Br J Clin Pharmacol.* 2012;74(1):180–8.

169. Cooper WO et al. Major congenital malformations after first-trimester exposure to ACE inhibitors. *N Engl J Med.* 2006;354(23):2443–51.

170. Bansal N et al. Chemotherapy-induced cardiotoxicity in children. *Expert Opin Drug Metab Toxicol.* 2017;13(8):817–32.

171. Bristow MR. Mechanism of action of beta-blocking agents in heart failure. *Am J Cardiol.* 1997;80(11):26L–40L.

172. Shaddy RE et al. Efficacy and safety of metoprolol in the treatment of doxorubicin-induced cardiomyopathy in pediatric patients. *Am Heart J.* 1995;129(1):197–9.

173. Noori A et al. β-Blockade in adriamycin-induced cardiomyopathy. *J Card Fail.* 2000;6(2):115–9.

174. Oliveira PJ et al. Carvedilol-mediated antioxidant protection against doxorubicin-induced cardiac mitochondrial toxicity. *Toxicol Appl Pharmacol.* 2004;200(2):159–68.

175. El-Shitany NA et al. Protective effect of carvedilol on adriamycin-induced left ventricular dysfunction in children with acute lymphoblastic leukemia. *J Card Fail.* 2012;18(8):607–13.

176. Nabati M et al. Cardioprotective effects of carvedilol in inhibiting doxorubicin-induced cardiotoxicity. *J Card Pharmacol.* 2017;69(5):279–85.

177. Simsir SA et al. Left ventricular assist device as destination therapy in doxorubicin-induced cardiomyopathy. *Ann Thorac Surg.* 2005;80(2):717–9.

178. Arico M et al. Heart transplantation in a child with doxorubicin-induced cardiomyopathy. *N Engl J Med.* 1988;319(20):1353.

179. Ward KM et al. Pediatric heart transplantation for anthracycline cardiomyopathy: Cancer recurrence is rare. *J Heart Lung Transplant.* 2004;23(9):1040–5.

180. Reulen RC et al. Long-term cause-specific mortality among survivors of childhood cancer. *JAMA.* 2010;304(2):172–9.

181. van der Pal HJ et al. High risk of symptomatic cardiac events in childhood cancer survivors. *J Clin Oncol.* 2012;30(13):1429–37.

182. Haddy N, Diallo S, El-Fayech C, Schwartz B, Pein F, Hawkins M et al. Cardiac Diseases Following Childhood Cancer Treatment: Cohort Study. *Circulation*. 2016;133(1):31–8.

183. Armstrong GT et al. Modifiable risk factors and major cardiac events among adult survivors of childhood cancer. *J Clin Oncol*. 2013;31(29):3673–80.

184. Chow EJ et al. Prediction of ischemic heart disease and stroke in survivors of childhood cancer. *J Clin Oncol*. 2017;36 (1):44–52.

185. Chow EJ et al. Obesity and hypertension among children after treatment for acute lymphoblastic leukemia. *Cancer*. 2007;110(10):2313–20.

186. Smith WA et al. Lifestyle and metabolic syndrome in adult survivors of childhood cancer: A report from the St. Jude Lifetime Cohort Study. *Cancer*. 2014;120(17):2742–50.

187. Maryna K-R et al. Health status of Polish children and adolescents after cancer treatment. *Eur J Pediatr*. 2018;177(3):437–447.

188. Marriott CJ et al. Body composition in long-term survivors of acute lymphoblastic leukemia diagnosed in childhood and adolescence: A focus on sarcopenic obesity. *Cancer*. 2018;124(6):1225–31.

189. Halvorsen JF et al. Health-related quality of life and psychological distress in young adult survivors of childhood cancer and their association with treatment, education, and demographic factors. *Qual Life Res*. 2018;27(2):529–37.

190. Lipshultz SE, Sallan SE. Cardiovascular abnormalities in long-term survivors of childhood malignancy. *J Clin Oncol*. 1993;11: 1199–203.

191. Adams MJ et al. Cardiovascular status in long-term survivors of Hodgkin's disease treated with chest radiotherapy. *J Clin Oncol*. 2004;22(15):3139–48.

192. Brosius FC, Waller BF, Roberts WC. Radiation heart disease. Analysis of 16 young (aged 15–33 years) necropsy patients who received over 3,500 rads to the heart. *Am J Med*. 1981;70(3):519–30.

193. Slama MS et al. Complete atrioventricular block following mediastinal irradiation: A report of six cases. *Pacing Clin Electrophysiol*. 1991;14:1112–8.

194. Morton DL et al. Management of patients with radiation-induced pericarditis with effusion: A note on the development of regurgitation in two of them. *Chest*. 1973;64:291–7.

195. Adams MJ, Constine LS, Lipshultz SE. Radiation. In: Crawford MH, DiMarco JP, eds. *Cardiology*. London: Mosby International Ltd. 2001; pp. 8.15.1–8.

10

Cardio-oncology case studies

GREGORY R. HARTLAGE, PALMER H. COLE, AARTI A. PATEL, HASSAN TARIQ, SHETAL AMIN, MILLEE SINGH, CESAR ALBERTO MORALES-PABON, KRISTINA CAHILL, ANITA RADHAKRISHNAN, AND ERIC E. HARRISON

OVERVIEW

Cardio-oncology is a novel field, focused on minimizing cardiovascular morbidity and mortality in cancer survivors (1). This field is growing rapidly due to recognition that many effective cancer therapies may leave survivors at heightened risk for cardiovascular disease (2). To reduce this risk, cancer patients should be assessed at baseline to define their risk of cardiotoxicity and then followed closely during and after chemotherapy to assess for early signs and symptoms of cardiovascular disease. Cardiac imaging plays an essential role in the baseline assessment and serial follow-up in this patient population. In this chapter, we will present three case studies of patients encountered in cardio-oncology specialty clinics.

CASE 1

GREGORY R. HARTLAGE, PALMER H. COLE, AARTI A. PATEL, CESAR ALBERTO MORALES-PABON, ANITA RADHAKRISHNAN, AND ERIC E. HARRISON

Introduction

Doxorubicin is one of the most commonly used chemotherapeutic agents that has been shown to improve survival in breast cancer and hematological malignancies. Its use, however, is limited by its potential cardiotoxic effects such as heart disease, arrhythmias and cardiomyopathy leading to congestive heart failure (3). This case highlights the potential late consequences of doxorubicin therapy on cardiovascular health.

Case presentation

A 66-year-old African American woman was diagnosed with a lymph node negative, estrogen receptor positive, human epidermal growth factor receptor (HER-2) negative infiltrating ductal carcinoma 6 years prior. She had a left modified radical mastectomy followed by six cycles of 5-fluorouracil, doxorubicin, and cyclophosphamide and 5 years of tamoxifen. She now presents with symptoms of chest discomfort lasting 3 weeks in duration. Her electrocardiogram (EKG) was abnormal showing nonspecific T wave abnormalities. An echocardiogram revealed normal left ventricular (LV) size and systolic function, left ventricular ejection fraction (LVEF) of 57%, moderate mitral regurgitation (MR), and normal right ventricular systolic pressures (RVSP). Subsequent stress echocardiography was normal, showing no echocardiographic evidence of inducible ischemia or infarction. The patient was monitored closely and had an echocardiogram performed 2 years after the initial presentation (9 years postanthracycline). This revealed moderate to severe MR, left atrial enlargement (LAE), mildly dilated left ventricle with mild LV systolic dysfunction, and RVSP of 48 mm Hg consistent with moderate pulmonary hypertension (Table 10.1). The patient was asymptomatic at that time, but medical therapy for LV dysfunction was initiated, with a beta-blocker and angiotensin receptor blockade. Over the following 6 months, the patient developed a decrease in exercise tolerance, orthopnea, paroxysmal nocturnal dyspnea, lower extremity edema, and symptoms consistent with New York Heart Association class III/IV congestive heart failure. A transesophageal echocardiogram (TEE) was performed to further assess the mechanism of her MR. The TEE revealed moderate to severe functional MR from LV dilation. There were no structural abnormalities of the mitral valve leaflets or chordal structures, and her LVEF was estimated to be 35% (Figure 10.1).

The patient was treated medically, but due to frequent heart failure (HF) exacerbations, she was evaluated for mitral valve repair. Preoperative cardiac catheterization confirmed moderate to severe MR, but no obstructive coronary artery disease. The patient underwent robotic invasive mitral valve repair with placement of a #29 American Thoracic Society (ATS) annuloplasty ring. Her immediate postoperative recovery was uncomplicated, and she was discharged on the fourth postoperative day. After surgery, a TTE showed stable LV systolic function with an LVEF of 49%. The patient started cardiac rehabilitation and her functional status improved. At 10 months postmitral valve repair (10 years postanthracycline), the patient was admitted to the hospital with exertional shortness of breath and congestive heart failure. TTE revealed an ejection fraction of 26% with global LV dysfunction, a well-repaired mitral valve with trace MR, and an RVSP of 45 mm Hg. The patient was instructed to continue valsartan and change atenolol to carvedilol. Aldactone was added to her therapy and there was up-titration of her diuretic regimen. The patient was monitored clinically every few months and by 2 years postmitral valve repair (12 years postanthracycline) her LVEF improved to 45% on medical therapy (Table 10.1). At 3 years postmitral valve repair (13 years postanthracycline), her LV systolic function had recovered and normalized

with a LVEF of 60% (Table 10.1). Her most recent echocardiogram, 20 years since her initial anthracycline exposure, revealed a preserved LV systolic function, with average peak global longitudinal strain of −16.5% (Figure 10.2).

Discussion

Doxorubicin cardiotoxicity can have an acute, subacute, or late presentation (4). Here, we present a classic example of late presentation valvular disease and cardiomyopathy. Six years after anthracycline exposure and a cumulative dose of 300 mg/m^2, the patient started showing signs of valvular dysfunction, although one can argue that diastolic dysfunction likely preceded this. The initial insult to her myocardium resulting in mild LV systolic dysfunction and abnormal myocardial contractile reserve was likely related to her anthracycline exposure. She subsequently developed functional secondary MR owing to a dilated left ventricle. Significant MR causes a low resistance pathway for LV systolic ejection owing to the relatively lower pressure in the left atrium compared to the aorta, which reduces overall LV afterload. Owing to the removal of the low resistance regurgitant lesion with surgical correction, LV afterload can increase significantly after mitral valve repair or replacement (5). The increase in LV afterload is likely what precipitated her subsequent decompensation with further reduction in LVEF after her mitral valve repair (6,7). Owing to the risk of overt cardiomyopathy with reduced LVEF after surgical MR correction, optimization of medical therapy prior to intervention is prudent. Left ventricular dysfunction can improve with aggressive goal directed medical therapy for heart failure with reduced ejection fraction (HFrEF), including aldosterone antagonists, in patients with anthracycline-induced cardiomyopathy.

The most commonly accepted pathophysiological mechanism of anthracycline-induced cardiotoxicity is related to topoisomerase (Top) 2-alpha (8). Top 2-alpha, which is overexpressed in tumors, is the cellular target for the drug's anticancer effect. DNA damage via Top2-beta (expressed in adult cardiomyocytes) leading to cardiomyocyte death has recently been implicated as a major mechanism of anthracycline-related cardiomyopathy. Cardiotoxicity is cumulative and typically occurs at an average total dose of 400 mg/m^2; however,

Table 10.1 Overview of changes from anthracycline exposure, MV repair, relevant echocardiography findings, medications, and changes to medications from June 2002 through April 2010

	06.14.2002	06.22.2004	12.14.2006	03.22.2007	07.02.2007	04.07.2008	08.25.2008	06.01.2009	04.13.2010
Time since AC exposure (months)	67	92	121	125	128	137	142	151	161
Time since MV repair (days)	–	–	–	–	11	291	431	711	1027
MR grade[a]	2+	1+	3+	3–4+	0	0–1+	2+	1+	0
LVEF	57%	50%	48%	48%	49%	26%	20%	45%	60%
LVEDD (mm)	50	52	60	52	48	53	52	42	38
LVESD (mm)	36	37	45	40	36	47	47	30	26
RSVP (mmHg)	37	37	32	43	–	45	–	42	30
Medications	Atenolol 50 mg	Atenolol 50 mg	Atenolol 50 mg	Atenolol 50 mg, Valsartan 80 mg	Atenolol 50 mg, Valsartan 80 mg	Atenolol 50 mg, Valsartan 80 mg	Carvedilol 25 mg BID, Valsartan 80 mg	Carvedilol 25 mg BID, Valsartan 80 mg, Spironolactone 25 mg	Carvedilol 25 mg BID, Valsartan 80 mg, Spironolactone 25 mg
Medication changes			Added Valsartan 80 mg			Changed atenolol to carvedilol 25 mg BID	Added spironolactone 25 mg		

Abbreviation: AC, anthracycline; LVEDD, left ventricular end diastolic diameter; LVEF, left ventricular ejection fraction; LVESD, left ventricular end systolic diameter; MR, mitral regurgitation; MV, mitral valve; RVSP, right ventricular systolic pressure.

a MR grading: 0—none, 1+—mild, 2+—moderate, 3+—moderate to severe, 4+—severe.

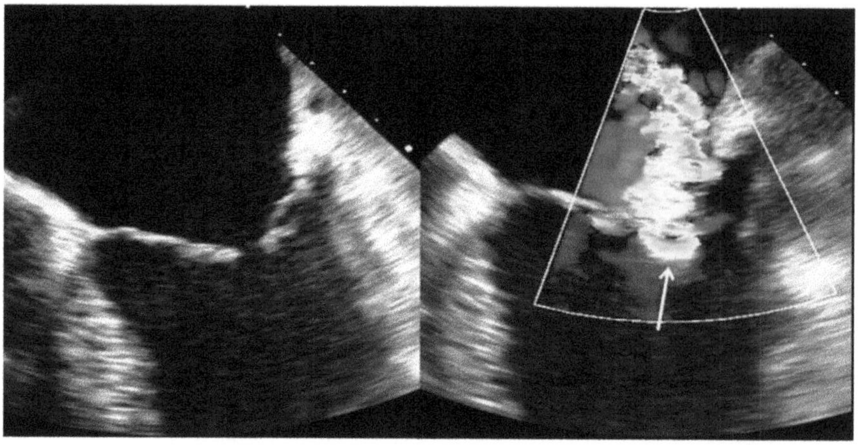

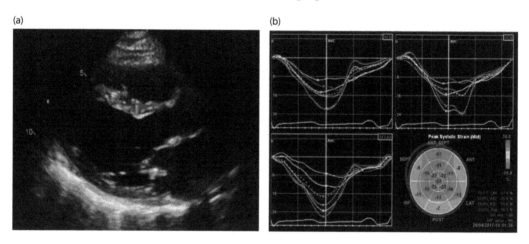

Figure 10.1 A mid-esophageal view illustrating functional mitral regurgitation owing to poor coaptation of the mitral leaflets. The arrow points to severe mitral regurgitation.

(a)

(b)

Figure 10.2 Panel (a): Parasternal long axis view showing reduction in LV size, s/p mitral valve annuloplasty ring from our patient. Panel (b): Strain profiles from three apical views. Speckle-tracking echocardiography analyses of three apical views in the apical 4, 2-chamber and apical long-axis view with the respective speckle-tracking echocardiography measurements. Strain (y-axis) plotted over time (x-axis) for each LV segment with a color-coded linear graphical display. Average peak global longitudinal strain of −16.5%.

studies (9) have shown that cardiotoxicity can occur at a cumulative dose of as low as 240 mg/m² (10).

Based on current guidelines, all patients should receive a baseline clinical cardiovascular assessment including history and physical examination, baseline cardiac risk factor modification, cardiac biomarkers including high sensitivity troponin and BNP, and LV function assessment by echocardiogram prior to initiation of anthracycline-based therapy. For patients with no history of HF with baseline LVEF ≥50%, the patient's cardiovascular status should be optimized with special attention to blood pressure control (11). For patients with current or past HFrEF (LVEF ≤45%), anthracycline

chemotherapy should generally be avoided. If the clinical benefit is felt to outweigh the risks, informed and shared decision-making with the patient should occur. Strategies to reduce cardiotoxicity should be considered with liposomal formulation of doxorubicin, continuous infusion or dexrazoxane. Medical management typically consists of an angiotensin-converting enzyme (ACE) inhibitor or angiotensin-receptor blocker (ARB) plus beta-blocker, ideally carvedilol (12). For patients who develop HF during chemotherapy with LVEF <50% or >5% decline in LVEF, guidelines recommend holding anthracyclines and treating with standard evidence-based guidelines for HF with reduced EF (13). For such patients, utilizing a nonanthracycline-based regimen for future treatment cycles may be considered. For asymptomatic patients with a decline in LVEF of at least 10% to <50% but >45%, HF medical therapy for secondary prevention as well as having a risk-benefit discussion regarding continued anthracyclines may be considered.

Anthracyclines are associated with cardiac dysfunction (14), causing myocyte destruction which may leads to clinical HF. Late detection of anthracycline induced cardiotoxicity is often irreversible (15). This case demonstrates that with aggressive medical therapy, and appropriate diagnostic monitoring, patients may experience some recovery of LV function.

CASE 2

ANITA RADHAKRISHNAN AND
ERIC E. HARRISON

Introduction

Human epidermal growth factor receptor (HER2)-targeted therapies such as trastuzumab, lapatinib, pertuzumab, and ado-trastuzumab emtansine (TDM-1) have revolutionized the management of HER2 positive breast cancer (16). The HER2 gene is overexpressed in 25%–30% of breast cancers (17), leading to high levels of HER2 protein in malignant cells , making the cancer more aggressive and subsequently threatening the patient's survival (18). Trastuzumab is a humanized monoclonal antibody targeted against the HER2 protein, which has dramatically improved disease-free and overall survival in patients with HER2-positive breast cancer (19).

Case summary

A 35-year-old Swedish woman presented to our clinic for monitoring of her cardiac function during her cancer treatment. In 2010, while 6 months pregnant, she noticed a breast lump that was red and tender in the inner upper quadrant of the right breast. Ultrasound-guided core biopsy yielded a grade III infiltrating ductal carcinoma (IDC) that was estrogen receptor (ER)-negative, progesterone receptor (PR)-negative, and HER2 positive by immunohistochemistry. Metastatic workup was negative. Clinically, she was diagnosed with stage IIIA right breast carcinoma. Prior to the initiation of her chemotherapy, she delivered a healthy baby. She was treated with neoadjuvant chemotherapy included two cycles of Adriamycin, radiation therapy for 5 weeks, followed by six cycles of TCH (docetaxel [T], carboplatin [C], trastuzumab [H]). After completion of her therapy, she underwent a modified radical mastectomy and right breast prosthesis implantation. Review of echocardiographic reports from her first round of chemotherapy revealed that her left ventricle was normal in size and she had mild to moderate LV systolic dysfunction with an ejection fraction of 40%–45%. The etiology of her mild LV systolic dysfunction was unclear and felt to be either pregnancy-related or preexisting. No images were available of her diagnostic studies performed at that time and the patient was not on medical therapy for LV dysfunction.

In May 2014, 3 years after finishing cancer therapy, she was found to have a enlarging left lower lobe nodule on routine imaging with Fluorodeoxyglucose positron emission tomography. She underwent CyberKnife radiation of the lung lesion and was placed on paclitaxel, trastuzumab, and pertuzumab therapy for six cycles.

While receiving dual anti-HER2 therapy with taxane-based chemotherapy, she had echocardiograms performed every 3–4 months. In July 2014, at the start of her first cycle, her echocardiogram revealed the left ventricle was mildly dilated with a LV ejection fraction of 42% on echocardiogram and cardiac magnetic resonance (CMR). Average global longitudinal strain was −16.5%. Table 10.2 illustrates the key diagnostic and imaging tests that were performed during her cancer treatment. At baseline, the patient was started on a low dose beta-blocker and ACE inhibitor. After six cycles of combined therapy, her paclitaxel was discontinued and her anti-HER2 targeted therapy was continued for 15 cycles. One year after chemotherapy, the patient developed asymptomatic LV systolic dysfunction with an LVEF of 17% and a change in average global longitudinal strain of –13.2%. At that time, the beta-blocker and ACE inhibitor were up-titrated, and HER2 targeted therapy was held (Figure 10.3). The echocardiogram was repeated 4 weeks later showing that her LV systolic function recovered to her baseline. A CMR was performed to confirm these findings (Figure 10.4). The patient

Table 10.2 Overview of echocardiographic changes from HER-2 targeted therapy—echocardiography findings, medications, and changes to targeted therapy from July 2014 to July 2016

Date	2D LVEF (%)	GLS (%)	CMR LVEF (%)	TnI ng/mL	BNP
Day 1	40 – Coreg 3.125 mg BID and Lisinopril 2.5 mg daily started	–	42	<0.01	15.6
1 month	44	−17.5	–	<0.01	19.6
3 months	42	−17	–	<0.01	
6 months	40	−18	–	0.02	66
12 months	17 (held targeted therapy) Coreg and Lisinoril uptitrated	−13.2		<0.01	41
13 months	40 (targeted therapy restarted)	−15.2	40	–	–
16 months	47 (targeted therapy completed)	−18	–	–	–
20 months	46	–	–	<0.01	10
24 months	50	−17	–	–	–

Note: (−) signifies no data available. Normal GLS is defined as −18%. Normal 2D LVEF in women is 54% and normal LVEF by CMR is 55%.

(a)   (b)

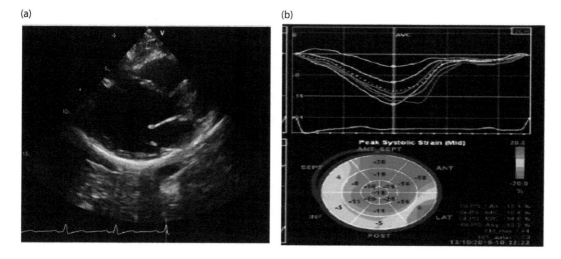

Figure 10.3 Panel (a): Parasternal long axis view revealing dilated left ventricle. Panel (b): Myocardial strain is a marker of deformation that can be measured in each myocardial segment and globally for the entire ventricle (Figure 10.2). It can be measured in systole or diastole, in three primary directions (longitudinal, radial, and circumferential), and is quantified as a change in length of a myocardial segment in relation to its initial length. Peak systolic global longitudinal strain (GLS; a measure of peak longitudinal myocardial deformation during systole) has been shown to identify myocardial dysfunction in patients who receive chemotherapy. Patient's GLS of –13.4%.

was reinitiated on her dual anti-HER2 targeted therapy and completed another three cycles. The patient had close clinical and echocardiographic monitoring during this time.

Discussion

The mechanism of trastuzumab cardiotoxicity remains unclear. HER2 is a tyrosine kinase inhibitor of the epidermal growth factor receptor, or ERBB family. NRG (neuregulin) is a ligand to the ERBB receptors, and NRG-ERBB signaling is involved in cardiac development and physiology (20). This pathway, when stressed with the use of this monoclonal antibody, may cause cardiomyopathy indirectly. This is more often associated with a loss of contractility, presumably a form of stunning or hibernation, that is less likely to be associated

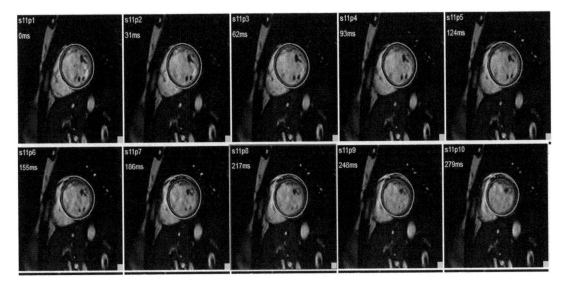

Figure 10.4 Short-axis, end-diastolic CMR cine image demonstrating quantitative approach to left ventricular volume measurement. Endocardial contour (red) is traced in a series of images encompassing the entire ventricle during cardiac cycle. Based on volumes calculations, her LVEF was 44%.

with myocyte death or clinical heart failure and is more likely to be reversible.

Previous or concurrent anthracycline use and prior LV dysfunction are the strongest risk factors for development of trastuzumab-related cardiotoxicity (21). Based on current guidelines, all patients should receive a baseline clinical cardiovascular assessment including history and physical examination, baseline cardiac risk factor modification, cardiac biomarkers including high sensitivity troponin and BNP, and LV function assessment by echocardiogram prior to initiation of HER2 targeted therapy. During treatment, cardiac imaging to assess LVEF and global longitudinal strain is recommended every 3 months while on therapy with high sensitivity troponin measurements. If a decline in LVEF <40% or LVEF decline of >10% from baseline, the targeted therapy should be held and cardiac medical therapy for heart failure with beta-blockers and ACE inhibitors should be initiated. LV function should be reevaluated again in 4 weeks, and the targeted therapy can be started again if the LVEF increases >40% (12). Targeted therapy should be discontinued if there is persistent decline in LVEF >8 weeks or if there has been a suspension of trastuzumab more than three times per the Food and Drug Administration labelling insert. After completion of targeted therapy, LV function assessment should be done at 6 months or 1 year, if EF remains abnormal, follow

American College of Cardiology/American Heart Association (ACC/AHA) HF guidelines (13).

This patient's case demonstrates the importance of guideline compliance. In this case study, the patient was at high risk for cardiotoxicity due to her prior anthracycline use and prior LV dysfunction. Her LVEF dropped by 24% and global longitudinal strain (GLS) dropped by 28% 1 year after targeted therapy. According to recent ACC Best Practice Guidelines, (12) LVEF decline of <40% are indications to interrupt targeted therapy, optimize heart failure therapy, and rechallenge if there is recovery of LV function. In this case, we followed current recommendations for cardiac monitoring, which resulted in a favorable outcome in this patient.

CASE 3

HASSAN TARIQ, SHETAL AMIN, MILLEE SINGH, CESAR ALBERTO MORALES-PABON, KRISTINA CAHILL, ANITA RADHAKRISHNAN, AND ERIC E. HARRISON

Introduction

Coronary artery disease (CAD) is a major cardiovascular complication of radiation therapy. Women with mediastinal radiation and higher doses of radiation are at high risk for CAD. This risk begins within the first 5 years after radiation therapy and continues until the third decade. This case presents accelerated CAD in a patient with history of non-Hodgkin's lymphoma (NHL). Here, we demonstrate the utility of CCTA and inflammatory protein markers for the evaluation of accelerated CAD and risk prediction of acute coronary events in a patient exposed to radiation therapy.

Case presentation

A 67-year-old Caucasian male with gastroesophageal reflux disease (GERD) and family history significant for hypertension was diagnosed with NHL in 1989. He was treated on a National Institute of Health (NIH) trial with mantle radiation to the chest (unclear radiation dose) and chemotherapy consisting of methotrexate, Adriamycin, cyclophosphamide, etoposide, mechlorethamine, vincristine (Oncovin), procarbazine, and prednisone (ProMACE-MOPP) with no evidence of recurrent disease.

In August 2013, the patient experienced an episode of left arm and left chest discomfort that awakened him from sleep and prompted a visit to the local emergency room. The pain was sharp, substernal, and had no relation to exertion, food, or emotion. At the hospital, the patient was administered nitroglycerin that did not alleviate his chest pain. He had a complete cardiac workup, which consisted of an EKG showing normal sinus rhythm and left axis deviation and a chest x-ray (CXR) showing a linear scar or atelectasis at the right lung base and elevation of the right hemidiaphragm. A transthoracic echocardiogram (TTE) showed left ventricular hypertrophy (LVH) with a normal systolic function and bicuspid aortic valve with moderate aortic regurgitation. An exercise myocardial perfusion single photon emission computed tomography (SPECT) was performed and revealed no perfusion defects consistent with infarction or ischemia. Lab results revealed troponin I of 0.031 ng/mL and creatinine phosphokinase (CPK) of 118 mcg/L. The patient was diagnosed with GERD exacerbation and was discharged home.

The patient was seen in a cardio-oncology clinic for further evaluation of his chest pain. His history and physical examination were unremarkable, and his only cardiac risk factors included his exposure to anterior chest radiation. Lab results indicated a total cholesterol of 252 mg/dL, high-density lipoprotein of 57 mg/dL, low-density lipoprotein of 121 mg/dL, and triglycerides of 79 mg/dL. The

patient's atherosclerotic cardiovascular disease (ASCVD) risk was 13%, and a moderate to high intensity statin was recommended. The patient refused a statin. Owing to the poor negative and positive predictive value of most community stress test nuclear scans, other than positron emission tomography—computed tomography (PET-CT), a CCTA was performed, and the images were processed with the Vital Images Vitrea Sure Plaque software for coronary plaque analysis. The Vitrea Sure Plaque software characterizes visualized plaque on coronary CTA and helps define the density of the composition in Hounsfield units. It quantifies plaque burden and coronary remodeling noninvasively. It characterizes a lesion in the vessel wall as either calcified or noncalcified and helps delineate a lipid core vs. a fibrous core (Figure 10.5).

Using this CCTA protocol, we identified 60% stenosis in the proximal dominant left circumflex (LCX) with a lipid-rich plaque that appeared to be high risk and vulnerable (Figure 10.6). No evidence of calcification was seen in this lesion. There were also moderate partially-calcified plaques seen in the proximal and distal left main coronary artery (LMCA), and proximal LCX. The nondominant right coronary artery (RCA) was found to have mild to moderate partially-calcified plaques with some evidence of positive remodeling. The coronary findings and the increased risk of an acute cardiac event involving the proximal LCX were discussed with the patient and maximum medical therapy with 81 mg aspirin, 40 mg atorvastatin, and a beta-blocker were started. Lifestyle modification with dietary changes, exercise, and weight loss was recommended, but unfortunately the patient was non-compliant.

Functional hemodynamics of coronary blood flow were measured by Heart Flow FFR-CT using Navier-Stokes Equations and a supercomputer (Figure 10.7). These revealed significant reductions in blood flow across the left anterior descending (LAD) artery and LCX artery. The importance of this is accentuated by the fact that the RCA was hypoplastic. The patient declined bypass surgery and unfortunately owing to statin myopathy the atorvastatin was switched to 5 mg pravastatin daily.

In April 2014, 6 months after the initial diagnosis of coronary artery disease, the patient presented to the emergency department with chest pain and was diagnosed with a myocardial infarction,

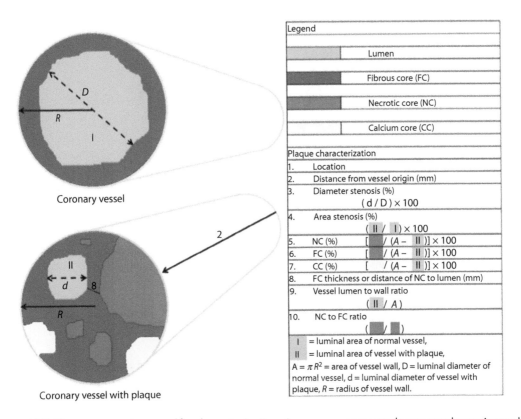

Figure 10.5 Plaque parameters used for characterization via coronary computed tomography angiography.

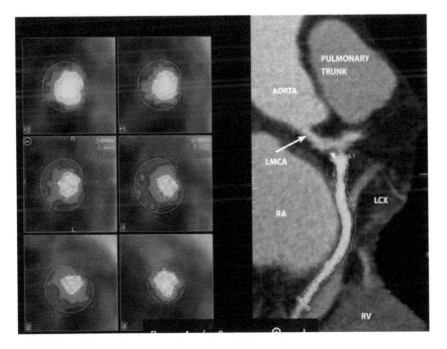

Figure 10.6 Vulnerable LCX artery plaque identified coronary CTA. Longitudinal view displaying the luminal narrowing at the vulnerable plaque site in LCX. Cross-sectional view of vulnerable plaque is shown on left. Red, necrotic core; blue: fibrotic core; yellow, calcium core.

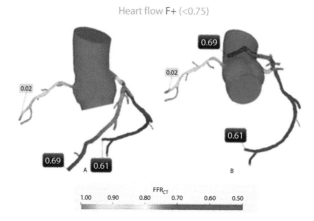

Figure 10.7 Functional hemodynamics of coronary blood flow was measured by heart flow CT FFR using Navier-Stokes equations and a supercomputer. These revealed significant reductions in blood flow across the LAD and LCX.

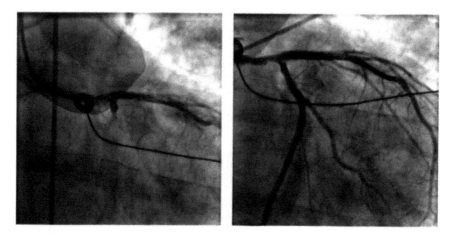

Figure 10.8 Cardiac cath showing 100% occlusion of the left circumflex artery at the same vulnerable site predicted using coronary CTA. Successful revascularization of the vulnerable LCX lesion.

complete heart block, and cardiogenic shock. His EKG revealed inferior ST segment elevation with reciprocal lateral changes. His cardiac catheterization revealed a 100% occlusion of the dominant LCX. He was found to have a 70% proximal RCA lesion, a 50% ostial LMCA lesion, and a 50% lesion in the first diagonal branch off LAD. In the catheterization lab, the patient underwent aspiration thrombectomy and a Xience stent placement (Figure 10.8). His hospital course was complicated by ventricular fibrillation arrest immediately postintervention, which led to intubation and an intra-aortic balloon pump placement. His hospital stay was prolonged, but he was eventually transitioned to optimal medical therapy, including

aspirin, pravastatin, clopidogrel bisulfate, furosemide, Ramipril, carvedilol, spironolactone, and a defibrillator vest. At discharge a repeat echocardiogram revealed a LVEF of 35% with severe lateral hypokinesis.

The patient reported to the cardiovascular clinic for follow-up and underwent a repeat CCTA to determine his residual plaque burden and assess the risk of another cardiac event. A significant noncalcified plaque of moderate range in the LMCA was identified that extended into the origin of the LCX, but ended before the start of the LCX stent. Furthermore, there appeared to be an area in the LMCA that had an ulcerated lipid-rich plaque (Figure 10.9). Besides the LMCA, there were

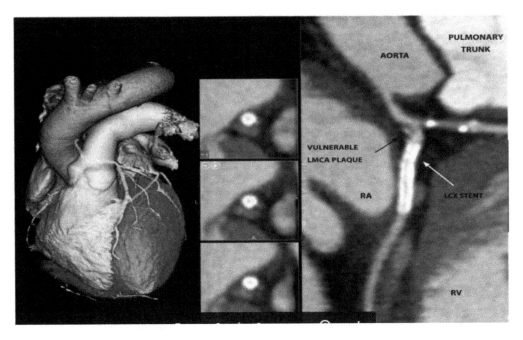

Figure 10.9 Residual coronary artery disease—noncalcified plaque of moderate range in the LMCA was identified that extended into the origin of the LCX, but ended before the start of the left circumflex stent.

calcified plaques with positive remodeling in the proximal LAD and proximal RCA. The patient was educated about his risk of a future cardiac event involving the LMCA and underwent up-titration of his aggressive medical therapy. The left internal mammary artery (LIMA) appeared intact and viable without distortion or narrowing from fibrosis.

The patient entered cardiac rehabilitation and developed jaw pain with significant ST segment depression while walking on the treadmill. The patient called from rehabilitation and came directly to the cardio-oncology clinic for a webinar with image review. We agreed that because of his history of chest radiation that he would not be a good candidate for conventional coronary bypass surgery, but would be an excellent candidate for an off pump hybrid procedure with an LIMA to the LAD from a keyhole with robotic harvesting of the LIMA graft to mobilize it for anastomosis to the distal LAD. The main left and proximal circumflex could be stented. The patient completed the hybrid procedure without problems or complications. He is now several years postsurgery without cardiac problems, but with immunological incompetence requiring intravenous immunoglobulin (IV IG) and continued follow-up at the NIH for newly developed chronic lymphocytic leukemia.

Discussion

Acute cardiac inflammation can occur at the time of radiotherapy or shortly afterwards, resulting in myocarditis or pericarditis (22). Late cardiovascular effects can manifest clinically years or even decades after treatment resulting in a variety of cardiovascular complications including myocardial fibrosis, valvular heart disease, systolic and diastolic heart failure, coronary artery disease, pericardial disease, and conduction system dysfunction.

The risk of developing CAD-associated events after chest irradiation (23) is augmented by several factors, including concomitant chemotherapy with anthracyclines (24), young age (25), high-fractionated doses, lack of thoracic shielding (26), cardiovascular risk factors, and established CAD. The risk of myocardial infarction in patients treated for Hodgkin's lymphoma is two- to seven-fold higher than in the general population, with a cumulative incidence of 10% at 30 years (27–29). Radiation induced vasculopathy manifests as both micro- and macrovascular disease and can be rapidly progressive, despite not being clinically apparent until years or even decades after radiotherapy. Radiation-induced endothelial damage may be because of reactive oxygen species, production of cytokines (30), and other inflammatory mediators. Endothelial cell damage, increased permeability, interstitial fibrin deposits, and platelet thrombin ultimately lead to fibrosis and therefore development of CAD. Owing to the location of epicardial coronary arteries and sustained inflammation, resulting from radiation exposure to heart, CAD will often involve the left main, ostial left anterior descending artery and the right coronary artery. Lesions are usually longer, concentric, and tubular, making cardiac revascularization more challenging. Newer radiation techniques, including deep inspiration breath-hold gating, accelerated partial breast irradiation, and use of modern 3D planning results in less radiation exposure to the heart, which may ameliorate cardiovascular complications. Management of radiation-induced CAD is the same as in nonradiation-related CAD. Medical therapy or revascularization is done depending upon symptoms, cancer stage, comorbidities, and expected survival. However, surgical intervention may be difficult sometimes owing to mediastinal fibrosis. In addition, the internal mammary artery may not be available for graft because of the irradiation of this vessel itself. Percutaneous intervention (PCI) for isolated CAD may be considered, but intervention can be difficult because the lesions are typically diffuse and extensively calcified (rather than discrete single vessel disease), making stenting less appropriate. When long-term PCI outcomes are compared with nonirradiated, matched controls, those with radiation-induced CAD have higher mortality and worse functional class (31).

Typically, screening for CAD should commence within 5 years of radiation exposure, based upon timing of major coronary events in breast cancer survivors (32). Multiple imaging modalities can be used such as stress tests, exercise stress echocardiography, and cardiac CTA. Nuclear stress interpretations have limitations owing to significant attenuation artifacts, especially breast cancer patients who frequently have breast prothesis implants. CT-FFR heart flow measurements are a newer tool that has revolutionized functional assessment. It uses computational fluid dynamics combined with anatomical models based on CCTA scans and provides information on the coronary flow and pressure. Functional hemodynamics of coronary stenosis are assessed noninvasively and validated when compared to invasive FFR in studies.

This is an excellent case of how coronary CTA with fractional flow reserve helped identify high-risk radiation-induced CAD that was missed by nuclear perfusion imaging. It is established that the CTA method of acquisition and of characterization with morphology and composition is appropriate to identify high-risk lesions that may lead to acute coronary events in vulnerable patients. CCTA remains the only modality that allows for reliable noninvasive visualization of coronary arteries and this makes it very useful for the evaluation of patient at risk for radiation induced cardiotoxicity.

REFERENCES

1. Albini A et al. Cardiotoxicity of anticancer drugs: The need for cardio-oncology and cardio-oncological prevention. *J the Nat Cancer Inst.* January 6, 2010;102(1):14–25.
2. Swain SM et al. Congestive heart failure in patients treated with doxorubicin. *Cancer.* June 1, 2003;97(11):2869–79.
3. Henderson IC et al. Improved outcomes from adding sequential paclitaxel but not from escalating doxorubicin dose in an adjuvant chemotherapy regimen for patients with node-positive primary breast cancer. *J Clin Oncol.* March 15, 2003;21(6):976–83.
4. Lipshultz SE et al. Sex and higher drug dose as risk factors for late cardiotoxic effects of doxorubicin therapy for childhood cancer. *N Engl J Med.* June 29, 1995;332(26):1738–44.
5. Crawford MH et al. Determinants of survival and left ventricular performance after mitral valve replacement. Department of veterans affairs cooperative study on valvular heart disease. *Circulation.* April 1, 1990;81(4):1173–81.
6. Rozich JD et al. Mitral valve replacement with and without chordal preservation in patients with chronic mitral regurgitation. Mechanisms for differences in postoperative ejection performance. *Circulation.* December 1, 1992;86(6):1718–26.
7. Clavel MA et al. Comparison between transcatheter and surgical prosthetic valve implantation in patients with severe aortic stenosis and reduced left ventricular ejection fraction. *Circulation.* November 9, 2010;122(19):1928–36.
8. Mordente A et al. Topoisomerases and anthracyclines: Recent advances and perspectives in anticancer therapy and prevention of cardiotoxicity. *Curr Med Chem.* May 1, 2017;24(15):1607–26.

9. Sawaya H et al. Early detection and prediction of cardiotoxicity in chemotherapy-treated patients. *Am J Cardiol.* May 1, 2011;107(9):1375–80.

10. Nysom K et al. Relationship between cumulative anthracycline dose and late cardiotoxicity in childhood acute lymphoblastic leukemia. *J Clin Oncol* 1998;16:545–50.

11. McMurray JJ et al. ESC Guidelines for the diagnosis and treatment of acute and chronic heart failure 2012. *Eur J Heart Fail.* August 1, 2012;14(8):803–69.

12. Chang H-M et al. Cardiovascular complications of cancer therapy—Best practices in diagnosis, prevention, and management: Part 1. *J Am Coll Cardiol.* November 14, 2017; 70(20):2536–2551

13. Yancy CW et al. 2013 ACCF/AHA guideline for the management of heart failure. *Circulation.* January 1, 2013;128:e240–e327.

14. Eschenhagen T et al. Cardiovascular side effects of cancer therapies: A position statement from the Heart Failure Association of the European Society of Cardiology. *Eur J Heart Fail.* January 1,2011 ;13(1):1–0.

15. Ferreira AL et al. Anthracycline-induced cardiotoxicity. *Cardiovasc Hematol Agents Med Chem (Formerly Current Med Chem-Cardiovasc Hematol Agents).* October 1, 2008;6(4):278–81.

16. Ahmed S et al. HER2–directed therapy: Current treatment options for HER2-positive breast cancer. *Breast Cancer.* March 1, 2015;22(2):101–16.

17. Baselga J et al. Recombinant humanized anti-HER2 antibody (Herceptin™) enhances the antitumor activity of paclitaxel and doxorubicin against HER2/neu overexpressing human breast cancer xenografts. *Cancer Res.* July 1,1998 ;58(13):2825–31.

18. Yarden Y et al. Biology of HER2 and its importance in breast cancer. *Oncology.* 2001;61(Suppl. 2):1–13.

19. Vogel CL et al. Efficacy and safety of trastuzumab as a single agent in first-line treatment of HER2–overexpressing metastatic breast cancer. *J Clin Oncol.* February 1, 2002;20(3):719–26.

20. Lemmens K et al. Role of neuregulin-1/ErbB signaling in cardiovascular physiology and disease. *Circulation.* August 21, 2007;116(8):954–60.

21. Cardinale D et al. Trastuzumab-induced cardiotoxicity: Clinical and prognostic implications of troponin I evaluation. *J Clin Oncol.* August 2, 2010;28(25):3910–6.

22. Gaya AM et al. Cardiac complications of radiation therapy. *Clin Oncol.* May 31, 2005;17(3):153–9.

23. Adams MJ et al. Radiation-associated cardiovascular disease. *Critical Rev Oncol/Hematol.* January 31, 2003;45(1):55–75.

24. Adams MJ et al. Pathophysiology of anthracycline-and radiation-associated cardiomyopathies: Implications for screening and prevention. *Pediatr Blood Cancer.* June 15, 2005;44(7):600–6.

25. Brosius FC et al. Radiation heart disease: Analysis of 16 young (aged 15 to 33 years) necropsy patients who received over 3,500 rads to the heart. *Am J Med.* March 31, 1981;70(3):519–30.

26. Om A et al. Radiation-induced coronary artery disease. *Am Heart J.* December 1, 1992;124(6):1598–602.

27. Swerdlow AJ et al. Myocardial infarction mortality risk after treatment for Hodgkin disease: A collaborative British cohort study. *J the Nat Cancer Inst.* February 7, 2007;99(3):206–14.

28. Hull MC et al. Valvular dysfunction and carotid, subclavian, and coronary artery disease in survivors of Hodgkin lymphoma treated with radiation therapy. *JAMA.* December 3, 2003;290(21):2831–7.

29. Aleman BM et al. Late cardiotoxicity after treatment for Hodgkin lymphoma. *Blood.* March 1, 2007;109(5):1878–86.

30. Rubin P et al. A perpetual cascade of cytokines postirradiation leads to pulmonary fibrosis. *Int J Radiat Oncol Biol Phys.* August 30, 1995;33(1):99–109.

31. Darby SC et al. Long-term mortality from heart disease and lung cancer after radiotherapy for early breast cancer: Prospective cohort study of about 300 000 women in US SEER cancer registries. *Lancet Oncol.* August 31, 2005;6(8):557–65.

32. Correa CR et al. Coronary artery findings after left-sided compared with right-sided radiation treatment for early-stage breast cancer. *J Clin Oncol.* July 20, 2007;25(21): 3031–7.

PART III

The cardio-oncology clinic

11

Establishing a cardio-oncology clinic

SUSAN F. DENT, MOIRA RUSHTON-MAROVAC, HEATHER LOUNDER,
JOSEE IVARS, JOYCE BOTROS, AND JOERG HERRMANN

INTRODUCTION

Improvements in early detection and cancer therapeutics have led to a significant increase in the number of people surviving a cancer diagnosis. In the USA, there are an estimated 15.5 million cancer survivors, a number expected to grow to 20.3 million by the year 2026 (1). Individuals with advanced cancers (e.g., melanoma, non-small cell lung cancer, and renal cell carcinoma), once facing a very poor prognosis after diagnosis, are now living with their disease for years due to novel cancer treatment strategies such as immunotherapy.

Cardiovascular (CV) disease and cancer are the two leading causes of mortality in the Western world (2–4). Both are complex diseases, sharing risk factors such as age, obesity, smoking, genetics, and various lifestyle factors. As the proportion of individuals greater than 65 years of age continues to increase in North America, so will the prevalence of individuals at risk of CV disease, cancer, or both. The interplay between these two common disease entities necessitates a collaborative and multidisciplinary approach by healthcare providers. Those

individuals who have survived a cancer diagnosis may develop CV diseases owing to the interplay of underlying CV risk factors or as a result of their cancer treatment. Individuals with heart disease may develop cancer and require life-saving or sustaining cancer treatment that could have a deleterious impact on their CV health. Cardio-oncology has emerged as a new subspecialty of medicine born from the need to provide optimal care for patients during and following completion of their cancer therapy without compromising CV health.

CARDIO-ONCOLOGY: THE NEED FOR A MULTIDISCIPLINARY APPROACH

Cancer treatment related cardiac dysfunction (CTRCD) can be seen with a wide variety of cancer therapeutics (5). While anthracycline-induced cardiomyopathy is the most widely known CV consequence of cancer treatment, the adoption of novel cancer therapeutics, including targeted agents and immunotherapy, could potentially have adverse effects on the CV system including hypertension, arrhythmias, thromboembolic events, QT prolongation, and in rare cases fulminant myocarditis (6,7).

Cardio-oncology has emerged as a subspeciality of medicine with the goal of maximizing cancer treatment while minimizing the negative implications on CV health. Increasing awareness by healthcare providers of the potential detrimental impact of cancer therapies on the CV health of patients during and/or following cancer therapy has led to the establishment of increasing numbers of dedicated cardio-oncology clinics across North America and around the world. There are currently no established guidelines that outline the components and infrastructure needed to establish cardio-oncology clinics or programs. In this chapter, we utilize the expertise of pioneers in the field of cardio-oncology to outline the components and structure necessary to establish a successful cardio-oncology clinic/program.

COMPONENTS OF A CARDIO-ONCOLOGY CLINIC

The development of a cardio-oncology clinic is a complex process involving multidisciplinary collaboration, administrative support and institutional resources. In order to ensure the success of a clinic, attention to detail in the initial planning stages is crucial. The exact needs at each stage must be identified and met in order to ensure all components are working in unison. Most importantly, any provider involved in the operation of a cardio-oncology clinic has to recognize the value and necessity of a cardio-oncology service.

The first step in developing a cardio-oncology clinic is to identify an individual or individuals who will champion and lead the program within the healthcare organization in which it will operate (see Figure 11.1). Since this is a collaborative specialty, having leaders from oncology as well as cardiology is essential to ensure the success of the clinic. These leaders should develop a proposal for their institution based on local patient needs and provider abilities.

Once leaders have been identified, they can use their expertise to review local patient data to establish the need for a dedicated cardio-oncology clinic. Concrete information and comprehensive data must be available in order to approach the practice leadership and administration for approval and endorsement. Information on number of patients being referred from oncology to cardiology each year, and delays in cancer therapy while awaiting cardiac assessment, can make a case for establishing a cardio-oncology clinic. Local healthcare providers who have an interest and expertise in managing the cardiac concerns of cancer patients are important in demonstrating the value of a cardio-oncology clinic to healthcare administration.

Once need has been established and recognized, the provider in charge of a cardio-oncology service is responsible for exploring and defining the practice landscape, and estimating clinic volume. This includes not only an assessment of how many patients one will encounter, but also which types of questions will be asked and which expectations are to be met. With this in mind, a review of referral patterns is very helpful. For instance, if cancer patients are repeatedly presenting at a cardiology practice for consultation related to their cancer history and treatment, the need for a joint practice may be more easily recognized and accepted. On the other hand, if the primary reason for cardiology referral is for a pretreatment cardiac optimization, a stronger case could be made for a cardiology clinic focused on cancer patients. At the outset of establishing a new clinic, there should be clear guidance on the appropriate reasons for referral to a cardio-oncology clinic. Once the patient populations are defined, patient volumes and the staffing needs can be estimated.

After these steps have been completed, a full clinical proposal can be developed including information on appropriate referrals, staffing requirements, physical space requirements, and cost estimates. In most situations, cardio-oncology programs are established within either a hospital or cancer center. Generally speaking, these

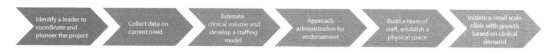

Figure 11.1 The cardio-oncology clinic set-up.

organizations have a leadership structure that has requirements for approval of new clinical programs. A detailed proposal should focus on the benefits to improving patient care.

Once approval and funding from administration has been granted, operations can commence. At this point it is important to distribute information to local providers in cardiology, oncology, and allied healthcare on the launch of the clinic. This should include referral forms with clearly identified reasons for referral to this clinic. The anticipated demand will determine how frequently the clinic will operate. Regular review of clinic performance (number of patients seen, time to referral, etc.) compared to data originally collected for establishing the clinic in the first place will allow for ongoing assessment of efficacy. These quality assurance metrics will likely be important for local administrators if they are to continue to support the clinic's existence.

Communication between oncology and cardiology is a key element for the establishment of any cardio-oncology clinic. Initially, it may be beneficial to establish a clinic with a narrow focus, for example, breast cancer patients with CV issues. Practitioners can then focus their attention on successfully establishing a cardio-oncology clinic on a small scale, allowing for the identification of any logistical issues that can then be addressed. It may be easier for a scheduling team to successfully adjust to this concept if the scope of the clinic is gradually increased over time. Naturally, the cardio-oncology practice will expand with demand, as other medical services gain interest in this highly collaborative approach.

OPERATION OF A CARDIO-ONCOLOGY CLINIC

Regarding the operational structure of a cardio-oncology program, a clinic can be staffed by cardiologists alone, or cardiologists and oncologists working together in the same physical space. Either model can be successful. In the former example, communication is paramount to ensure the success of the program. A practical tool to aid communication can be the establishment of multidisciplinary rounds where all involved healthcare providers are invited to discuss cardio-oncology cases. This exchange and sharing of ideas will continually educate and involve all members of the team in current cardio-oncology topics relating to real patient care (8).

The cardio-oncology clinic should have timely access to a range of cardiac imaging modalities so that assessments and interventions can be made with minimal disruption to cancer therapy. In many cases, patients may have baseline cardiac disease that needs optimization prior to initiation of cancer therapy, while in others, treatment and management of complications owing to cancer therapy need to be initiated. The main advantage of multidisciplinary care is the interaction among specialists which allows the cardiologist to inform oncologists on best practices to manage cardiac risks and complications, while the oncologist can inform on the relative importance of anticancer therapeutics and absolute benefit to the patient on a case by case basis.

There are currently no established benchmarks to guide clinicians with regard to timely access and assessment of patients who experience CTRCD. Wait times to be assessed in a cardio-oncology clinic need to be balanced with the urgency of impending cancer treatments. The patient receiving active cancer treatment will generally require more urgent access (1–2 weeks), while it might be appropriate for patients not receiving active therapy (e.g., surveillance) to be seen in a less timely fashion (weeks to months) (9). Cancer patients should be referred for an urgent consult (within 7 days) if they have symptoms of heart failure, or their cancer treatment has been placed on hold owing to cardiotoxicity (e.g., left ventricular ejection fraction [LVEF] <50%). All patients referred to a cardio-oncology clinic should have a clinical assessment (history and physical examination) performed with particular attention to patients' comorbidities, such as coronary artery disease (CAD) and hypertension. CV investigations prior to, and during the administration of chemotherapy, known to be associated with significant cardiotoxicity, will be driven by the specific cancer therapy prescribed (e.g., sunitinib and risk of hypertension) and the patient's underlying CV risk factors. Optimal treatment of preexisting conditions (e.g., diabetes, hypertension) should be incorporated into the patient care plan. Patients receiving cancer therapy who are at high risk, or who have experienced cancer therapy-related cardiac dysfunction, should be discussed by the cardio-oncology team at multidisciplinary cardio-oncology rounds. The discussion should focus on the balance between the individual's potential benefits of cancer treatment vs. CV risk. In patients with metastatic disease receiving cancer treatment with palliative intent, the risk of cardiac complications and related symptoms, which may compromise quality of life, may not be acceptable. For cancer patients being treated with curative intent, the occurrence of symptoms due to CTRCD, may be tolerable if the toxicity is fully reversible and manageable.

THE CARDIO-ONCOLOGY TEAM

Typically, the cardio-oncology team will consist of a group of healthcare professionals who are driven to meet the needs of patients in this specific field (see Figure 11.2). By definition, cardio-oncologists are medical providers who are focused on the CV health of cancer patients prior to, during, and after completion of their cancer treatment. They help ensure that optimal cancer therapy is administered by preventing, or at least mitigating, treatment-related cardiotoxicity whenever possible. They are responsible for managing CV complications to avoid limiting effective cancer therapy. They also play a role in the management and treatment of any CV effects that either exists prior to treatment or that occur as a result of cancer therapy, or the cancer itself. Cardio-oncologists also

endeavor to improve clinical CV care, enhance education, and promote research for patients who have an active or prior history of malignancy (10). Cardio-oncologists with a cardiology background should facilitate timely access to appropriate cardiac imaging and prescribe cardiac medications to prevent or alleviate cancer therapy-related cardiac dysfunction. Cardio-oncologists with an oncology background should actively screen cancer patients, during and following completion of cancer therapy, for CV risk factors, and refer to cardiologists, when appropriate, in a timely manner. They should have an understanding of the potential CV complications of established and novel cancer treatments, and work closely with cardiologists to maintain an open line of effective communication in order to ensure optimization of cancer treatment while maintaining CV health.

Allied healthcare providers

In successful cardio-oncology programs, allied healthcare providers play a key role in coordinating multidisciplinary care for cancer patients. Pharmacists are important members of the multidisciplinary team. They provide coordinated documentation of cancer treatment (chemotherapy/targeted therapy), medication adjustments, and dose updates, as well as patient education and

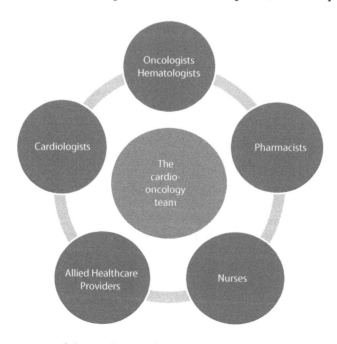

Figure 11.2 The components of the cardio-oncology team.

engagement. They can review possible drug-drug interactions that may potentiate the impact of potential cardiotoxic cancer drugs (e.g., QTc prolongation and cyclin-dependent kinase (CDK) 4/6 inhibitors). Clinic nurses and physician extenders (nurse practitioners/physician assistants), provide coordination of cardio-oncology appointments and other cancer care, including chemotherapy, radiology studies, oncology, and surgical appointments. They can assist in patient health assessments, patient educational needs, as well as patient and family support. Extended healthcare providers can facilitate timely scheduling of serial cardiac imaging and/or laboratory investigations. Nurses and physician assistants can see more stable patients, freeing up time for the cardio-oncologist to incorporate more complex patients into their clinic schedule (11). All team members assume responsibility to be aware of changes in cancer treatment plans (e.g., curative vs. palliative treatment) and/or changes in a patient's CV status. Nurses and extended healthcare providers can play a significant role in ensuring effective communication takes place between all other team members.

WHO SHOULD BE REFERRED TO A CARDIO-ONCOLOGY CLINIC

Cardio-oncology clinics should develop standardized referral forms to facilitate the delivery of care for cancer patients at risk of, or who have developed cardiotoxicity from cancer therapy. Cancer patients may benefit from referral to a cardio-oncology clinic at different stages in their treatment, depending on the cancer therapy planned and their underlying CV risk factors (see Figure 11.3). Pretreatment assessment—to assess risk of cardiotoxicity—is especially important in the presence of preexisting CV risk factors including smoking, hypertension, diabetes, dyslipidemia, obesity, age greater than 60 years, borderline low cardiac function (LVEF 50%–55%), history of myocardial infarction (MI), and at least moderate valvular disease (12). Similar to a preoperative cardiac assessment, this type of encounter would serve to manage undiagnosed or undertreated cardiac disease to optimize patients' chances of successfully completing their cancer treatment without serious cardiac complications. Patients with known CV disease should be referred for consideration of preventive strategies (primary or secondary) depending on the type of cancer therapy planned. Cancer patients who experience cardiac complications during their cancer treatment (e.g., left ventricular dysfunction) should be referred promptly to a cardio-oncologist for management of cardiotoxicity. These patients often need more complex cardiac workup, cardiac interventions, and medical management in order to continue their cancer therapy.

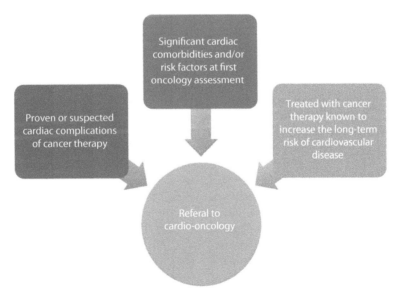

Figure 11.3 Decision making for cardio-oncology referral.

In addition, patients who have been treated with cancer therapy that places them at long-term risk of cardiac disease, should be considered for cardio-oncology clinic referral. Patients who have received high-dose anthracycline chemotherapy and chest irradiation remain at risk of CV disease for many years after completion of treatment. The following cancer treatment regimens are considered high risk (12):

- High-dose anthracycline (e.g., doxorubicin at ≥250 mg/m², epirubicin at ≥600 mg/m²)
- High-dose radiotherapy (≥30 Gy) where the heart is in the treatment field
- Lower-dose anthracycline (e.g., doxorubicin at <250 mg/m², epirubicin at <600 mg/m²) in combination with lower-dose radiotherapy (<30 Gy) where the heart is in the treatment field (12)
- Lower-dose anthraycline (e.g., <250 mg/m² doxorubucin) or trastuzumab alone and presence of any of the other cardiac risk factors including:
  - Multiple (≥2) CV risk factors: smoking, diabetes, hypertension, dyslipidemia, obesity
  - Older age (>60 years old) at time of cancer treatment
  - Compromised cardiac function (e.g., borderline LV function (LVEF 50%–55%), history of myocardial infarction, ≥ moderate valvular heart disease

These patients may warrant closer surveillance and risk modification by a cardio-oncologist.

DO CARDIO-ONCOLOGY CLINICS IMPROVE PATIENT CARE?

There are currently no prospective studies that have evaluated the impact of referral to a cardio-oncology clinic on patient outcomes. This raises the question: "do cardio-oncology clinics really improve patient care?" Conceptually, cardio-oncology clinics are established with the intention that they lead to superior care and better clinical outcomes. Sulpher et.al in a retrospective cohort study, reported high completion rates of planned chemotherapy for patients referred to a cardio-oncology clinic, however there was no comparison cohort and long-term outcomes, such as decreases in CV mortality, were not evaluated (13). Historically, cancer patients have been referred to

cardiologists who had little understanding of cancer treatments and associated cardiac dysfunction. Lack of understanding of the potential benefits of cancer therapy often led cardiologists to recommend discontinuation of potentially life-sustaining or curative cancer therapy in patients experiencing cardiac dysfunction. Oncologists have been hesitant to refer cancer patients with cancer therapy-related dysfunction to cardiologists, in part owing to prolonged wait times for referrals (weeks to months). It is intuitive that those familiar with cardio-oncology are better at balancing risks and benefits, advising appropriately on discontinuation or continuation of therapies, and recommending preventive strategies. It is important that patients feel that their care is in the hands of the most knowledgeable and capable professional. The opinion of cardio-oncologists, who are knowledgeable about the CV complications of cancer therapy and best treatment strategies, should lead to better patient care. Research is needed to objectively quantify these clinical outcomes.

There has been some progress in the field of cardio-oncology and its impact on patient care. There is increasing evidence to support a protocolized approach for detecting patients at high risk of cardiotoxicity from cancer therapies. Risk stratification for development of cardiotoxicity has been most extensively studied in breast cancer patients treated with anthracycline-based chemotherapy with or without trastuzumab (see Chapter 3). Clinical risk factors, cardiac biomarkers such as troponin, and cardiac imaging either alone or in combination, can determine which patients are at highest risk for cardiotoxicity (14–17). As we learn more about cardiotoxicity from other cancer therapies, cancer therapy-specific protocols can be implemented to risk-stratify patients for cardiotoxicity from these treatments. The goal of such an approach is to identify patients at high risk for cardiotoxicity and triage them for prompt referral to a cardio-oncology clinic or a healthcare provider, with the aim of instituting measures to prevent cancer therapy-related cardiac dysfunction.

HOW TO DEFINE SUCCESS OF A CARDIO-ONCOLOGY CLINIC/ PROGRAM

There are currently no standardized cardio-oncology metrics that can easily be measured to define the success of a cardio-oncology clinic. Delays in treatment due to cardiac dysfunction, cancer therapy completion rates, and cardiac safety (especially compared to historical controls) could be used to determine benefit in terms of delivering effective cancer therapy without harming the heart. The success of a cardio-oncology clinic will be self-defined, not necessarily by its own standards but by its demand. If the clinic is successful in what it aims to accomplish, the demand will grow. If the cardio-oncology clinic meets the needs of the patients and the referring providers in addition to markedly improving clinical outcomes, it can be expected that the clinic will see increasing numbers of requests for consultation. The leader of the cardio-oncology program is invested in its success and needs to devote time and effort continuously, in this service line, staying up to date with demands and advances in the field, incorporating changes and striving toward best possible practice.

A pilot study during the first year of clinic operations could be launched to compare outcomes between patients managed before and after a cardio-oncology clinic. Incorporating quality control projects into the workflow of cardio-oncology clinics, along with formal research projects outside the clinic, could provide further support for the existence of the clinic. In this way, administrators can examine the clinic from a quality improvement perspective. Patient testimonials indicating how referral to a cardio-oncology clinic helped them get through their cancer treatment, despite cardiac issues, can serve as a powerful and tangible metric for hospital administrators.

The standards for becoming a cardio-oncology care provider are largely undefined. Any healthcare provider working in a "cardio-oncology clinic" can be regarded as a "cardio-oncologist." Specialty boards and credentialing bodies for this discipline do not exist; however, the last several years has seen a concerted effort by pioneers in cardio-oncology to remedy this field. A proposal for training requirements for healthcare providers with an interest in cardio-oncology (18) has provided some context for trainees as well as junior and senior healthcare providers. Efforts are currently underway to develop tools to assess healthcare providers' knowledge in cardio-oncology, which could eventually lead to a certificate-based program. These are important steps in defining

the field of cardio-oncology; however, clearly more efforts in this area are needed.

CONCLUSION

Modern treatment strategies have led to an improvement in surviving a diagnosis of cancer; however, cancer treatments may have a detrimental impact on CV health either during or following completion of therapy. The recognition and need to optimize CV health prior to and during cancer therapy has led to the development of the new subspecialty of cardio-oncology and the establishment of cardio-oncology clinics. The organization of cardio-oncology clinics is a complex process involving multidisciplinary collaboration as well as administrative support and institutional resources. Cardio-oncology clinics should strive to facilitate the delivery of "state of the art" cancer care while maintaining the highest levels of cardiac safety. Beyond clinical care delivery, cardio-oncology clinics can serve to educate patients and healthcare providers on the optimization of CV health prior to, during, and following completion of cancer treatment. Research defining which cancer patients are at greatest risk of cancer therapy-related cardiac dysfunction, prevention strategies, and optimization of cardiac testing and management should ultimately be incorporated into cardio-oncology programs. Cardio-oncology clinics that can implement protocols which improve cancer therapy effectiveness, enhance cardiac safety, and streamline health care costs would be welcomed in any healthcare system.

REFERENCES

1. Bluethmann SM, Mariotto AB, Rowland, JH. Anticipating the "silver tsunami": Prevalence trajectories and comorbidity burden among older cancer survivors in the United States. *Cancer Epidemiol Biomarkers Prev.* 2016;25: 1029–36.
2. Leading causes of death, total population, by age. 2016. Retrieved from https://www150.statcan.gc.ca/t1/tbl1/en/tv.action?pid=1310039401
3. Causes of death statistics. Retrieved from http://ec.europa.eu/eurostat/statistics-explained/index.php/Causes_of_death_statistics

4. Causes of death. 2018, May 22. Retrieved from http://www.who.int/gho/mortality_burden_disease/causes_death/en/

5. Dong J, Chen H. Cardiotoxicity of anticancer therapeutics. *Front Cardiovasc Med.* 2018;5:9. PMID 29473044, Doi:10.3389/fcvm.2018.00009.

6. Maurea N et al. Pathophysiology of cardiotoxicity from target therapy and angiogenesis inhibitors. *J Cardiovasc Med.* 2016;17. doi:10.2459/jcm.0000000000000377

7. Varricchi G et al. Antineoplastic drug-induced cardiotoxicity: A redox perspective. *Frontiers Physiol.* 2018;9. doi:10.3389/fphys.2018.00167

8. Wright F, Vito CD, Langer B, Hunter A. Multidisciplinary cancer conferences: A systematic review and development of practice standards. *Eur J Cancer.* 2007;43(6):1002–10. doi:10.1016/j.ejca.2007.01.025

9. Virani SA et al. Canadian cardiovascular society guidelines for evaluation and management of cardiovascular complications of cancer therapy. *Can J Cardiol.* 2016;32(7):831–41.

10. Lenihan DJ, Westcott G. Cardio-oncology: A tremendous opportunity to improve patient care. *Future Oncol.* 2015;11(14):2007–10.

11. Okwuosa TM, Barac A. Burgeoning cardio-oncology programs. *J Am Coll Cardiol.* 2015;66(10):1193–7. Available from: http://linkinghub.elsevier.com/retrieve/pii/S0735109715045702

12. Armenian SH et al. Prevention and monitoring of cardiac dysfunction in survivors of adult cancers: American Society of Clinical Oncology Clinical Practice Guideline. *J Clin Oncol.* 2017;35(8):893–911.

13. Sulpher J et al. Clinical experience of patients referred to a multidisciplinary cardiac oncology clinic: An observational study. *J Oncol.* 2015;2015:671232.

14. Thavendiranathan P, Poulin F, Lim K-D, Plana JC, Woo A, Marwick TH. Use of myocardial strain imaging by echocardiography for the early detection of cardiotoxicity in patients during and after cancer chemotherapy: A systematic review. *J Am Coll Cardiol.* 2014;63(25Pt. A):2751–68.

15. Sawaya H et al. Assessment of echocardiography and biomarkers for the extended prediction of cardiotoxicity in patients treated with anthracyclines, taxanes, and trastuzumab. *Circ Cardiovasc Imaging.* 2012;5(5):596–603.

16. Ezaz G, Long JB, Gross CP, Chen J. Risk prediction model for heart failure and cardiomyopathy after adjuvant trastuzumab therapy for breast cancer. *J Am Heart Assoc.* 2014;3:e000472.

17. Cardinale D et al. Prognostic value of troponin I in cardiac risk stratification of cancer patients undergoing high-dose chemotherapy. *Circulation* 2004;109(22):2749–2754.

18. Lenihan D et al. Cardio-oncology training: A proposal from the international cardioncology society and canadian cardiac oncology network for a new multidisciplinary specialty. *J Card Fail.* March 2016;22(6).

12

Cardio-oncology training

SARJU GANATRA AND MICHAEL G. FRADLEY

INTRODUCTION

Over the last decade, there has been explosive development in novel cancer therapeutics (1). With improved understanding of cancer biology, targeted treatments affecting tumor cell growth and proliferation have led to substantially improved patients outcomes (2). The 5 year survival rate for many cancers have increased dramatically over the last several decades owing in part to improved cancer therapies and screening. While the number of patients with cancer is expected to increase over the next decade, the number of cancer survivors is also expected to increase dramatically, from an estimated 14 million in 2014 to over 22 million by 2024 (3). It is increasingly recognized, however, that many cancer treatments have off target cardiovascular (CV) side effects. These cardiotoxicities can have a unique impact on a cancer patient's overall survival and quality of life. For example, a recent study utilizing data from the Surveillance, Epidemiology, and End Results-Medicare database in the USA demonstrated a cancer cohort treated from 2002 to 2007 to had a 3-year incidence of heart failure (HF) or left ventricular (LV) dysfunction of up to 42%, depending on the treatment. This is significantly higher when compared to the matched general population (4). Furthermore, managing CV disease and cardiotoxicities in cancer patients and survivors poses many unique

challenges. The multidisciplinary field of cardio-oncology was developed to provide optimal CV care to this population (5).

While there has been significant momentum in developing the field of cardio-oncology, there remains inconsistency in the diagnostic and treatment algorithms that are offered to patients, often as a result of practitioners' variable exposure and knowledge of different therapeutics and disease states. For example, in a recent survey of adult and pediatric cardiology division chiefs and fellowship directors, 52% believed that a dedicated cardio-oncology program would improve patient care and yet only 11% included cardio-oncology lectures as part of their core curriculum (6). Since completion of that survey, there has been substantial interest in creating formal educational requirements that are incorporated into traditional cardiology and oncology fellowship training programs, as well as developing dedicated cardio-oncology fellowships (7). Cardio-oncology fellows are expected to have an immersive educational experience such that they can provide expert CV care to cancer patients after completion of their training (8). Nonetheless, there are substantial challenges to the widespread implementation of cardio-oncology fellowships ranging from deficiencies in the number of expert educators and adequate training facilities, to the lack of a standardized curriculum and established training requirements (Figure 12.1).

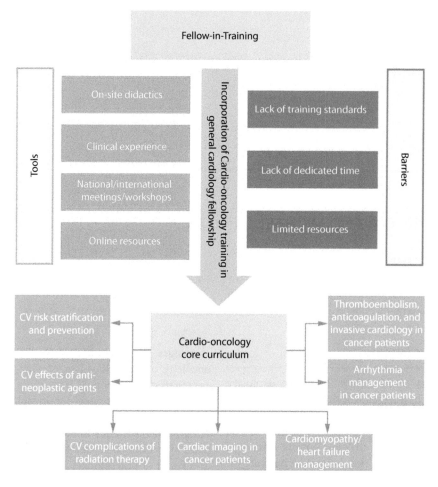

Figure 12.1 Cardio-oncology training recommendations, CV = cardiovascular.

CURRICULUM

Curriculum and training requirements

Management of patients inflicted with a dual diagnosis of cancer and CV disease is particularly challenging and mandates a thorough understanding of the complex pathophysiology of these diseases, as well as the antineoplastic treatments (9). Familiarity with the modalities to stratify risk and detect the early CV effects of cancer treatment are among the skills required for optimal care of the cancer patient. While there is no consensus or uniformity regarding the curriculum or training standards of a cardio-oncology fellowship, we propose the following topics as necessary components for the adequate training of the cardio-oncologist. With the rapidly evolving nature of cancer therapeutics, a stagnant list of topics may prove to be incomplete and continual reexamination is always necessary.

1. *Pretherapeutic CV risk factor stratification and management:* Significant overlap between comorbid CV disease and cancer is expected with the aging population and the growing number of cancer survivors (10). As such, risk stratification and optimization of CV risk factors prior to initiation of anticancer therapy is increasingly important (11). Additionally, understanding the potential cardiotoxicities of cancer therapies can lead to utilization of specific prevention strategies for patients at high-risk for the development of CV complications (12).

2. *Antineoplastic therapy-related cardiotoxicity:* Chemotherapeutic agents associated with

a short- and long-term cardiotoxic effects include anthracyclines, 5-fluorouracil (5-FU), cyclophosphamide, tyrosine kinase inhibitors (TKIs), vascular endothelial growth factor (VEGF) inhibitors, immune checkpoint inhibitors (ICIs), HER-2 antagonists, and radiation therapy. Cardiomyopathy and heart failure related to anthracycline and HER-2 antagonists are the classic examples; however, a myriad of CV effects, extending from arrhythmias, to malignant hypertension, valvular heart disease, arterial and venous thrombosis, coronary ischemia, and myocarditis, are observed with novel antineoplastic agents, warranting a thorough understanding of pathophysiology, monitoring, prevention, and treatment strategies (4,13–18).

3. *CV complications of radiation therapy:* Mediastinal radiation therapy is known to increase the risk of premature coronary artery disease, valvular disease, cardiomyopathy, conduction system disease, arrhythmia, pericardial disease, and autonomic dysfunction (17,19). In addition to a baseline assessment, ongoing surveillance is essential as most radiation-induced CV complications occur years after the initial exposure. The American Society of Echocardiography (ASE) recommends annual CV assessment and stress echocardiogram 5 years after completion of radiation therapy even for asymptomatic patients (20). Management of radiation therapy-related CV complications can be complex, requiring unique and individualized treatment strategies.

4. *Cardiac imaging in patients with cancer:* Cardiac imaging is the primary tool for prompt detection of cardiotoxicity, which in turn may improve the clinical outcome with the early initiation of cardioprotective medications (21). Multiple imaging modalities are available such as 2D echocardiography, strain echocardiography, 3D echocardiography, multigated acquisition (MUGA) scans, and cardiac magnetic resonance imaging (MRI) for baseline assessment of cardiac structure and function, cardiotoxicity surveillance, early diagnosis, and treatment-related decisions. Additionally, cardiac computed tomography (CT) scan, particularly coronary CT angiogram can be useful for the noninvasive assessment of coronary arteries. Indications, advantages, and shortcomings

of each modality in this patient population should be incorporated into the curriculum (9).

5. *Management of cardiomyopathy in patients with cancer:* Although the treatment of chemotherapy-induced cardiomyopathy and heart failure is similar to any other etiology, cancer patients frequently experience episodes of hypotension, fluctuation in kidney function, and drug interactions, making management more challenging. Short- or long-term advanced mechanical support and heart transplantation in this population requires special consideration in light of the patient's diagnosis and prognosis (22).

6. *Management of arrhythmias and QT prolongation in patients with cancer:* Arrhythmias are commonly observed in cancer patients and are due to multiple factors including surgery, chronic inflammation, autonomic nervous system imbalance, paraneoplastic manifestations, metabolic abnormalities, cardiac metastasis, or chemotherapy (23). Atrial fibrillation (AF) is especially common in cancer patients and is associated with a significantly higher risk of heart failure and thromboembolism, even after adjusting for known risk factors. Treatment of AF and other arrhythmias can be challenging in cancer patients due to excess bleeding risks and the potential for drug interactions. One prime example is ibrutinib, a medication used for the treatment of variety of B-cell lymphomas. Its use is associated with significantly increased incidence of AF; however, it also inhibits platelet activation leading to increased bleeding complications. Ibrutinib's interaction with calcium channel blockers, digoxin, amiodarone, and various anticoagulants can result in drug-related toxicity and careful selection and dose adjustment may be needed (24,25).

QT prolongation in cancer patients can be related to the antineoplastic therapies themselves (i.e., arsenic, nilotinib, ribociclib, etc.), as well as the concomitant use of other QT prolonging medications such as antidepressants and antimicrobials. Patient-specific factors such as electrolyte imbalances or underlying CV disease may also have an impact (26). While QT prolongation is commonly observed in the cancer patient population, rates of associated malignant ventricular arrhythmias are low (27).

As such, trainees must be adept at accurately monitoring and measuring the QT interval in order to ensure patient safety while minimizing unnecessary treatment disruptions.

7. *Arterial and venous thromboembolism in patients with cancer:* Although the incidence of arterial and venous thromboembolic events varies based on the type of cancer and antineoplastic therapy, a higher burden of morbidity and mortality is noted across the spectrum when thromboembolic events occur in this population. Patients with cancer also have a significantly higher risk of bleeding with anticoagulation, especially in the setting of thrombocytopenia or coagulopathy. In patients with cancer, the choice of anticoagulant and/or invasive interventions such as inferior vena cava filter insertion, as well as duration of therapy, requires complex decision making balancing risk with potential benefits.

8. *Percutaneous coronary interventions (PCI), length of dual antiplatelet therapy, and choice of stent:* Evidence increasingly shows that cancer and coronary artery disease (CAD) are interlinked through common risk factors, co-occurrence in an aging population, and through the deleterious effects of cancer treatment on cardiovascular health (28,29). Furthermore, acute myocardial infarction in patients with a history of cancer is associated with a higher incidence of cardiogenic shock, in-hospital mortality, and long-term mortality when compared to patients without cancer (30). Additionally, the treatment of CAD in this population is challenging for several reasons given the potentially increased rates of bleeding as well as hypercoagulability. This issue poses a unique challenge in the setting of PCI, as individualized risk profiles have a tremendous impact on the options for stenting and antiplatelet therapy. Although bare metal stents (BMS) have been traditionally preferred in patients with cancer due to a perceived need for shorter dual antiplatelet therapy (DAPT), several drug-eluting stent (DES) options are emerging, which may be more efficacious than traditional BMS, with the advantage of shorter-duration of DAPT when compared to traditional DES (31). More emphasis is also required on reducing the risk of bleeding in the peri-procedural period by using radial artery access when feasible and the routine use of ultrasound when femoral artery access is required (32).

TRAINING REQUIREMENTS

There are a growing number of cardio-oncology training programs, the majority of which are located at tertiary/quaternary referral centers with both comprehensive cancer and CV centers (7). However there remains a great degree of variation in core curricula, training duration and environment, institutional infrastructure, research opportunities, and degree of collaboration between cardiology and oncology. There is also no consensus regarding prerequisite experience prior to entering such programs or for assessing competency at the completion of the training, which is largely due to lack of predefined training standards and regulatory oversight.

Currently, the Core Cardiology Training Statement (COCATS-4) does not include dedicated time for cardio-oncology exposure and training during general CV fellowship programs (33). Conversely, the European Society of Cardiology Committee for Education has incorporated formal cardio-oncology exposure and assessment into its training recommendations for the general cardiologist (34). While the 3-year length of CV training programs should allow for incorporating exposure to cardio-oncology, the better solution would be recognition and incorporation of cardio-oncology as a part of the core curriculum by the upcoming COCATS-5 Task Force (9).

In order to standardize the training experience and to ensure high quality training in cardio-oncology, the Accreditation Council for Graduate Medical Education (ACGME), the Core Cardiology Training Statement (COCATS) by American College of Cardiology, and the various oncology societies need to form a consensus on curriculum and training requirements. Eventually, board certification after dedicated training in this subspecialty will be helpful given the complexity of this rapidly developing field. To this end, the International Cardio-Oncology Society (ICOS) and the Canadian Cardiac Oncology Network (CCON) have proposed a conceptual framework with comprehensive training goals and standards for this growing subspecialty (8). They recommend the following requirements for high quality level III training in cardio-oncology.

Pre-requisite for enrollment in training program

Successful completion of training in an ACGME accredited cardiology or hematology-oncology fellowship program (36 months). It is important to note that although cardio-oncology subspecialty training can be pursued after a hematology-oncology fellowship, such candidates may require additional training about CV disease and various diagnostic and management modalities.

Duration of training: One year

TRAINING ENVIRONMENT

In order to provide adequate instruction in cardio-oncology (for both dedicated cardio-oncology fellows and other trainees), the facilities must be of appropriate size and volume to provide sufficient exposure to all aspects of cardio-oncology. At a minimum, training must occur at a facility with both oncology and cardiology services. The oncology program should be comprehensive including treatment of solid and liquid tumors, stem cell transplantation, oncologic surgery, radiation therapy (including proton therapy if available), and exposure to modern treatments including chemotherapy, targeted cancer therapeutics, and immunotherapies (checkpoint inhibitors, chimeric antigen receptor therapy, etc.). In addition, it is recommended that the center have a robust clinical trials and research program, as cardio-oncology trainees can derive significant educational benefit from these complex patient scenarios (29,35).

From a CV perspective, a robust cardio-oncology program requires a unique integration of CV imaging, bio-marker testing and invasive evaluations including cardiac catheterizations, cardiac biopsies, and electrophysiology procedures. Cardio-oncology patients may present unique challenges when considering these different diagnostic modalities. As such, trainees must be given adequate exposure to the various CV procedures in order to understand their best utilization in this unique population. In particular, CV imaging must be emphasized. There should be immediate availability of 2D echocardiography and the laboratory must focus on accurate and precise reproducibility of studies. In addition, 3D echocardiography and measures of ventricular strain should be integrated into routine evaluations readily available as these modalities play a significant role in the care of the cardio-oncology patient. Access to advanced imaging modalities including cardiac CT and cardiac MRI is strongly recommended (21,36–38).

PERSONNEL REQUIREMENT

The cardio-oncology trainee benefits from a robust, multidisciplinary group of educators including cardiologists, hematologist-oncologists, pharmacists, and nurses dedicated to the mission of academic training and instruction. Cardiologists with particular interest in the field of cardio-oncology must play a primary role in the education of the trainee and be readily available to provide expeditious care to cancer patients. The cardio-oncologist needs to have sufficient understanding of various cancer therapeutics and their potential cardiotoxic effects, as well as experience in the management of common CV diseases. Ideally, subspecialists including interventional cardiologists, electrophysiologists, and heart failure and transplant cardiologists with an interest in the field of cardio-oncology should be identified to augment the training experience. Cardiologists and trainees should routinely participate in oncology tumor boards and other committee meetings in which complex decision making that can have an impact on CV health is discussed. Similarly, oncologists should be invited to CV meetings to provide their perspective when discussing issues related to anticoagulation and antiplatelet initiation, as well as the use of invasive CV procedures in cancer patients. Interdisciplinary education also includes joint participation in case conferences, journal clubs, and cardio-oncology focused grand rounds. Pharmacists can be an especially useful resource to help provide refined knowledge about different cancer therapeutics and nurse navigators help ensure patients understand the complexities and interplay of cancer and their CV health (7,8,29, 35).

CLINICAL EXPERIENCE

There is no consensus on the minimum amount of clinical experience required during 1 year of training. The ICOS/CCON consensus statement recommends a minimum of 100 unique patient encounters per year who are survivors of cancer treatment or undergoing active cancer therapy. However, over the last decade, there has been a progressive move toward competency-based training, where the evaluation is focused on specific learner outcomes rather than mere number of patients/procedure encounters (33). Currently there is an unmet need to delineate the specific components of competency within the subspecialty, to define the tools necessary to assess training, and to establish milestones that should be met as fellows progress toward independence. As the field of cardio-oncology and the number of training programs grow, objective assessment of predefined core competencies and milestones set by the ACGME and American Board of Medical Specialties should be easier to define and adopt. A trainee should be provided an opportunity to work on both outpatient and inpatient cardio-oncology consult services. Experience should also be inclusive of exposure to cardiac imaging, heart failure, arrhythmia, and other common CV disease management pertinent to this population.

RESEARCH OPPORTUNITIES

Clinical and translational research is the key for the advancement of the field. Regardless of the eventual career path of a trainee, a robust research infrastructure is a necessary component of a successful cardio-oncology program. Research provides increased recognition and growth of the program and trainees should expect to devote significant time to scholarly cardio-oncology activities. Trainees should be encouraged to pursue clinical, translational or basic science research based on their unique cardio-oncology interests. Trainees should be expected to present their research at national meetings as well as publish their findings in peer reviewed journals. As the field of cardio-oncology continues to grow and with an established research infrastructure, there may be opportunities to obtain National Institute of Health (NIH) funded T-32 training grants focusing on various scientific areas relevant to cardio-oncology (39–42).

BARRIERS

Here we briefly describe the major barriers to the successful implementation of cardio-oncology training programs and potential ways to overcome them.

1. *Cardio-oncology remains an ill-defined field,* with an unclear scope of practice and a poorly defined field. As the field evolves, objective assessment of predefined core competencies and milestones set by the ACGME and American Board of Medical Specialties (ABMS) should be easier to define and adopt. Eventual accreditation by both the ACGME and ABMS will help to sustain the programs and to ensure high quality standardized education.

2. *Lack of recognition as a separate subspecialty* is a major barrier. Most experts practicing cardio-oncology are trained cardiologists though few have received dedicated cardio-oncology training. Although several major societies including American College of Cardiology (ACC), American Heart Association (AHA), and American Society of Clinical Oncology (ASCO) have acknowledged the importance of this field, cardio-oncology is not yet recognized as a separate, individual subspecialty which is a typical challenge faced by most emerging specialties in the early days of development. Cardio-oncology specialists need to mobilize the major medical societies and advocacy groups to achieve the recognition as a distinguished subspecialty. While this process may take years, it is important to establish both clinical and training programs to provide excellent patient care and also to attain institutional recognition.

3. *Limited and variable resource availability* is a barrier in establishing and achieving uniformity among the cardio-oncology training programs. Major academic institutions with both comprehensive cancer centers and heart failure/cardiac imaging/interventional cardiology/electrophysiology programs can be an ideal place to initiate such programs. However, there are only few such centers across the nation (USA) and with a growing demand for experts in this field, alternative arrangements may need to be explored. There is also a greater need to incorporate basic cardio-oncology experience into general CV fellowship training. While the current Core Cardiology Training Statement (COCATS-4) does not recognize or include cardio-oncology as a part of the core-curriculum (33), the ultimate solution would be recognition and incorporation of cardio-oncology by the upcoming COCATS-5 task force (9).

4. *Lack of institutional and financial support* represents a major barrier for successful development of both clinical and training programs. This is largely driven by all the factors previously mentioned including lack of formal recognition as a subspecialty by both academic governing bodies and insurance/payer networks, limited resources with other competing financial investment interests, the ill-defined nature of the field without clear guidelines, and the lack of definitive evidence that cardio-oncology improves overall outcomes/patient care. A collaborative work environment will invariably increase the patient

volume and appropriate CV testing in order to ensure financial viability. Research grant funding (e.g., NIH T32 teaching grants, industry support grants, foundation support, etc.) may help to ensure sustainability of the mission of the fellowship. Finally, increased awareness among cancer patients and survivors of potential cardiotoxicities associated with antineoplastic therapy will result in increased demand for experts in cardio-oncology thereby increasing the need for training programs.

FUTURE DIRECTIONS

For the development and continuous growth of any field, formalized training and education is vital. Interdisciplinary collaboration of cardiology with oncology, radiation oncology, survivorship experts, and primary care physicians is the key to the successful development of dedicated cardio-oncology subspecialty training programs. It is also important that the major CV and oncology profession societies provide guidance for the development of unified training standards to care for this growing cohort of patients. Subspecialization in this field after general CV fellowship and board certification will be helpful given the complex and rapidly changing field. Eventual recognition as a separate subspecialty by ACGME, ABMS, and large insurance payer networks (including Centers for Medicare and Medicaid Services [CMS]) is essential.

REFERENCES

1. Guha A, Armanious M, Fradley MG. Update on cardio-oncology: Novel cancer therapeutics and associated cardiotoxicities. *Trends Cardiovasc Med.* 2019 January;29(1):29–39.
2. Krause DS, Van Etten RA. Tyrosine kinases as targets for cancer therapy. *N Engl J Med.* 2005;353(2):172–87.
3. Miller KD et al. Cancer treatment and survivorship statistics, 2016. *CA Cancer J Clin.* 2016;66(4):271–89.
4. Chen J, Long JB, Hurria A, Owusu C, Steingart RM, Gross CP. Incidence of heart failure or cardiomyopathy after adjuvant trastuzumab therapy for breast cancer. *J Am Coll Cardiol.* 2012;60(24):2504–12.
5. Albini A, Pennesi G, Donatelli F, Cammarota R, De Flora S, Noonan DM. Cardiotoxicity of anticancer drugs: The need for cardio-oncology and cardio-oncological prevention. *J Natl Cancer Inst.* 2010;102(1):14–25.
6. Barac A et al. Cardiovascular health of patients with cancer and cancer survivors: A roadmap to the next level. *J Am Coll Cardiol.* 2015;65(25):2739–46.
7. Johnson MN, Steingart R, Carver J. How to develop a cardio-oncology fellowship. *Heart Fail Clin.* 2017;13(2):361–6.
8. Lenihan DJ et al. Cardio-oncology training: A proposal from the International Cardioncology Society and Canadian Cardiac Oncology Network for a new multidisciplinary specialty. *J Card Fail.* 2016;22(6):465–71.
9. Ganatra S, Hayek SS. Cardio-oncology for GenNext: A missing piece of the training puzzle. *J Am Coll Cardiol.* 2018;71(25):2977–81.
10. DeSantis CE et al. Cancer treatment and survivorship statistics, 2014. *CA Cancer J Clin.* 2014;64(4):252–71.
11. Koene RJ, Prizment AE, Blaes A, Konety SH. Shared risk factors in cardiovascular disease and cancer. *Circulation.* 2016;133(11):1104–14.
12. Cardinale D et al. Early detection of anthracycline cardiotoxicity and improvement with heart failure therapy. *Circulation.* 2015;131(22):1981–8.
13. Lipshultz SE, Alvarez JA, Scully RE. Anthracycline associated cardiotoxicity in survivors of childhood cancer. *Heart.* 2008;94(4):525–33.
14. Moslehi JJ, Deininger M. Tyrosine kinase inhibitor-associated cardiovascular toxicity in chronic myeloid leukemia. *J Clin Oncol.* 2015;33(35):4210–8.
15. Mahmood SS et al. Myocarditis in patients treated with immune checkpoint inhibitors. *J Am Coll Cardiol.* 2018;71(16):1755–64.
16. Murbraech K et al. Valvular dysfunction in lymphoma survivors treated with autologous stem cell transplantation: A national cross-sectional study. *JACC Cardiovasc Imaging.* 2016;9(3):230–9.
17. Groarke JD, Nguyen PL, Nohria A, Ferrari R, Cheng S, Moslehi J. Cardiovascular complications of radiation therapy for thoracic

malignancies: The role for non-invasive imaging for detection of cardiovascular disease. *Eur Heart J.* 2014;35(10):612–23.

18. Ganatra S, Neilan TG. Immune checkpoint inhibitor associated myocarditis. *Oncologist.* 2018;23:518–23.

19. Darby SC et al. Risk of ischemic heart disease in women after radiotherapy for breast cancer. *N Engl J Med.* 2013;368(11):987–98.

20. Lancellotti P et al. Expert consensus for multi-modality imaging evaluation of cardiovascular complications of radiotherapy in adults: A report from the European Association of Cardiovascular Imaging and the American Society of Echocardiography. *J Am Soc Echocardiogr.* 2013;26(9):1013–32.

21. Plana JC et al. Expert consensus for multimodality imaging evaluation of adult patients during and after cancer therapy: A report from the American Society of Echocardiography and the European Association of Cardiovascular Imaging. *J Am Soc Echocardiogr.* 2014;27(9):911–39.

22. Shah S, Nohria A. Advanced heart failure due to cancer therapy. *Curr Cardiol Rep.* 2015;17(4):16.

23. Armanious MA, Mishra S, Fradley MG. Electrophysiologic toxicity of chemoradiation. *Curr Oncol Rep.* 2018;20(6):45.

24. Ganatra S, Majithia A, Shah S. Challenges in ibrutinib associated atrial fibrillation. *J Am Coll Cardiol.* 2017;11(69):2308.

25. Ganatra S et al. Ibrutinib-associated atrial fibrillation. *JACC Clin Electrophysiol.* 2018 December;4(12):1491–1500.

26. Fradley MG, Moslehi J. QT prolongation and oncology drug development. *Card Electrophysiol Clin.* 2015;7(2):341–55.

27. Naing A et al. Electrocardiograms (ECGs) in phase I anticancer drug development: The MD Anderson Cancer Center experience with 8518 ECGs. *Ann Oncol.* 2012;23(11):2960–3.

28. Ganatra S. Cardio-oncology: A tale of two diseases. *Cardiovasc Pharm Open Access.* 2017;6(6):e136.

29. Okwuosa TM, Barac A. Burgeoning cardio-oncology programs: Challenges and opportunities for early career cardiologists/faculty directors. *J Am Coll Cardiol.* 2015;66(10):1193–7.

30. Wang F et al. Cancer history portends worse acute and long-term noncardiac (but not cardiac) mortality after primary percutaneous coronary intervention for acute ST-segment elevation myocardial infarction. *Mayo Clin Proc.* 2016;91(12):1680–92.

31. Ganatra S, Sharma A, Levy MS. Re-evaluating the safety of drug-eluting stents in cancer patients. *JACC Cardiovasc Interv.* 2017;10(22):2334–7.

32. Iliescu CA et al. SCAI Expert consensus statement: Evaluation, management, and special considerations of cardio-oncology patients in the cardiac catheterization laboratory (endorsed by the cardiological society of India, and Sociedad Latino Americana de Cardiologia Intervencionista). *Catheter Cardiovasc Interv.* 2016;87(5):E202–23.

33. Fuster V et al. COCATS 4 task force 1: Training in ambulatory, consultative, and longitudinal cardiovascular care. *J Am Coll Cardiol.* 2015;65(17):1734–53.

34. Gillebert TC et al. ESC core curriculum for the general cardiologist (2013). *Eur Heart J.* 2013;34(30):2381–411.

35. Fradley MG et al. Developing a comprehensive cardio-oncology program at a cancer institute: The Moffitt Cancer Center experience. *Oncol Rev.* 2017;11(2):340.

36. Stanton T, Jenkins C, Haluska BA, Marwick TH. Association of outcome with left ventricular parameters measured by two-dimensional and three-dimensional echocardiography in patients at high cardiovascular risk. *J Am Soc Echocardiogr.* 2014;27(1):65–73.

37. Thavendiranathan P, Grant AD, Negishi T, Plana JC, Popovic ZB, Marwick TH. Reproducibility of echocardiographic techniques for sequential assessment of left ventricular ejection fraction and volumes: Application to patients undergoing cancer chemotherapy. *J Am Coll Cardiol.* 2013;61(1):77–84.

38. Kongbundansuk S, Hundley WG. Noninvasive imaging of cardiovascular injury related to the treatment of cancer. *JACC Cardiovasc Imaging.* 2014;7(8):824–38.

39. Shelburne N et al. Cancer treatment-related cardiotoxicity: Current state of knowledge and future research priorities. *J Natl Cancer Inst.* 2014;106(9).

40. Kobashigawa J et al. Report from a consensus conference on antibody-mediated rejection in heart transplantation. *J Heart Lung Transplant*. 2011;30(3):252–69.

41. Narahari AK et al. Cardiothoracic surgery training grants provide protected research time vital to the development of academic surgeons. *J Thorac Cardiovasc Surg*. 2018;155(5):2050–6.

42. Ky B, Vejpongsa P, Yeh ET, Force T, Moslehi JJ. Emerging paradigms in cardiomyopathies associated with cancer therapies. *Circ Res*. 2013;113(6):754–64.

13

Cardio-oncology nursing

ANECITA FADOL

INTRODUCTION

Cardio-oncology nursing is a rapidly emerging area of great clinical need, and one of the most challenging and rewarding fields in nursing that transcends across the continuum of cancer care. With the introduction of new anticancer treatments, improvements in patient survival, and an aging population, the clinical significance of cardiac toxicity has markedly increased. Following cancer treatments in many patients, the risk of cardiovascular death may be higher than the actual risk of tumor recurrence (1). In the era of both traditional and targeted cancer therapies, oncology care providers face complex decisions on a daily basis, whether before, during, or following definitive cancer treatments. Management of these patients is challenging. In particular, the presence of multiple comorbidities in older adults with cancer complicates coordination of cancer treatment. Adjuvant cancer treatments including chemotherapy and radiation therapy are associated with de novo and latent effects on the cardiovascular system resulting in "cardiotoxicity," which may result from the direct effects of cancer treatment on heart function and structure, or may be due to

accelerated development of cardiovascular disease, especially in the presence of traditional cardiovascular risk factors (2). Providing comprehensive care to these patients requires a multidisciplinary team, which led to the new discipline of onco-cardiology or cardio-oncology.

Multidisciplinary programs in oncology and cardiology have been associated with enhanced patient well-being and improved clinical outcomes (3). The goals of cardio-oncology programs are to support cancer patients through the early identification of and management of cardiac risk factors, the treatment of preexisting and de novo cardiac issues, and cardiac surveillance during and after cancer treatments (1). The cardio-oncology team include cardiologists, medical oncologists, advanced practice providers (nurse practitioners, physician assistants), pharmacists, nurses, dieticians, and social workers. This chapter will discuss the emerging role of cardio-oncology nursing as an integral component of the multidisciplinary team in the management of common cardiovascular toxicities associated with cancer therapy. The multifaceted role of the cardio-oncology nurse from cancer diagnosis, cancer treatment, and survivorship to end-of-life care will be discussed.

THE ROLE OF THE CARDIO-ONCOLOGY NURSE IN THE CARDIO-ONCOLOGY PROGRAM

The nurse is at the "heart of patient care" in the cardio-oncology multidisciplinary team. Nurses bridge the gap between cardiologists and oncologists/specialists and the interdisciplinary team to provide seamless care for patients with cancer with multiple comorbidities, including concurrent cardiovascular disease. The cardio-oncology nurses assume the role by happenstance because of their place of employment, where patients committed to the nurses' care may have cancer and concurrent cardiovascular disease. A majority of cardio-oncology nurses are employed in cancer centers, but many work in different healthcare settings, including community health clinics.

The roles of cardio-oncology nurses are diverse, depending on their scope of responsibility, and include bedside clinicians, advanced practice providers, educators, or managers. A majority of their roles involve coordination of patient care and providing education to patients, families, caregivers, and others in the healthcare team from diagnosis and treatment to survivorship and end-of-life care. Effective performance of these roles requires a knowledge of both cardiology and oncology. However, dedicated cardio-oncology content is lacking in the basic nursing curriculum for the education of nurses, and there is not a required certification to practice cardio-oncology nursing. Postgraduate education required for nurse practitioners may include a focus on oncology or cardiology nursing as a specialty; however, a degree in cardio-oncology nursing as a specialty is not available at this time. Physicians have dedicated cardi-oncology fellowships in universities affiliated with academic medical centers. This has created physician leaders who will champion patient care, educate other healthcare providers, and conduct research to expand knowledge in the evolving specialty of cardio-oncology. Nurses interested in advancing their knowledge and skills in cardio-oncology may do so through attending continuing education offerings and conferences, such as those offered by the cardio-oncology section of the American College of Cardiology, the International Cardio-Oncology Society, and the American Society of Clinical Oncology. However, notwithstanding a lack of specialized training in cardio-oncology nursing, nurses combine their scientific knowledge, technical skills, and caring abilities to help people living with cancer and cardiovascular disease and their families throughout the cancer journey.

Current practices in cardio-oncology are largely extrapolated from existing cardiology and oncology literature, while research specific to cardio-oncology is ongoing to support evidence-based practice. Multidisciplinary team members collectively have multiple areas of expertise relevant to cardio-oncology, thereby reducing the knowledge gaps and improving consistency in patient care.

CARDIO-ONCOLOGY NURSES AS COORDINATORS OF PATIENT CARE

Cardio-oncology nurses are at the forefront of patient-centered care. With the transformation of the healthcare system, care coordination is now being highlighted by hospitals and health systems as a key tool in improving patient health and satisfaction, as well as controlling healthcare costs. Care coordination has been a core professional standard and competency for nurses. As integral members of the multidisciplinary team, cardio-oncology nurses are responsible for coordinating the various patient care activities prescribed by the multidisciplinary healthcare team. In traditional care models, shared patients are seen individually by cardiologists and oncologists, which may result in fragmented care with consequent suboptimal outcomes. Oncologists are focused on cancer care, and might not assess for preexisting cardiac disease or screen for related risk factors, thereby missing the opportunity to prevent cardiovascular events (4). Similarly, cardiologists might fail to detect early signs of cancer resulting in delayed diagnosis, increased risk of disease progression, and poorer oncologic outcomes (3). With the increasing complexity of the multimodality cancer treatment options, it is imperative for the cardio-oncology team to devise detailed and organized interdisciplinary care plans that seek to avoid, detect, monitor, and manage a growing array of potential oncologic and cardiovascular interactions and complications (4–7). Cardio-oncology nurses and nurse practitioners coordinate the implementation of the multidisciplinary care plans, inform patients, monitor adverse events, evaluate outcomes, and notify cardiologists and oncologists

Table 13.1 Nursing management and patient education for common cardiotoxicities of cancer therapy

Cardiovascular toxicity	Nursing assessment	Monitoring/Management	Patient education
Atrial fibrillation			
Atrial fibrillation (AF) is the most commonly observed atrial dysrhythmia associated with cancer treatment.	1. Obtain a baseline ECG. 2. Compare apical and peripheral heart rate. 3. Assess patient's history for known medical conditions or medications that may precipitate AF. 4. Maintain ongoing monitoring (continuous or intermittent) of ECG rhythm. 5. Clinical assessment of the risk for stroke utilizing the CHA_2DS_2-VASc score (13,14) is essential, particularly as age increases and the prospect of the development of comorbidities becomes more likely (13,15–17).	1. Perform follow-up assessments of vital signs and symptoms of dyspnea, hypoxemia (shown as low oxygen saturation), hypotension, or chest discomfort (18). 2. If patient is on diuretics, emphasize adherence to supplemental potassium replacement therapy to prevent dysrhythmias related to hypokalemia. 3. Replace electrolytes and maintain within normal ranges, particularly potassium and magnesium. 4. Emphasize importance of periodic evaluation of laboratory values and ECG when at risk for dysrhythmias.	1. Teach patients and families the symptoms of AF (palpitations) and the potential urgency of treatment. 2. Patients need to know potential causes of their AF, how it will affect their life and what the therapeutic options are. 3. Patients need to be aware of their risk of stroke (13,15,17,19). 4. Teach patients of the potential harms of medications used to treat AF (e.g., beta-blockers, antidysrhythmic), which can include hypotension and bradycardia. 5. Patients need to be aware that late recurrences of AF after cardioversion and/or catheter ablation are a possibility and that more than one procedure may be required.

(Continued)

Table 13.1 (Continued) Nursing management and patient education for common cardiotoxicities of cancer therapy

Cardiovascular toxicity	Nursing assessment	Monitoring/Management	Patient education
			6. Patients need to know what they have been prescribed and why they are taking it, how to take the medication (dose, frequency, timings, with/before/after food, with other tablets, etc.), what will happen if they fail to adhere as prescribed, any factors that may modify drug efficacy, any possible side effects, and the likelihood of treatment success or failure, to enable realistic treatment expectations. 7. Teach preventive strategies such as hydration or electrolyte replacement. Emphasize that vomiting or diarrhea may disrupt fluid or electrolyte balance. *(Continued)*

Table 13.1 (Continued) Nursing management and patient education for common cardiotoxicities of cancer therapy

Cardiovascular toxicity	Nursing assessment	Monitoring/Management	Patient education
QT prolongation Definition: QT prolongation is defined as an increased duration of the QT interval (>450 ms [males] and >460 ms [females]). The QT interval represents the duration of electrical depolarization and repolarization of the ventricles (20), beginning at the initiation of the QRS complex and ending where the T wave returns to isoelectric baseline. The QT interval is inversely correlated with heart rate; therefore, QT interval is shorter with more rapid heart rates and longer with slower rates. Because of its inverse relationship to heart rate, the QT interval is routinely transformed into a heart rate–dependent "corrected" value known as the QTc interval. The QTc interval is intended to represent the QT interval at a standardized heart rate of 60 bpm. QTc prolongation >500 ms or a QT change from baseline of >60 ms (21) should be of particular concern because it can predispose patients to torsade de pointes (TdP).	1. Identify the etiology of the QT prolongation, resulting from toxic substances or other metabolic abnormalities, or from those associated with primary or structural abnormalities of the heart itself. 2. Obtain a 12-lead ECG. 3. Assess electrolytes, particularly the magnesium levels.	1. Monitor electrolytes, particularly potassium and magnesium levels; supplement as needed. 2. Correct contributing factors such as hypoxemia, anemia, fluid imbalance, and electrolyte abnormalities. 3. Administer electrolyte replacement to a goal potassium value >4 mEq/L and magnesium value >2 mEq/L (18,26,27). 4. Prior to starting medications with potential for QT prolongation, obtain a baseline ECG with QT measurement, and subsequent electrocardiogram monitoring for QT intervals as indicated by the drug's prescribing information. 5. In patients with excessive corrected QT interval prolongation (>500 ms), QT-prolonging cancer drugs should not be started, and potential causes or contributing factors should be evaluated and corrected. 6. Concomitant treatment with QT-prolonging drugs (e.g., certain antiarrhythmic, antibiotic, and antifungal agents) should be avoided.	1. Patients need to understand the importance of maintaining magnesium levels within normal limits. 2. Patients need to be aware if they are on medications that can result in QT prolongation.

(Continued)

Table 13.1 (Continued) Nursing management and patient education for common cardiotoxicities of cancer therapy

Cardiovascular toxicity	Nursing assessment	Monitoring/Management	Patient education
TdP is a polymorphic ventricular tachyarrhythmia characterized by a continuous twisting of the vector of the QRS complex around the isoelectric baseline. TdP may degenerate into ventricular fibrillation, leading to sudden cardiac death (22). A feature of TdP is pronounced prolongation of the QT interval in the supraventricular beat preceding the arrhythmia. Factors contributing to the development of QT prolongation include: 1. Anticancer medications including 5-fluorouracil (5-FU), arsenic trioxide, dasatinib, lapatinib, nilotinib, pazopanib, sunitinib, tamoxifen, temsirolimus, and vorinostat (21–25). 2. Presence of multiple comorbidities (e.g., preexisting cardiac disease). 3. Polypharmacy with concomitant QT-prolonging agents (e.g., antiemetics, antidepressants, and antibiotics). 4. Electrolyte disturbances (particularly hypokalemia and hypomagnesemia), and other metabolic abnormalities.			

(Continued)

Table 13.1 (Continued) Nursing management and patient education for common cardiotoxicities of cancer therapy

Cardiovascular toxicity	Nursing assessment	Monitoring/Management	Patient education
Hypertension Definition: Hypertension (HTN) is defined as a blood pressure (BP) >140/90, based on average of 2 or more BP readings on 2 or more visits (43). HTN is classified in two stages. Stage I HTN is defined as a systolic blood pressure (SBP) of 130–139 mm Hg or a diastolic blood pressure (DBP) of 80–89 mm Hg, while stage II is defined as SBP ≥140 mm Hg or a DBP ≥90 mm Hg (28). In the general population of adults 60 years and older, pharmacologic treatment should be initiated when the systolic pressure is 150 mm Hg or higher, or when the diastolic pressure is 90 mm Hg or higher. For individuals younger than 60 years, pharmacologic treatment should be initiated when the systolic pressure is 140 mm Hg or higher, or when the diastolic pressure is 90 mm Hg or higher.	1. Obtain a comprehensive patient history to establish baseline. 2. Assess for medications (e.g., sinus or cold remedies) or clinical conditions that may contribute to altered blood pressure. 3. Laboratory evaluation to determine specific cardiovascular (CV) risk factors prior to starting tyrosine kinase inhibitors (TKIs) (24). BP assessment should have a minimum of 2 standardized BP measurements and set a goal BP of <140/90 mm Hg for most patients, in accordance with recommendations for all adults.	1. Early diagnosis and controlling blood pressure to recommended guideline parameters to allow for effective antiangiogenic therapy for optimal cancer treatment (29). 2. A baseline BP and regular monitoring is recommended while patient is receiving vascular endothelial growth factor (VEGF) inhibitors, especially during the first cycle of chemotherapy when most patients experience an elevation in BP. 3. Actively monitor BP weekly during the first cycle of VEGF signaling pathway (VSP) inhibitor therapy and then at least every 2–3 weeks for the duration of treatment. 4. Patients with preexisting hypertension and on multiple antihypertensive agents should be evaluated for renal function and proteinuria.	1. Teach patients that hypertension can be life-threatening and cause stroke. 2. Teach patients to recognize signs of a hypertensive crisis or stroke which may include the following: memory lapses, blackouts or near syncope, visual abnormalities, persistent headache, slurred words, numbness or tingling of an extremity, and facial droop. 3. Patients should be aware that many antihypertensive agents can cause immediate orthostasis, dizziness, nausea, and risk of falling.

(Continued)

Table 13.1 (Continued) Nursing management and patient education for common cardiotoxicities of cancer therapy

Cardiovascular toxicity	Nursing assessment	Monitoring/Management	Patient education
	4. Higher-risk patients, including those with diabetes and/or chronic kidney disease, should achieve a lower BP goal (e.g., 130/80 mm Hg). 5. Evaluation of pain control which may be contributory to hypertension. 6. Assess for stress management, and other medications used in these patients (e.g., steroids, nonsteroidal anti-inflammatory drugs, and erythropoietin) that can cause hypertension are necessary for adequate estimation of blood pressure.	5. The choice of antihypertensive therapy must be individualized according to the patient's medical history and the specific properties of different classes of antihypertensive agents (24,30,31). 6. Antihypertensive agent classes that have been specifically prescribed to control hypertension associated with VSP inhibitor therapy include thiazide diuretics, beta-blockers, dihydropyridine calcium channel blockers, angiotensin-converting enzyme inhibitors, and angiotensin-receptor blockers (24,32). 7. Some agents may be preferable (e.g., renin–angiotensin or sympathetic system inhibitors) over others to minimize the risk of electrolyte depletion (e.g., thiazide diuretics). 8. Hypertension associated with TKIs is commonly quite manageable with appropriate therapy, and early intervention is key to minimizing additional cardiovascular adverse effects such as heart failure (24). 9. Patients should keep a BP measurement log especially during the first week of treatment because the magnitude of BP elevation is unpredictable.	4. Patients should be instructed to use a validated, automated oscillometric device that measures blood pressure in the brachial artery (upper arm) and to perform measurements in a quiet room after 5 minutes of rest in the seated position with the back and arm supported. 5. Blood pressure generally should be checked in both arms to determine if there is a difference. It is important to use an appropriate-sized arm cuff. 6. Adherence to taking the medications as prescribed should be emphasized to patients. 7. Patients should be aware of the potential side effects of the medications and when to report to their healthcare provider. *(Continued)*

Table 13.1 (Continued) Nursing management and patient education for common cardiotoxicities of cancer therapy

Cardiovascular toxicity	Nursing assessment	Monitoring/Management	Patient education
		10. The target BP should be based on Joint National Committee (JNC) 8 classification and guidelines (33). 11. Antihypertensive therapy should be adjusted accordingly based on associated comorbidities (e.g., <140/90 mm Hg) in patients with diabetes or chronic kidney disease.	8. Before starting TKIs, patients need to have a baseline measurement of their BP and be aware of what the target BP should be.
Myocardial infarction/ischemia Definition: Myocardial infarction (MI) or acute coronary syndrome, commonly known as a "heart attack," is the death of the heart muscle from a sudden blockage of a coronary artery usually caused by a blood clot (23,34). A diagnosis of an MI is based on a combination of clinical features, including electrocardiographic (ECG) findings, elevated values of biochemical markers (biomarkers) of myocardial necrosis, and by imaging, or may be defined by pathology. MI may be the first manifestation of coronary artery disease (CAD) or it may occur, repeatedly, in patients with established disease. The World	1. Initial evaluation which should be done within 10 minutes of clinical presentation or occurrence of signs and symptoms. 2. Obtain a cardiac-focused history and physical examination 3. Obtain 12-lead ECG. 4. Send blood specimen for serum cardiac enzymes (creatine kinase phosphokinase- Creatine-kinase muscle/ brain MB Creatine- kinase muscle/brain), troponin I, or troponin T, which are elevated when myocardial injury occurs (36).	1. Initiate medical treatment as appropriate (e.g., supplemental oxygen; morphine 2–4 mg IV PRN for analgesia; nitroglycerin sublingually PRN for chest pains). 2. Administer O_2 at a rate sufficient to maintain O_2 saturation above 90% unless otherwise contraindicated. 3. Implement cardiac monitoring: observe for dysrhythmias and ischemic changes, low oxygen saturation, or extremes in BP measurements. 4. Obtain order for aspirin 325 mg to be chewed as soon as 12-lead ECG is performed and ST changes are present. Caution in patients with low platelet counts and brain metastases. 5. Consider patient candidacy for reperfusion strategies such as cardiac catheterization with angioplasty, stent placement, or intracoronary/IV thrombolysis (37).	1. Explain to patient and family the disease process, diagnostic tests, and medications. 2. Provide emotional support to patients and families to lower the patient and family's level of anxiety, which can reduce heart rate and myocardial oxygen demand. 3. Provide instruction regarding risk factor modification (46,47). 4. Reportable symptoms: chest discomfort, left arm or neck pain, dyspnea.

(Continued)

Table 13.1 (Continued) Nursing management and patient education for common cardiotoxicities of cancer therapy

Cardiovascular toxicity	Nursing assessment	Monitoring/Management	Patient education
Health Organization's definition of MI involves at least two of the following criteria: (1) a history of ischemic-type chest pain symptoms; (2) evolutionary ECG changes; and (3) a rise and fall in serial cardiac biomarkers (35).	5. Request for an echocardiogram or multigated acquisition (MUGA) scan to evaluate for left ventricular function. 6. Initiate medical treatment as appropriate (e.g., supplemental oxygen; morphine 2–4 mg IV PRN for analgesia; nitroglycerin sublingually PRN for chest pains). 7. Request for chest x-ray to rule out any chest abnormalities.	6. Consider ischemia-reducing or myocardial preservation strategies such as administration of nitrates, beta-blockers, or statins (38,39). 7. Maintain potassium >4 mEq/L, magnesium >2 mEq/L, and ionized calcium >1 mEq/L (40). 8. Consider discontinuation of antineoplastic agents such as fluoropyrimidines, oxaliplatin, sorafenib, or tamoxifen that are thought to cause cardiac ischemia or infarction (41–43). 9. Determine need for follow-up assessment of coronary arteries and myocardial function with exercise stress testing, cardiac catheterization, echocardiogram, or MUGA scan (44,45). 10. Aggressively manage cardiac risk factors (e.g., tobacco use, high blood pressure, high cholesterol, alcohol use, obesity, physical inactivity, hypertension, hyperlipidemia).	5. Management of risks for cardiac ischemia that are specific to oncology (e.g., anemia, cardiac demands of infection, electrolyte disturbances). 6. Cardiac medications and unique considerations in oncology care (e.g., risk for low BP, increased when febrile, electrolyte disturbances with nausea and vomiting may contribute to cardiac dysrhythmias). 7. Referral and education regarding cardiac rehabilitation programs (48).

(Continued)

Table 13.1 (Continued) Nursing management and patient education for common cardiotoxicities of cancer therapy

Cardiovascular toxicity	Nursing assessment	Monitoring/Management	Patient education
Left ventricular dysfunction/heart failure			
Definition: A consensus definition for cardiotoxicity-induced cardiomyopathy (CMP) and heart failure (HF) is still lacking. The Common Terminology Criteria for Adverse Events (CTCAE) (53) Version 4 defines left ventricular dysfunction (LVD) and HF based on severity (grades 1–5), with a change in left ventricular ejection fraction (LVEF) to below the lower limit of normal (LLN) or LVEF <50% ("NCI. Common Terminology Criteria for Adverse Events (CTCAE)," 2009). The Cardiac Review and Evaluation Committee (CREC) supervising trastuzumab clinical trials defined drug-related cardiotoxicity as one or more of the following: (1) CMP characterized by a decrease in LVEF, either global or more severe in the septum; (2) symptoms associated with congestive heart failure (CHF); (3) signs associated with CHF (e.g., S3 gallop, tachycardia or both);	1. Perform a comprehensive history and physical assessment 2. Obtain history of treatments received for cancer therapy 3. Determine the etiology of heart failure (e.g., ischemic vs. nonischemic) 4. Classify the presenting syndrome (e.g., acute vs. chronic; systolic versus diastolic). 5. Identify concomitant disease relevant to HF (e.g., amyloidosis, hemochromatosis). 6. Evaluate for presence of coronary artery disease and valvular problems. 7. Assess severity of symptoms. 8. Perform diagnostic and interventional procedures as needed (e.g., cardiac catheterization).	1. Identify precipitating factors for acute decompensated HF including: (1) patient-related factors (e.g., nonadherence to medications, excessive salt intake, physical and environmental stressors); (2) cardiac-related factors (e.g., cardiac arrhythmias [e.g., AF, ventricular fibrillation, bradyarrhythmia], uncontrolled HTN, acute MI, valvular disease, worsening mitral regurgitation); (3) adverse effects of anticancer treatment (e.g., steroids, chemotherapy [e.g., doxorubicin, cyclophosphamide], nonsteroidal anti-inflammatory drugs, thiazolidinediones). 2. Prepare patient for diagnostic tests and procedures to establish diagnosis of LVD/HF (e.g., echocardiography, nuclear imaging, endomyocardial biopsy, left and right heart catheterizations). 3. Evaluate for other causes of signs and symptoms that can mimic HF (e.g., pulmonary edema, pleural effusion). 4. Monitor thyroid profile to evaluate for hypothyroidism, hyperthyroidism as HF etiology. 5. Send blood specimen to check for viral titers to evaluate causes of myocarditis, endocarditis, and pericarditis, and iron studies to evaluate for hemochromatosis resulting in HF.	1. Dietary modifications. Instructions on sodium restriction to 2000 mg/day to prevent volume overload (34). 2. Encourage physical activity except during periods of acute exacerbation when physical rest is recommended. 3. Weight monitoring. Patients should be advised on daily weight monitoring and notify their provider in case of a sudden unexpected weight gain (more than 2 lbs. per day for 2 consecutive days or more than 5 lbs. per week for possible adjustment of diuretic dose.

(Continued)

Table 13.1 (Continued) Nursing management and patient education for common cardiotoxicities of cancer therapy

Cardiovascular toxicity	Nursing assessment	Monitoring/Management	Patient education
or (4) reduction in LVEF from baseline of <5% to <55% with accompanying signs or symptoms of CHF, or a reduction in LVEF of >10% to <55%, without accompanying signs or symptoms (49).		6. Initiate clinical guideline–recommended pharmacologic therapies for HF including: (a) angiotensin-converting enzyme inhibitors (ACE-I); (b) angiotensin receptor blockers; (c) aldosterone antagonists; (d) cardiac glycosides; (e) direct-acting vasodilator.	4. Alcohol intake. Moderate intake (1 drink per day for females and 2 drinks per day for males) is permitted except in cases of alcoholic cardiomyopathy. 5. Smoking cessation is encouraged.
Venous thromboembolism (VTE) Definition: A blood clot that forms in a vein and migrates to another location. VTE is a serious and life-threatening disorder and is the second leading cause of death in hospitalized patients with cancer (50). Cancer treatment with chemotherapy and biotherapy agents, including bevacizumab, cisplatin, erlotinib, lenalidomide, tamoxifen, thalidomide, and vorinostat (51) can increase the risk of developing VTE. The risk of VTE in patients with cancer ranges from 1.9%–11% based on a variety of risk factors. The addition of thalidomide increases this risk to as high as 30%, and antiangiogenic agents increase the risk up to 30%, even in lower-risk individuals (52).	1. Obtain health history at every clinic or hospital visit. 2. Assess patients for signs and symptoms of VTE, such as pain, redness, and swelling of extremities, especially unilaterally.	1. Refer patients for diagnostic testing (e.g., venous Doppler study). 2. Initiate anticoagulant therapy when indicated, and monitor therapeutic levels when necessary. 3. Discontinue medications thought to contribute to VTE.	1. Teach patients the signs and symptoms of vascular complications. 2. Teach lifestyle changes, such as smoking cessation, low-fat diet, moderate exercise, and stress management, that may reduce incidence and severity of vascular complications. 3. Advise patients to report symptoms to care provider so that assessment and preventive strategies can be implemented early.

as necessary. In addition, nurses develop nursing care plans guided by patients' needs and preferences, educate patients and their families prior to discharge, and facilitate continuity of care across settings and among providers. Nurses play a key role in the success of multidisciplinary teams. A meta-analysis of randomized trials for patients with heart failure reported that multidisciplinary clinics are associated with reductions in mortality and hospitalizations (5).

CARDIO-ONCOLOGY NURSES AS EDUCATORS

Cardio-oncology nurses play many roles in patient care, but one of the most important and lasting roles is that of patient educator. A patient with a new diagnosis of cancer often comes with a whirlwind of emotions: overwhelmed, frightened, and full of questions. Medical jargon and complex procedures can only worsen the situation. Words like "autoimmune," "chronic," and "adjuvant therapy" may be familiar to clinicians, but are foreign and scary to many patients. Cardio-oncology nurses can help patients, families, and their loved ones by providing thorough patient education. The role of patient education spans across the continuum of care, from the initial diagnosis, to treatments, to cancer survivorship. Patient education includes teaching patients about their illness, helping patients understand their treatments and potential adverse effects, and how their life will be different after recovery.

INITIAL DIAGNOSIS

After patients are informed of their cancer diagnosis, patient education should initially focus on what the diagnosis means for the patient. The patient's reactions to the initial cancer diagnosis are dependent on several factors, including past experiences and the individual's psychosocial makeup. Cardio-oncology nurses should assess the patient's current knowledge about their condition. Some patients need time to adjust to new information, and what the diagnosis means in terms of a prognosis. Cardio-oncology nurses provide emotional support through providing information with empathy and compassion.

Patients with cancer and cardiovascular disease have complex healthcare issues. It is essential that patients understand their treatment plan in order to improve clinical outcomes. Educating patients about their disease and motivating and monitoring their adherence to a course of therapy are critical components in promoting positive outcomes (6).

TREATMENT

Receiving a cancer diagnosis can be overwhelming, but sometimes the treatment process can even be more daunting. Cancer treatments may include surgery, chemotherapy, immunotherapy, and/or transplantation. Some of the treatment protocols for cancer treatment can be arduous. By educating patients about their specific treatment plan, cardio-oncology nurses can dispel many fears and help to ensure the greatest success for their patients. Patient education should be ongoing and thorough with any of these treatment options. Cardio-oncology nurses should inform patients of any preparations for the procedure, such as not eating or drinking the night before a procedure, making lifestyle changes to accommodate chemotherapy treatment, and potential adverse effects of treatment. Involvement of patients in their treatment is critical in order to achieve positive outcomes.

Cancer treatment delivery is undergoing a shift from intravenous to oral treatment. In fact, it is projected that the use of oral chemotherapy will more than double in the next several years (7). Patient education is vital to promote patient safety, optimal dosing, and adherence to the treatment plan. Several studies show that patients on long-term medications geared toward decreasing mortality, such as oral chemotherapy, have a low adherence rate of 42% (8). Cardio-oncology nurses need to tailor their patient education efforts to the individual needs of each patient and use resources such as medication information sheets to reinforce teaching. Patients must be taught when to take their medications, if they should take their medications with or without food, if they should avoid alcohol, and if they should look out for any serious side effects. Along the way, nurses must check in with patients to ensure they are following their medication protocols accurately and that they are not experiencing any adverse symptoms.

SURVIVORSHIP

For many patients, survivorship follows completion of cancer treatment. Following treatment, patients may experience great relief from their symptoms, but they may also experience a new set of symptoms caused by the treatment. Cardio-oncology nurses are at the forefront of patient-centered care to ensure that patients with all prognoses are able to plan for their future accordingly. Patient education should address the patient's quality of life, health promotion, and long-term care. Long-term survivorship care requires three components: (1) comprehensive coordination; (2) follow-up and transitional care; and (3) ongoing discussions about care planning, coping skills, and health behavior to mitigate the long-term risks of having a cancer history and being treated for cancer (9).

Developing educational strategies to inform patients, and to encourage their active participation during this phase of care can be an effective surveillance tool for cancer recurrence and secondary cancers. These strategies may also enhance the management of long-term late effects and co-morbid conditions as the cardiovascular complications of cancer therapy. To date, evidence-based strategies to address this need have been lacking.

For cancer survivors with chronic conditions such as cardiovascular disease, or who received cancer treatment with potential cardiotoxicity, nurses must provide a great deal of information in an easy-to-understand manner. Many cancer survivors do not optimally receive necessary cancer screenings or adopt protective health behaviors (e.g., smoking cessation, physical activity) known to prevent and detect new or recurrent disease. This is despite their increased risk for future illnesses (10). Whether it is teaching patients how to monitor for signs and symptoms of cardiomyopathy or how to test their blood glucose levels, or educating them about proper diet and exercise to reduce cholesterol, it is up to the nurse to simplify the experience and give actionable information to each patient. In addition, comprehensive education regarding lifestyle modification, polypharmacy review, social support, pain control, and discussion of end-of-life issues should be included (11).

Educating cancer survivors on the early identification of cardiotoxicity is paramount for timely initiation of pharmacologic therapy. Actual patients' characteristics clearly differ from those in clinical trials (e.g., presence of comorbidities, risk factors, borderline cardiac parameters), and late effects of cardiovascular toxicity may occur, which was not previously identified in clinical trials. Long-term monitoring of the cardiovascular complications of

cancer therapy is needed as several novel targeted drugs are entering the pipeline (12).

The most common cardiotoxicities of cancer therapy that may occur acutely, during cancer treatment, or as late effects in cancer survivorship are listed in Table 13.1. A brief definition for each condition, the corresponding nursing assessment, monitoring/management strategies, and patient education are summarized.

CONCLUSION

Cardio-oncology nursing is an emerging field of nursing practice that spans the cancer care continuum. The role of cardio-oncology nurses is essential in the multidisciplinary approach to manage the complex healthcare issues of patients with cancer and after antineoplastic treatment. This is necessary in order to reduced morbidity and mortality in cancer patients and survivors. To prepare the next generation of nurses, cardio-oncology topics should be integrated within the undergraduate nursing curriculums and for all members of the interdisciplinary healthcare team. Cardio-oncology nurses must not only be aware of the potential side effects of cancer treatment on the cardiovascular system, but they must also be adept at conducting careful serial symptom review, and consider risk reduction and cancer rehabilitation strategies. Teamwork is essential for optimal management of patients with cancer and cardiovascular disease.

REFERENCES

1. Yeh ET. Cardiotoxicity induced by chemotherapy and antibody therapy. *Annu Rev Med.* 2006;57:485–98.
2. Armstrong GT, Ross JD. Late cardiotoxicity in aging adult survivors of childhood cancer. *Prog Pediatr Cardiol.* 2014;36(1–2):19–26.
3. Parent S, Pituskin E, Paterson DI. The cardio-oncology program: A multidisciplinary approach to the care of cancer patients with cardiovascular disease. *Can J Cardiol.* 2016;32(7):847–51.
4. Albini A, Pennesi G, Donatelli F, Cammarota R, De Flora S, Noonan DM. Cardiotoxicity of anticancer drugs: The need for cardio-oncology and cardio-oncological prevention. *J Natl Cancer Inst.* 2010;102(1):14–25.

5. McAlister FA, Stewart S, Ferrua S, McMurray JJ. Multidisciplinary strategies for the management of heart failure patients at high risk for admission: A systematic review of randomized trials. *J Am Coll Cardiol.* 2004;44(4):810–9.

6. Kutzleb J, Reiner D. The impact of nurse-directed patient education on quality of life and functional capacity in people with heart failure. *J Am Acad Nurse Pract.* 2006;18(3):116–23.

7. Moody M, Jackowski J. Are patients on oral chemotherapy in your practice setting safe? *Clin J Oncol Nurs.* 2010;14(3):339–46.

8. Wood L. A review on adherence management in patients on oral cancer therapies. *Eur J Oncol Nurs.* 2012;16(4):432–8.

9. Hewitt M. *From Cancer Patient to Cancer Survivor: Lost in Transition.* National Academies Press; 2006.

10. Underwood JM et al. Surveillance of demographic characteristics and health behaviors among adult cancer survivors—Behavioral risk factor surveillance system, United States, 2009. *MMWR Surveill Summ.* 2012;61(1):1–23.

11. Pituskin E, Haykowsky M, McNeely M, Mackey J, Chua N, Paterson I. Rationale and design of the multidisciplinary Team IntervenTion in cArdio-oNcology study (TITAN). *BMC Cancer.* 2016;16(1):733.

12. Cheng H, Force T. Molecular mechanisms of cardiovascular toxicity of targeted cancer therapeutics. *Circ Res.* 2010;106(1):21–34.

13. Lane DA, Barker RV, Lip GY. Best practice for atrial fibrillation patient education. *Curr Pharm Des.* 2015;21(5):533–43.

14. Lip GY, Nieuwlaat R, Pisters R, Lane DA, Crijns HJ. Refining clinical risk stratification for predicting stroke and thromboembolism in atrial fibrillation using a novel risk factor-based approach: The euro heart survey on atrial fibrillation. *Chest.* 2010;137(2):263–72.

15. Olesen JB, Torp-Pedersen C, Hansen ML, Lip GY. The value of the CHA2DS2-VASc score for refining stroke risk stratification in patients with atrial fibrillation with a CHADS2 score 0–1: A nationwide cohort study. *Thromb Haemost.* 2012;107(6):1172–9.

16. Potpara TS, Lip GY. Lone atrial fibrillation: What is known and what is to come. *Int J Clin Pract.* 2011;65(4):446–57.

17. Potpara TS et al. A 12-year follow-up study of patients with newly diagnosed lone atrial fibrillation: Implications of arrhythmia progression on prognosis: The Belgrade atrial fibrillation study. *Chest.* 2012;141(2):339–47.

18. Hazinski M, Samson R, Schexnayder S. 2010. *Handbook of Emergency Cardiovascular Care for Healthcare Providers.* Dallas, Texas: American Heart Association; 2010.

19. Deremer DL, Ustun C, Natarajan K. Nilotinib: A second-generation tyrosine kinase inhibitor for the treatment of chronic myelogenous leukemia. *Clin Ther.* 2008;30(11):1956–75.

20. Strevel EL, Ing DJ, Siu LL. Molecularly targeted oncology therapeutics and prolongation of the QT interval. *J Clin Oncol.* 2007;25(22):3362–71.

21. Guglin M, Aljayeh M, Saiyad S, Ali R, Curtis AB. Introducing a new entity: Chemotherapy-induced arrhythmia. *Europace.* 2009;11(12):1579–86.

22. Kim PY, Ewer MS. Chemotherapy and QT prolongation: Overview with clinical perspective. *Curr Treat Options Cardiovasc Med.* 2014;16(5):303.

23. Fadol A, Lech T. Cardiovascular adverse events associated with cancer therapy. *J Adv Pract Oncol.* 2011;2(4):229–42.

24. Lenihan DJ, Kowey PR. Overview and management of cardiac adverse events associated with tyrosine kinase inhibitors. *Oncologist.* 2013;18(8):900–8.

25. Kubota T, Shimizu W, Kamakura S, Horie M. Hypokalemia-induced long QT syndrome with an underlying novel missense mutation in S4-S5 linker of KCNQ1. *J Cardiovasc Electrophysiol.* 2000;11(9):1048–54.

26. Hinkle C. Electrolyte disorders in the cardiac patient. *Crit Care Nurs Clin N Am.* 2011;23(4):635–43.

27. Pepin J, Shields C. Advances in diagnosis and management of hypokalemic and hyperkalemic emergencies. *Emerg Med Pract.* 2012;14(2):1–7; quiz-8.

28. Whelton PK et al. 2017 ACC/AHA/AAPA/ABC/ACPM/AGS/APhA/ASH/ASPC/NMA/PCNA guideline for the prevention, detection, evaluation, and management of high blood pressure in adults: A report of the American College of Cardiology/American Heart Association Task Force on Clinical Practice Guidelines. *Circulation.* 2018 October 23;138(17):e484-e594. doi:10.1161/CIR.0000000000000596.

29. Ranpura V, Pulipati B, Chu D, Zhu X, Wu S. Increased risk of high-grade hypertension with bevacizumab in cancer patients: A meta-analysis. *Am J Hypertens.* 2010;23(5):460–8.

30. Mancia G, Grassi G. Individualization of antihypertensive drug treatment. *Diabetes Care.* 2013;36 Suppl 2:S301–6.

31. Mancia G et al. 2013 ESH/ESC guidelines for the management of arterial hypertension: The Task Force for the Management of Arterial Hypertension of the European Society of Hypertension (ESH) and of the European Society of Cardiology (ESC). *Eur Heart J.* 2013;34(28):2159–219.

32. Maitland ML et al. Initial assessment, surveillance, and management of blood pressure in patients receiving vascular endothelial growth factor signaling pathway inhibitors. *J Natl Cancer Inst.* 2010;102(9):596–604.

33. James PA et al. 2014 evidence-based guideline for the management of high blood pressure in adults: Report from the panel members appointed to the Eighth Joint National Committee (JNC 8). *JAMA.* 2014;311(5):507–20.

34. Fadol A. *Cardiac Complications of Cancer Therapy.* Pittsburgh, Pennsylvania: Oncology Nursing Society; 2013.

35. Antman EM. ST-segment elevation myocardial infarction: Pathology, pathophysiology, and clinical features. In: Bonow RO, Zipres DP, Libby J, eds. *Braunwald's Heart Disease: A Textbook of Cardiovascular Medicine.* 9th ed. Philadelphia, PA: Elsevier Saunders; 2012. p. 1087–1109.

36. Gaze DC. The perils, pitfalls and opportunities of using high sensitivity cardiac troponin. *Curr Med Chem.* 2011;18(23):3442–5.

37. Iyengar SS, Godbole GS. Thrombolysis in the era of intervention. *JJ Assoc Physicians India.* 2011;59 Suppl:26–30.

38. Ferreira JC, Mochly-Rosen D. Nitroglycerin use in myocardial infarction patients. *Circ J.* 2012;76(1):15–21.

39. Gerczuk PZ, Kloner RA. An update on cardioprotection: A review of the latest adjunctive therapies to limit myocardial infarction size in clinical trials. *J Am Coll Cardiol.* 2012;59(11):969–78.

40. Akhtar MI, Ullah H, Hamid M. Magnesium, a drug of diverse use. *J Pak Med Assoc.* 2011;61(12):1220–5.

41. Basselin C et al. 5-Fluorouracil-induced Tako-Tsubo-like syndrome. *Pharmacotherapy.* 2011;31(2):226.

42. Chang PH, Hung MJ, Yeh KY, Yang SY, Wang CH. Oxaliplatin-induced coronary vasospasm manifesting as Kounis syndrome: A case report. *J Clin Oncol.* 2011;29(31):e776–8.

43. Shah NR, Shah A, Rather A. Ventricular fibrillation as a likely consequence of capecitabine-induced coronary vasospasm. *J Oncol Pharm Pract.* 2012;18(1):132–5.

44. Al-Zaiti SS, Pelter MM, Carey MG. Exercise stress treadmill testing. *Am J Crit Care.* 2011;20(3):259–60.

45. Arrighi JA, Dilsizian V. Multimodality imaging for assessment of myocardial viability: Nuclear, echocardiography, MR, and CT. *Curr Cardiol Rep.* 2012;14(2):234–43.

46. Brown JP, Clark AM, Dalal H, Welch K, Taylor RS. Patient education in the management of coronary heart disease. *Cochrane Database Syst Rev.* 2011(12):CD008895.

47. Crumlish CM, Magel CT. Patient education on heart attack response: Is rehearsal the critical factor in knowledge retention? *Medsurg Nurs.* 2011;20(6):310–7.

48. Heran BS et al. Exercise-based cardiac rehabilitation for coronary heart disease. *Cochrane Database Syst Rev.* 2011 July 6;7:CD001800. doi:10.1002/14651858.CD001800.pub2.

49. Raschi E, De Ponti F. Cardiovascular toxicity of anticancer-targeted therapy: Emerging issues in the era of cardio-oncology. *Intern Emerg Med.* 2012;7(2):113–31.

50. Lyman GH et al. American Society of Clinical Oncology guideline: Recommendations for venous thromboembolism prophylaxis and treatment in patients with cancer. *J Clin Oncol.* 2007;25(34):5490–505.

51. Zangari M, Berno T, Zhan F, Tricot G, Fink L. Mechanisms of thrombosis in paraproteinemias: The effects of immunomodulatory drugs. *Semin Thromb Hemost.* 2012;38(8):768–79.

52. Yusuf SW, Razeghi P, Yeh ET. The diagnosis and management of cardiovascular disease in cancer patients. *Curr Probl Cardiol.* 2008;33(4):163–96.

53. Common Terminology Criteria for Adverse Events (CTCAE). 2009. https://evs.nci.nih.gov/ftp1/CTCAE/CTCAE_4.03/CTCAE_4.03_2010-06-14_QuickReference_8.5x11.pdf

14

Treating the cardio-oncology patient

SEBASTIAN SZMIT

INTRODUCTION: DEFINING THE ROLE OF CARDIO-ONCOLOGY IN CARING FOR THE PATIENT WITH CANCER

Patients seen in a cardio-oncology clinic are those who need the combined expertise of oncologists and cardiologists in their care planning. While cardio-oncology clinics have emerged across the globe, few have defined the population of patients commonly referred. Two broad categories of patients to be considered are those who have pre-existing cardiovascular disease (1) and those who experience cardiovascular complications as a result of their cancer or its treatment (2). Occasionally, cancer involves the heart (cardiac tumors, cardiac metastasis, cardiac amyloidosis, pericardial effusion, vascular or pericardium infiltration, etc.) (3). The multidisciplinary care afforded by a cardio-oncology program is paramount to the patient's survival, but more often, referred patients either have ongoing cardiac dysfunction after treatment or require monitoring because they are at high risk of late cardiovascular toxicity (4–7). Nine main categories of cardiotoxicity were defined

by the 2016 European Society of Cardiology (ESC) Position Paper on Cancer Treatments and Cardiovascular Toxicity including (8):

- Myocardial dysfunction and heart failure (HF)
- Coronary artery disease (CAD)
- Valvular disease
- Arrhythmias, especially those induced by QT-prolonging drugs
- Arterial hypertension
- Thromboembolic disease
- Peripheral vascular disease and stroke
- Pulmonary hypertension
- Pericardial complications

The main purpose of the new scientific discipline of cardio-oncology is to define and minimize causes of cardiovascular (CV) disease in cancer patients in order to prolong survival and improve quality of life (9).

Figure 14.1 outlines the roles of cardiology and oncology, confirming the purpose and importance of creating a cardiology clinic. In the cardio-oncology clinic, there is collaboration between disciplines, with the oncologist recognizing the

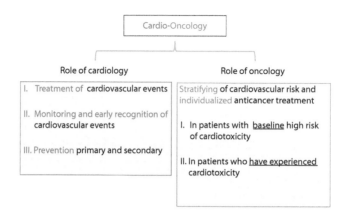

Figure 14.1 The main activities of each discipline relating to the cardio-oncology patient.

potential threat of CV disease and complications of therapy, and the cardiologist optimizing CV health to permit effective treatment of the cancer (10,11). In this field, we are also beginning to see specialists who have particular expertise in the new discipline of cardio-oncology. These specialists can be trained cardiologists with interest, or extra training in oncology, trained oncologists with extra training in cardiology or, more rarely, dual-trained specialists in oncology and cardiology.

Cardio-oncology is a young subspecialty. Where high-level scientific evidence is lacking, consultants make recommendations based on clinical experience. The shared knowledge of the two disciplines can lead to a more favorable prognosis for the patient, both from a cardiac and oncologic perspective. The task of cardio-oncology consultants should be to optimize cardiac management using drugs and interventions with confirmed efficacy in the cancer population. Equally important, the cardio-oncology consultation should take into account the prescribed anticancer therapy in the context of CV risk factors or disease so that the expected benefit of the proposed cancer treatment is higher than the risk of possible CV complications (including premature cardiac death).

CARDIAC ASSESSMENT BEFORE ANTICANCER THERAPY: IDENTIFYING THE PATIENT WHO IS AT HIGH RISK OF CV COMPLICATIONS FROM CANCER THERAPY

The main purpose of cardiac assessment in patients with cancer should be to identify patients at high risk of short- and long-term CV events. In order to minimize CV morbidity and mortality in patients with cancer, baseline evaluation should include the following:

- An assessment of the planned anticancer regimen with respect to type and severity of CV toxicity and the risk of that toxicity in the patient. History of previous anticancer therapy (especially cumulative doses of anthracyclines and chest radiotherapy).
- Recognition of preexisting CV disease (especially coronary artery disease with complications: myocardial infarction, status of revascularization, etc.).
- Identification of classical risk factors for developing HF (hypertension, diabetes, older age, dyslipidemias, obesity, etc.).
- Echocardiographic cardiac assessment in selected patients (the European Society of Cardiology Position Paper suggests this for all patients before initiation of potentially cardiotoxic cancer treatment, irrespective of clinical history, in order to confirm baseline adequacy of heart function [8]).

It is also important to assess exercise tolerance (especially in patients with heart disease), general performance status (especially in the geriatric population), and cancer-related life expectancy, with or without cancer treatment. A history of prior CV events may increase the risk of cardiotoxicity such that cancer therapy is contraindicated. In cases where there are few options for therapy, cardio-oncologists may consider aggressive modification of risk factors and treatment of CV disease in order to make cancer treatment possible. In addition, patients' preferences need to be included in weighing the risks and benefits of treatment.

The type of anticancer therapy may contribute to the development of new CV events or aggravation of previous CV disease. According to the American Society of Clinical Oncology guidelines (12), the following are associated with an increased risk for developing cardiac dysfunction:

1. Doxorubicin $\geq$250 mg/m^2, epirubicin $\geq$600 mg/m^2
2. Radiotherapy $\geq$30 Gy where the heart is in the treatment field
3. Lower-dose anthracycline (e.g., <250 mg/m^2) in combination with lower-dose radiotherapy (<30 Gy)
4. Lower-dose anthracycline followed by trastuzumab (sequential therapy)
5. Lower-dose anthracycline or trastuzumab alone and presence of any of the following risk factors:
   a. Multiple CV risk factors (at least two risk factors), including smoking, hypertension, diabetes, dyslipidemia, and obesity, during or after completion of therapy
   b. Older age ($\geq$60 years) at cancer treatment
   c. Compromised cardiac function (e.g., borderline low left ventricular ejection fraction [LVEF] in the range of 50%–55%, history of myocardial infarction, at least moderate valvular heart disease) at any time before or during treatment

INDIVIDUALIZED CARDIO-ONCOLOGY MANAGEMENT IN RELATION TO BASELINE RISK

A modified plan for anticancer therapy and close clinical and cardiac monitoring is necessary in cancer patients who are deemed to be at high risk of cardiotoxicity from anticancer treatment. The American Society of Clinical Oncology guidelines recommend that potentially cardiotoxic therapies should be avoided or minimized in situations where equally effective alternatives exist. For example, a woman with HER2-positive breast cancer who is deemed high risk for cardiotoxicity might be treated with the docetaxel, carboplatin, trastuzumab (TCH) regimen (13) or a taxane-based regimen (14) rather than anthracycline-based regimens; or, a woman with metastatic breast cancer might receive liposomal doxorubicin instead of conventional doxorubicin (15).

Cancer patients at high risk of cardiotoxicity often receive more rigorous cardiac monitoring—yet there is no supporting scientific evidence with regard to the benefit of performing more frequent echocardiography (or other cardiac imaging) in these patients (16). Cardiac monitoring has been studied in women receiving trastuzumab for early-stage HER2-positive breast cancer. Per protocol, these women had cardiac imaging every 3 months during trastuzumab therapy, which is the current recommendation (17). The American Society of Clinical Oncology guidelines state that the frequency of surveillance for patients who have completed cancer therapy including anthracyclines should be determined by the healthcare providers based on clinical judgment and patient circumstances. The European Society of Cardiology Position Paper provides more detailed recommendations (8):

- For low-risk patients (normal baseline echocardiogram, no clinical risk factors), surveillance should be considered with echocardiography:
  - Every four cycles (especially in adjuvant setting) while receiving anti-HER2 treatment
  - After 240 mg/m^2 of doxorubicin (or equivalent) from the beginning of treatment with anthracyclines.
- More frequent surveillance may be considered for patients with abnormal baseline echocardiography (e.g., reduced or low normal LVEF, structural heart disease) and those with higher baseline clinical risk (e.g., prior anthracyclines, previous myocardial infarction [MI], treated HF).
- Survivors who have completed higher-dose anthracycline-containing chemotherapy ($\geq$300 mg/m^2 of doxorubicin or equivalent) or who have developed cardiotoxicity (e.g., left ventricular [LV] impairment) requiring treatment during chemotherapy may be considered for follow-up surveillance echocardiography at 1 and 5 years after completion of cancer treatment.

URGENT CARDIO-ONCOLOGY TREATMENT

Urgent cardio-oncology consultation may be required for patients who experience CV decompensation during treatment that directly threatens their life and, therefore, requires immediate treatment such as acute pulmonary embolism, acute HF, acute coronary syndromes, or symptomatic arrhythmias. Less common, but equally serious events include pericardial complications, superior vena cava syndrome, pulmonary hypertension, symptomatic cardiac tumors, and hypotension.

Patients with an acute pulmonary embolism may be considered for hospitalization, especially those with a high Pulmonary Embolism Severity Index (PESI) scores (18–20). Hemodynamic parameters must always be monitored as cardiogenic shock is a strong indicator for thrombolysis or more invasive procedures. Cardiac surgery is necessary when clots are observed in the right ventricular cavity. Concomitant deep vein thrombosis can increase the risk of death (21). The initial treatment of a venous thromboembolism, regardless of cancer diagnosis, includes the use of either low-molecular-weight heparin or unfractionated heparin (intravenous infusion under activated partial thromboplastin time [aPTT] control). Low-molecular-weight heparins may be superior to unfractionated heparin as initial (5–10 days) antithromboembolic therapy in the absence of severe renal insufficiency (creatinine clearance <30 mL/min.) (22,23). Asymptomatic episodes of pulmonary embolism should be treated in the same way as symptomatic events (24). Filter implantation into the inferior vena cava should be considered in cancer patients with a venous thromboembolism of the lower extremity and a contraindication to optimal anticoagulant therapy owing to risk of bleeding or need for urgent cancer treatment, including surgery.

Acute HF may require hospitalization if patients present with severe dyspnea, hemodynamic instability, and/or fluid overload (25). The etiology of HF should be evaluated and treated as this will impact the ability to deliver anticancer therapy. Treatment should be in accordance with current guidelines (26). Cardinale et al. demonstrated that negative predictors for efficacy of treatment for HF were the occurrence of symptoms in New York Heart Association (NYHA) class III or IV as well as any delay in cardiac treatment, which meant a longer period (>2 months) from anthracycline-based chemotherapy completion (27). Newer data confirmed that patients who did not recover had a higher NYHA class and were less likely to tolerate the association of enalapril and beta-blockers (28). Intravenous diuretics are often needed for HF attributed to anthracycline use, while beta-blockers

and digoxin are used for HF observed during anti-HER2 therapy (trastuzumab) (29). Even severe acute HF related to trastuzumab can be effectively treated (30,31); however, patients with elevated troponin have worse outcomes (32).

Acute coronary syndromes can also be a direct threat to life, most often presenting as chest pain or shortness of breath. Additionally, electrocardiogram (ECG) changes, disturbances in contractility in echocardiography and troponin increase are observed. Identification of these abnormalities is the basis for the diagnosis of MI. In cancer patients, it is always necessary to exclude other causes of ECG abnormalities and elevated troponin levels since cardiotoxicity and nephrotoxicity may be responsible for such results. Moreover, in a cancer patient, the potential benefits of cardiac invasive procedures should be considered. First, if anticancer therapy is still possible and valuable for the patient's prognosis, coronary angiography is necessary to determine whether the current episode is a type I or type II MI. Although in both cases acute myocardial ischemia is noticed, type I is associated with endothelial damage and arterial thromboembolic event, whereas type II is usually associated with vasospastic reaction (33). Knowledge of this fact determines whether oncologists can continue, for example, cisplatin or antiangiogenic drug, which are usually responsible for type I MI (34,35). Vasospastic reaction, on the other hand, is an indication for the use of vasodilators such as nitrates or calcium channel blockers (e.g., diltiazem). Second, the prognosis of the patient from a cancer perspective should be taken into account. When this timeframe is <1 year, more invasive approaches such as coronary angiography and revascularization should be considered individually. Coronary procedures are recommended in patients with STEMI (ST-elevation myocardial infarction) and high-risk patients with observed NSTE ACS (no ST-elevation acute coronary syndrome). Coronary angiography is necessary in differential diagnosis of stress-induced cardiomyopathy, which is reported more and more frequently in cancer patients. Cancer patients have higher risk of any bleeding and for stent thrombosis; therefore, the duration of a dual antiplatelet therapy after stent placement depends on cancer prognosis (36). Current literature shows, however, that cancer patients do benefit from revascularization and standard pharmacotherapy, including beta-blockers, aspirin, and statins after acute coronary events (37). The benefit of aspirin, in particular, is seen even if there is coexisting thrombocytopenia (38). In patients where dual antiplatelet therapy is contraindicated (platelet count [PLT] <30,000/uL), or who require urgent noncardiac surgical intervention, balloon angioplasty should be considered. Coronary artery bypass grafting (CABG) is reserved for patients with slow progressive or radically treated cancer disease (39). It has been shown, however, that compared to noncancer patients, cancer patients have higher in-hospital mortality (odds ratio [OR] = 3.2; 95% confidence interval [CI]: 1.12–9.4) and higher mortality rates during the first year (OR = 2.15; 95% CI 1.3–3.4) after percutaneous coronary intervention (PCI) (40).

Chemotherapy-induced arrhythmias include a heterogeneous group of electrophysiologic problems, including both ventricular and atrial arrhythmias (41). Ventricular tachycardia (VT), which can cause sudden cardiac death, can be induced directly by anticancer drugs or supportive therapies. VT has been described as occurring in cancer patients as a result of prolongation of the QT interval, either in the setting of preexisting heart disease or electrolyte imbalance. Atrial fibrillation, with rapid ventricular rate, is the most common clinical problem in clinical oncology and thoracic surgery (42). It may cause an exacerbation of HF or tachyarrhythmic cardiomyopathy. Treatment of atrial fibrillation aims to control either cardiac rhythm or heart rate (43). Atrial fibrillation increases risk of thrombotic events, including stroke, so antithrombotic prophylaxis should be considered.

There is a special consideration needed for cancer patients whose electronic cardiac device is within a radiation field. Electronic malfunction of a cardiac pacemaker or intracardiac defibrillator (ICD) from radiotherapy to the device has been reported (44). Malfunction of the device may lead to symptomatic bradycardia in pacemaker-dependent patients or inadequate ICD discharges and death in patients with an ICD (45). Unexpected return of the cardiac device to the factory settings is also a frequent complication; hence the electrophysiological control after radiotherapy is always necessary (46,47). Sometimes it is reasonable to move the device outside the radiotherapy field.

Pericardial complications, including pericarditis and pericardial effusion, can be well visualized with echocardiography. Prognosis and treatment of pericardial disease in cancer patients is dependent on the underlying cause (48). Pericarditis may be a direct complication of anticancer treatment, especially radiotherapy (49). Pericardial effusion may be a manifestation of the progression of cancer, especially lung cancer (50,51). In some centers the standard treatment for pericardial effusions is pericardiocentesis, with prolonged drainage and subsequent chemotherapy administered to the pericardial space (52). A pericardial window is a palliative cardiac surgical procedure to create a communication from the pericardial space to the pleural cavity. It is performed to avoid recurrent large effusions or cardiac tamponade when the risk for pericardiectomy is high, or when the patients' life expectancy is short (e.g., end-stage malignancy).

Vena cava superior syndrome in cancer patients is a result of tumor compression or thrombotic occlusion of the superior vena cava, which impairs blood flow from the head and upper limbs to the right heart and is considered an urgent clinical situation. Chemotherapy and radiotherapy are effective for selected types of tumors (e.g., small cell lung cancer); anticoagulation is necessary if the cause is thromboembolic (53,54). In cases where severe neurological or hemodynamic symptoms are present, more invasive interventions may be indicated, specifically angioplasty with stent implantation, (55,56).

Pulmonary hypertension has several causes in cancer patients. It may be a sign of cancer progression, such as a progressive myeloproliferative disease (57). It may also be caused by cancer therapy (58). For instance, dasatinib therapy, used to treat chronic myelogenous leukemia and acute lymphoblastic leukemia, has been associated with pulmonary hypertension; dasatinib-related pulmonary hypertension can be treated with sildenafil (59,60). The veno-occlusive form of pulmonary hypertension may be associated with alkylating agents, but medical management of this form of pulmonary hypertension is usually unsatisfactory (61). Chronic thromboembolic pulmonary hypertension may be observed in cancer patients and must be distinguished from pulmonary hypertension associated with HF or lung diseases (62).

Symptomatic malignant cardiac tumors are rare but always associated with poor prognosis (63). Management options depend on the type of tumor and can include surgery or chemotherapy. Cardiac surgery should be considered in the presence of symptoms of hemodynamic instability. Chemotherapy use depends on the histopathological diagnosis. Patients with tumors located in the left heart usually have symptoms of mitral stenosis or subacute endocarditis, frequent HF, arrhythmias, chest pain, cyanosis and dyspnea, recurrent fever, progressive weight loss, syncope, hemoptysis, or thromboembolic complications in peripheral arteries. The risk of sudden cardiac death is high (64). Patients with tumors located in the right heart experience symptoms of tricuspid regurgitation, and often have pulmonary emboli or pulmonary hypertension (65).

OUTPATIENT TREATMENT

The American College of Cardiology and the American Heart Association state that patients receiving potentially cardiotoxic anticancer therapy should be considered as having Stage A HF (66). It is reasonable, therefore, to consider primary prevention or early secondary prevention strategies (67).

The goal of the ambulatory cardio-oncology service is to manage all possible CV risk factors and to provide effective secondary cardiac prevention in cancer patients at risk of, or with established cancer therapy–related cardiac dysfunction (68). Cancer patients should be referred to this service if they are at a high risk of developing cardiac complications or have been hospitalized for a CV complication of cancer therapy. An early secondary strategy should be based on the recognition of subclinical forms of cardiotoxicity, either by assessing biochemical markers (such as natriuretic peptide or troponin) or using modern cardiac imaging tools.

Cardioprotective interventions are considered when there are abnormal increases in biomarkers of myocardial damage (especially troponin) or early echocardiographic abnormalities, such as a decline in global longitudinal strain (GLS) (69). The European Society of Cardiology Position Paper states that if LVEF decreases >10 points to a value below the lower limit of normal (considered as an LVEF <50%), angiotensin-converting enzyme (ACE) inhibitors (or angiotensin-receptor blockers [ARBs]) in combination with beta-blockers are recommended to prevent further LV dysfunction or the development of symptomatic HF independent

of the type of cancer or anticancer therapy (8). Ammon et al. showed that in patients with iatrogenic myocardial dysfunction (defined as LVEF ≤45%), guideline-recommended HF medication can have a beneficial effect for overall survival (70).

Classical modifiable clinical risk factors (such as arterial hypertension, diabetes mellitus, obesity, dyslipidemia) for development of myocardial dysfunction/HF should be well-controlled; however, detailed therapeutic goals are undefined in cancer patients. The American Society of Clinical Oncology guidelines recommend that clinicians should screen for, and actively manage, modifiable CV risk factors (smoking, hypertension, diabetes, dyslipidemia, obesity) in all patients receiving potentially cardiotoxic treatments (12). It is assumed that the treatment of coronary heart disease and hypertension in cancer patients should be the same as in the general population, but it is necessary to consider potential interactions with anticancer drugs and medications used as supportive care in cancer patients. Each therapeutic option should be considered and implemented with the intention of prolonging and improving quality of life. The optimal antihypertensive treatment is particularly important in patients receiving inhibitors of the vascular endothelial growth factor signaling pathway. The occurrence of arterial hypertension correlates with the effectiveness of this therapy—longer progression-free survival and lower mortality (71,72). The dose reduction of antivascular endothelial growth factor (VEGF) drugs should only be considered if there are other types of toxicity affecting the clinical condition of a patient (73). When blood pressure levels are well controlled through home monitoring, temporary discontinuation of anticancer drugs rarely become necessary. Discontinuation of anticancer drugs (at least temporarily) may be warranted if despite the administration of several antihypertensive drugs, patients experience hypertensive symptoms. ACE inhibitors or ARBs, beta-blockers (with vasodilatory effects: nebivolol, carvedilol) and dihydropyridine calcium channel blockers are the preferred antihypertensive drugs for use in patients receiving anticancer VEGF inhibitors.

Venous thromboembolic disease needs lifetime treatment in patients with metastatic cancer. After an acute episode, administration of low-molecular-weight heparin for at least 3–6 months is recommended, with a dose of 75%–80% of the

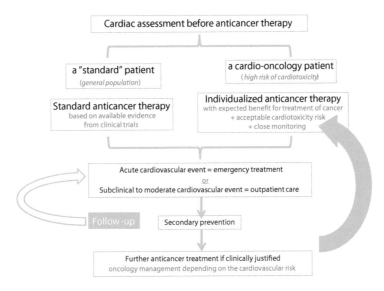

Figure 14.2 The principles of management of a cardio-oncology patient.

therapeutic dose administered once a day (74–77). At present, new oral anticoagulants are being evaluated as an alternative (78). The decision to continue anticoagulant therapy over 3–6 months should be made individually for a specific patient, taking into account the prothrombotic risk as well as bleeding risk, therapy costs, quality of life, expected survival time, and patient preferences. Further active anticancer treatment is the most important reason for long-term anticoagulation.

SUMMARY

The main goal of the subspecialty of cardio-oncology is to improve the prognosis and quality of life of patients with cancer. This can only be achieved if the best available and obtainable anticancer treatments are offered in parallel with optimization of CV health (Figure 14.2). As our population ages, the prevalence of cancer and CV disease will continue to increase, highlighting the importance of this collaborative approach.

REFERENCES

1. Al-Kindi SG, Oliveira GH. Prevalence of pre-existing cardiovascular disease in patients with different types of cancer: The unmet need for onco-cardiology. *Mayo Clin Proc.* 2016;91(1):81–3.
2. Yeh ET, Bickford CL. Cardiovascular complications of cancer therapy: Incidence, pathogenesis, diagnosis, and management. *J Am Coll Cardiol.* 2009;53(24):2231–47.
3. Moslehi JJ. Cardiovascular toxic effects of targeted cancer therapies. *N Engl J Med.* 2016;375(15):1457–67.
4. Haugnes HS, Wethal T, Aass N, Dahl O, Klepp O, Langberg CW, Wilsgaard T, Bremnes RM, Fosså SD. Cardiovascular risk factors and morbidity in long-term survivors of testicular cancer: A 20-year follow-up study. *J Clin Oncol.* 2010;28(30):4649–57.
5. Daher IN, Daigle TR, Bhatia N, Durand JB. The prevention of cardiovascular disease in cancer survivors. *Tex Heart Inst J.* 2012;39(2):190–8.
6. Singla A, Kumar G, Bardia A. Personalizing cardiovascular disease prevention among breast cancer survivors. *Curr Opin Cardiol.* 2012;27(5):515–24.
7. Mulrooney DA et al. Cardiac outcomes in adult survivors of childhood cancer exposed to cardiotoxic therapy: A cross-sectional study. *Ann Intern Med.* 2016;164(2):93–101.
8. Zamorano JL et al. Task Force Members; ESC Committee for Practice Guidelines (CPG). 2016 ESC Position Paper on cancer treatments and cardiovascular toxicity developed under the auspices of the ESC Committee for Practice Guidelines: The Task Force for cancer treatments and cardiovascular toxicity of the European Society of Cardiology (ESC). *Eur Heart J.* 2016;37(36):2768–801.

9. Lenihan DJ, Cardinale D, Cipolla CM. The compelling need for a cardiology and oncology partnership and the birth of the International Cardio-Oncology Society. *Prog Cardiovasc Dis.* 2010;53(2):88–93.

10. Sulpher J, Mathur S, Graham N, Crawley F, Turek M, Johnson C, Stadnick E, Law A, Wentzell J, Dent S. Clinical experience of patients referred to a multidisciplinary cardiac oncology clinic: An observational study. *J Oncol.* 2015;2015:671232.

11. Snipelisky D, Park JY, Lerman A, Mulvagh S, Lin G, Pereira N, Rodriguez-Porcel M, Villarraga HR, Herrmann J. How to develop a cardio-oncology clinic. *Heart Fail Clin.* 2017;13(2):347–59.

12. Armenian SH et al. Prevention and monitoring of cardiac dysfunction in survivors of adult cancers: American Society of Clinical Oncology Clinical Practice Guideline. *J Clin Oncol.* 2017;35(8):893–911.

13. Au HJ et al. Translational Research in Oncology BCIRG 006 Trial Investigators. Health-related quality of life with adjuvant docetaxel- and trastuzumab-based regimens in patients with node-positive and high-risk node-negative, HER2-positive early breast cancer: Results from the BCIRG 006 Study. *Oncologist.* 2013;18(7):812–8.

14. Jones S et al. Docetaxel with cyclophosphamide is associated with an overall survival benefit compared with doxorubicin and cyclophosphamide: 7-year follow-up of US oncology research trial 9735. *J Clin Oncol.* 2009;27(8):1177–83.

15. Batist G et al. Reduced cardiotoxicity and preserved antitumor efficacy of liposome-encapsulated doxorubicin and cyclophosphamide compared with conventional doxorubicin and cyclophosphamide in a randomized, multicenter trial of metastatic breast cancer. *J Clin Oncol.* 2001;19(5):1444–54.

16. Tilemann LM, Heckmann MB, Katus HA, Lehmann LH, Müller OJ. Cardio-oncology: Conflicting priorities of anticancer treatment and cardiovascular outcome. *Clin Res Cardiol.* 2018;107(4):271–80.

17. Mehta LS et al. American Heart Association Cardiovascular Disease in Women and Special Populations Committee of the Council on Clinical Cardiology; Council on Cardiovascular and Stroke Nursing; and Council on Quality of Care and Outcomes Research. Cardiovascular disease and breast cancer: Where these entities intersect: A scientific statement from the American Heart Association. *Circulation.* 2018;137(8):e30–66.

18. Konstantinides SV et al. Task Force for the Diagnosis and Management of Acute Pulmonary Embolism of the European Society of Cardiology (ESC). 2014 ESC guidelines on the diagnosis and management of acute pulmonary embolism. *Eur Heart J.* 2014;35(43):3033–69, 3069a–3069k.

19. Aujesky D, Obrosky DS, Stone RA, Auble TE, Perrier A, Cornuz J, Roy PM, Fine MJ. Derivation and validation of a prognostic model for pulmonary embolism. *Am J Respir Crit Care Med.* 2005;172(8):1041–6.

20. Jiménez D, Aujesky D, Moores L, Gómez V, Lobo JL, Uresandi F, Otero R, Monreal M, Muriel A, Yusen RD; RIETE Investigators. Simplification of the pulmonary embolism severity index for prognostication in patients with acute symptomatic pulmonary embolism. *Arch Intern Med.* 2010;170(15):1383–9.

21. Becattini C, Cohen AT, Agnelli G, Howard L, Castejón B, Trujillo-Santos J, Monreal M, Perrier A, Yusen RD, Jiménez D. Risk stratification of patients with acute symptomatic pulmonary embolism based on presence or absence of lower extremity DVT: Systematic review and meta-analysis. *Chest.* 2016;149(1):192–200.

22. Lyman GH et al. American Society of Clinical Oncology Clinical Practice. Venous thromboembolism prophylaxis and treatment in patients with cancer: American Society of Clinical Oncology clinical practice guideline update. *J Clin Oncol.* 2013;31(17):2189–204.

23. Akl EA, Kahale L, Neumann I, Barba M, Sperati F, Terrenato I, Muti P, Schünemann H. Anticoagulation for the initial treatment of venous thromboembolism in patients with cancer. *Cochrane Database Syst Rev.* 2014;6:CD006649.

24. den Exter PL, Hooijer J, Dekkers OM, Huisman MV. Risk of recurrent venous thromboembolism and mortality in patients with cancer incidentally diagnosed with pulmonary embolism: A comparison with symptomatic patients. *J Clin Oncol.* 2011;29(17):2405–9.

25. Finet JE. Management of heart failure in cancer patients and cancer survivors. *Heart Fail Clin.* 2017;13(2):253–88.

26. Ponikowski P et al. Authors/Task Force Members; Document Reviewers. 2016 ESC Guidelines for the diagnosis and treatment of acute and chronic heart failure: The Task Force for the diagnosis and treatment of acute and chronic heart failure of the European Society of Cardiology (ESC). Developed with the special contribution of the Heart Failure Association (HFA) of the ESC. *Eur J Heart Fail.* 2016;18(8):891–975.

27. Cardinale D, Colombo A, Lamantia G, Colombo N, Civelli M, De Giacomi G, Rubino M, Veglia F, Fiorentini C, Cipolla CM. Anthracycline-induced cardiomyopathy: Clinical relevance and response to pharmacologic therapy. *J Am Coll Cardiol.* 2010;55(3):213–20.

28. Cardinale D et al. Early detection of anthracycline cardiotoxicity and improvement with heart failure therapy. *Circulation.* 2015;131(22):1981–8.

29. Russell SD, Blackwell KL, Lawrence J, Pippen JE Jr, Roe MT, Wood F, Paton V, Holmgren E, Mahaffey KW. Independent adjudication of symptomatic heart failure with the use of doxorubicin and cyclophosphamide followed by trastuzumab adjuvant therapy: A combined review of cardiac data from the National Surgical Adjuvant Breast and Bowel Project B-31 and the North Central Cancer Treatment Group N9831 clinical trials. *J Clin Oncol.* 2010;28(21):3416–21.

30. Ewer MS, Vooletich MT, Durand JB, Woods ML, Davis JR, Valero V, Lenihan DJ. Reversibility of trastuzumab-related cardiotoxicity: New insights based on clinical course and response to medical treatment. *J Clin Oncol.* November 1, 2005;23(31):7820–6.

31. Szmit S, Kurzyna M, Główczynska R, Grabowski M, Kober J, Czerniawska J, Filipiak KJ, Opolski G, Szczylik C. Manageability of acute severe heart failure complicated with left ventricular thrombosis during therapy for breast cancer. *Int Heart J.* 2010;51(2):141–5.

32. Cardinale D et al. Trastuzumab-induced cardiotoxicity: Clinical and prognostic implications of troponin I evaluation. *J Clin Oncol.* September 1, 2010;28(25):3910–6.

33. Herrmann J, Yang EH, Iliescu CA, Cilingiroglu M, Charitakis K, Hakeem A, Toutouzas K, Leesar MA, Grines CL, Marmagkiolis K. Vascular toxicities of cancer therapies: The old and the new—An evolving avenue. *Circulation.* 2016;133(13):1272–89.

34. Ito D et al. Primary percutaneous coronary intervention and intravascular ultrasound imaging for coronary thrombosis after cisplatin-based chemotherapy. *Heart Vessels.* 2012;27:634–8.

35. Lewandowski T, Szmit S. Bevacizumab—cardiovascular side effects in daily practice. *Oncol Clin Pract.* 2016;12(4):136–43.

36. Binder RK, Lüscher TF. Duration of dual antiplatelet therapy after coronary artery stenting: Where is the sweet spot between ischaemia and bleeding? *Eur Heart J.* 2015;36(20):1207–11.

37. Yusuf SW, Daraban N, Abbasi N, Lei X, Durand JB, Daher IN. Treatment and outcomes of acute coronary syndrome in the cancer population. *Clin Cardiol.* 2012;35(7):443–50.

38. Sarkiss MG, Yusuf SW, Warneke CL, Botz G, Lakkis N, Hirch-Ginsburg C, Champion JC, Swafford J, Shaw AD, Lenihan DJ, Durand JB. Impact of aspirin therapy in cancer patients with thrombocytopenia and acute coronary syndromes. *Cancer.* 2007;109(3):621–7.

39. Vieira RD et al. Cancer-related deaths among different treatment options in chronic coronary artery disease: Results of a 6-year follow-up of the MASS II study. *Coron Artery Dis.* 2012;23:79–84.

40. Abbott JD, Ahmed HN, Vlachos HA, Selzer F, Williams DO. Comparison of outcome in patients with ST-elevation versus non-ST-elevation acute myocardial infarction treated with percutaneous coronary intervention (from the National Heart, Lung, and Blood Institute Dynamic Registry). *Am J Cardiol.* 2007;100:190–5.

41. Guglin M, Aljayeh M, Saiyad S, Ali R, Curtis AB. Introducing a new entity: Chemotherapy-induced arrhythmia. *Europace.* 2009;11 (12):1579–86.

42. Imperatori A, Mariscalco G, Riganti G, Rotolo N, Conti V, Dominioni L. Atrial fibrillation after pulmonary lobectomy for lung cancer affects long-term survival in a prospective single-center study. *J Cardiothorac Surg.* 2012;7:4.

43. Farmakis D, Parissis J, Filippatos G. Insights into onco-cardiology: Atrial fibrillation in cancer. *J Am Coll Cardiol.* 2014;63(10):945–53.

44. Tajstra M, Gadula-Gacek E, Buchta P, Blamek S, Gasior M, Kosiuk J. Effect of therapeutic ionizing radiation on implantable electronic devices: Systematic review and practical guidance. *J Cardiovasc Electrophysiol.* 2016;27(10):1247–51.

45. Grant JD, Jensen GL, Tang C, Pollard JM, Kry SF, Krishnan S, Dougherty AH, Gomez DR, Rozner MA. Radiotherapy-induced malfunction in contemporary cardiovascular implantable electronic devices: Clinical incidence and predictors. *JAMA Oncol.* 2015;1(5):624–32.

46. Opolski G et al. Task Force of National Consultants in Cardiology and Clinical Oncology. Recommendations of National Team of Cardiologic and Oncologic Supervision on cardiologic safety of patients with breast cancer. The prevention and treatment of cardiovascular complications in breast cancer. The Task Force of National Consultants in Cardiology and Clinical Oncology for the elaboration of recommendations of cardiologic proceeding with patients with breast cancer. *Kardiol Pol.* 2011;69(5):520–30.

47. Zecchin M et al. Malfunction of cardiac devices after radiotherapy without direct exposure to ionizing radiation: Mechanisms and experimental data. *Europace.* 2016; 18(2):288–93.

48. Adler Y et al. European Society of Cardiology (ESC). 2015 ESC Guidelines for the diagnosis and management of pericardial diseases: The Task Force for the Diagnosis and Management of Pericardial Diseases of the European Society of Cardiology (ESC) endorsed by: The European Association for Cardio-Thoracic Surgery (EACTS). *Eur Heart J.* 2015;36(42):2921–64.

49. Darby SC et al. Radiation-related heart disease: Current knowledge and future prospects. *Int J Radiat Oncol Biol Phys.* 2010;76(3):656–65.

50. Vaitkus PT, Herrmann HC, LeWinter MM. Treatment of malignant pericardial effusion. *JAMA.* 1994;272(1):59–64.

51. Tsang TS, Seward JB, Barnes ME, Bailey KR, Sinak LJ, Urban LH, Hayes SN. Outcomes of primary and secondary treatment of pericardial effusion in patients with malignancy. *Mayo Clin Proc.* 2000;75(3):248–53.

52. Darocha S, Wilk M, Walaszkowska-Czyż A, Kępski J, Mańczak R, Kurzyna M, Torbicki A, Szmit S. Determinants of survival after emergency intrapericardial cisplatin treatment in cancer patients with recurrent hemodynamic instability after pericardiocentesis. *In Vivo.* 2018;32(2):373–9.

53. Donato V, Bonfili P, Bulzonetti N, Santarelli M, Osti MF, Tombolini V, Banelli E, Enrici RM. Radiation therapy for oncological emergencies. *Anticancer Res.* 2001;21(3C):2219–24.

54. Rowell NP, Gleeson FV. Steroids, radiotherapy, chemotherapy and stents for superior vena caval obstruction in carcinoma of the bronchus: A systematic review. *Clin Oncol (R Coll Radiol).* 2002;14:338–51.

55. Darocha S, Szmit S, Pietura R, Kurzyna M. Percutaneous vena cava superior angioplasty and stenting as an effective method of treatment in vena cava superior syndrome in the course of lung cancer. *OncoReview.* 2014;3(15):108–12.

56. Darocha S, Szmit S, Pietura R, Torbicki A, Kurzyna M. Vena cava superior stenting for rescue treatment of critical stenosis related to progressing cancer disease. *Kardiol Pol.* 2016;74(6):601.

57. Adir Y, Humbert M. Pulmonary hypertension in patients with chronic myeloproliferative disorders. *Eur Respir J.* 2010;35(6):1396–406.

58. Galiè N et al. 2015 ESC/ERS Guidelines for the diagnosis and treatment of pulmonary hypertension: The Joint Task Force for the Diagnosis and Treatment of Pulmonary Hypertension of the European Society of Cardiology (ESC) and the European Respiratory Society (ERS): Endorsed by: Association for European Paediatric and Congenital Cardiology (AEPC), International Society for Heart and Lung Transplantation (ISHLT). *Eur Heart J.* January 1, 2016;37(1):67–119.

59. Shah NP, Wallis N, Farber HW, Mauro MJ, Wolf RA, Mattei D, Guha M, Rea D, Peacock A. Clinical features of pulmonary arterial hypertension in patients receiving dasatinib. *Am J Hematol.* November 2015;90(11):1060–4.

60. Szmit S. Is dasatinib-related pulmonary hypertension a clinical concern? *Future Oncol.* 2015;11(18):2491–4.

61. Ranchoux B et al. Chemotherapy-induced pulmonary hypertension: Role of alkylating agents. *Am J Pathol.* 2015;185(2):356–71.

62. Bonderman D et al. Risk factors for chronic thromboembolic pulmonary hypertension. *Eur Respir J.* 2009;33(2):325–31.

63. Chrissos DN, Stougiannos PN, Mytas DZ, Katsaros AA, Andrikopoulos GK, Kallikazaros IE. Multiple cardiac metastases from a malignant melanoma. *Eur J Echocardiogr.* 2008;9(3):391–2.

64. Shapiro LM. Cardiac tumours: Diagnosis and management. *Heart.* 2001;85(2):218–22.

65. Symbas PN, Hatcher CR Jr, Gravanis MB. Myxoma of the heart: Clinical and experimental observations. *Ann Surg.* 1976;183(5):470–5.

66. Schocken DD, Benjamin EJ, Fonarow GC, Krumholz HM, Levy D, Mensah GA, Narula J, Shor ES, Young JB, Hong Y; American Heart Association Council on Epidemiology and Prevention; American Heart Association Council on Clinical Cardiology; American Heart Association Council on Cardiovascular Nursing; American Heart Association Council on High Blood Pressure Research; Quality of Care and Outcomes Research Interdisciplinary Working Group; Functional Genomics and Translational Biology Interdisciplinary Working Group. Prevention of heart failure: A scientific statement from the American Heart Association Councils on Epidemiology and Prevention, Clinical Cardiology, Cardiovascular Nursing, and High Blood Pressure Research; Quality of Care and Outcomes Research Interdisciplinary Working Group; and Functional Genomics and Translational Biology Interdisciplinary Working Group. *Circulation.* 2008;117(19):2544–65.

67. Salvatorelli E, Menna P, Cantalupo E, Chello M, Covino E, Wolf FI, Minotti G. The concomitant management of cancer therapy and cardiac therapy. *Biochim Biophys Acta.* 2015;1848(10 Pt B):2727–37.

68. Herrmann J, Lerman A, Sandhu NP, Villarraga HR, Mulvagh SL, Kohli M. Evaluation and management of patients with heart disease and cancer: Cardio-oncology. *Mayo Clin Proc.* 2014;89(9):1287–306.

69. Plana JC et al. Expert consensus for multimodality imaging evaluation of adult patients during and after cancer therapy: A report from the American Society of Echocardiography and the European Association of Cardiovascular Imaging. *Eur Heart J Cardiovasc Imaging.* 2014;15(10):1063–93.

70. Ammon M, Arenja N, Leibundgut G, Buechel RR, Kuster GM, Kaufmann BA, Pfister O. Cardiovascular management of cancer patients with chemotherapy-associated left ventricular systolic dysfunction in real-world clinical practice. *J Card Fail.* 2013;19(9):629–34.

71. Rini BI, Cohen DP, Lu DR, Chen I, Hariharan S, Gore ME, Figlin RA, Baum MS, Motzer RJ. Hypertension as a biomarker of efficacy in patients with metastatic renal cell carcinoma treated with sunitinib. *J Natl Cancer Inst.* 2011;103(9):763–73.

72. Szmit S, Zaborowska M, Waśko-Grabowska A, Żołnierek J, Nurzyński P, Filipiak KJ, Opolski G, Szczylik C. Cardiovascular comorbidities for prediction of progression-free survival in patients with metastatic renal cell carcinoma treated with sorafenib. *Kidney Blood Press Res.* 2012;35(6):468–76.

73. Wilk M, Szmit S. Cardiovascular complications of antiangiogenic therapy in ovarian cancer patients. *Oncol Clin Pract.* 2017;13(2):49–56.

74. Mandalà M, Falanga A, Roila F; ESMO Guidelines Working Group. Management of venous thromboembolism (VTE) in cancer patients: ESMO Clinical Practice Guidelines. *Ann Oncol.* 2011;22(Suppl 6):vi85–92.

75. Lee AY, Levine MN, Baker RI, Bowden C, Kakkar AK, Prins M, Rickles FR, Julian JA, Haley S, Kovacs MJ, Gent M; Randomized Comparison of Low-Molecular-Weight Heparin versus Oral Anticoagulant Therapy for the Prevention of Recurrent Venous Thromboembolism in Patients with Cancer (CLOT) Investigators. Low-molecular-weight heparin versus a coumarin for the prevention of recurrent venous thromboembolism in patients with cancer. *N Engl J Med.* 2003;349(2):146–53.

76. Meyer G, Marjanovic Z, Valcke J, Lorcerie B, Gruel Y, Solal-Celigny P, Le Maignan C, Extra JM, Cottu P, Farge D. Comparison of low-molecular-weight heparin and warfarin for

the secondary prevention of venous thromboembolism in patients with cancer: A randomized controlled study. *Arch Intern Med.* 2002;162(15):1729–35.

77. Akl EA, Labedi N, Barba M, Terrenato I, Sperati F, Muti P, Schünemann H. Anticoagulation for the long-term treatment of venous thromboembolism in patients with cancer. *Cochrane Database Syst Rev.* June 15, 2011;(6):CD006650.

78. Khorana AA, Noble S, Lee AYY, Soff G, Meyer G, O'Connell C, Carrier M. Role of direct oral anticoagulants in the treatment of cancer-associated venous thromboembolism: Guidance from the SSC of the ISTH. *J Thromb Haemost.* 2018;16:1891–4.

PART IV

The future of cardio-oncology

15

Future directions in cardio-oncology research

LI-LING TAN, SEAN ZHENG, AND ALEXANDER R. LYON

BIOMARKERS

Current landscape

Circulating cardiac biomarkers play an increasingly important role in the detection of cancer therapy–related cardiotoxicity. Serum cardiac biomarkers are popular as they involve a simple blood draw that is minimally invasive, fast, and convenient.

However, there are several drawbacks associated with the current available biomarkers, cardiac troponin and brain natriuretic peptides. The wide heterogeneity in trial methodology has led to inconsistent results; hence a fair comparison across various studies cannot be made. The lack of fixed biomarker reference ranges, small patient cohort size, and short duration of follow-up complicate matters further. In addition, biomarker elevations can occur in noncardiac conditions and should be interpreted in the appropriate clinical context.

Randomized prospective studies analyzing the diagnostic and prognostic roles of cardiac troponin, particularly with high-sensitivity assays and natriuretic peptides, with large populations followed up for long periods are necessary. Trial protocols should be comparable in terms of patient malignancy profile, treatment regimens, and more importantly, the biomarker assay, time points measured, and frequency of biomarker sampling.

Novel biomarkers

There is a need for novel biomarkers with greater sensitivity and specificity. Age, gender, and renal dysfunction can influence natriuretic peptide levels (1–3). Conventional troponin assays may fail to detect elevations in cancer therapeutics–related cardiotoxicity given that elevations are usually small (4). Although this problem is circumvented by high-sensitivity troponin assays that can accurately measure troponin concentration up to 100 times lower, this comes at a price of reduced specificity (5). Moreover, the presence of troponin elevation signifies that myocardial injury has already occurred; hence the need for new biomarkers that can detect myocardial cell death even earlier.

MicroRNAs and ceramides are examples of promising new biomarkers.

MicroRNAs

MicroRNAs are small, noncoding RNA molecules that regulate post-transcription gene expression and have been implicated in cardiovascular diseases such as myocardial ischemia and heart failure (HF) (6,7). MicroRNAs are present in multiple body fluids (8), can withstand extreme temperatures and pH, and can be measured using various quantitative methods (9). The utility of microRNAs in cancer therapeutics–related cardiotoxicity has been demonstrated in animal models. Horie et al. showed an increase in miR-146a in neonatal cardiac rat models following doxorubicin treatment (10). MiR-1 was superior to troponin in predicting cardiotoxicity risk in breast cancer patients receiving anthracycline (11).

CERAMIDES

Ceramides are important lipid messengers found within cell walls and are involved in cellular signaling processes that lead to cell survival or death. Studies have demonstrated an early accumulation of ceramides within rat cardiomyocytes after doxorubicin exposure, which precedes the apoptosis of cardiomyocytes (12). This suggests that ceramides are involved in the pathophysiology of anthracycline cardiotoxicity and can potentially be a biomarker to detect very early myocardial injury.

Role of biomarkers in cardioprotective strategies

Apart from the detection of cardiotoxicity, biomarkers can be used to guide cardioprotective treatment strategies. Cardinale et al. identified 114 high-risk cancer patients based on troponin elevation after high-dose chemotherapy and randomized them to receive either enalapril for a year or no treatment (control group) (13). The enalapril group had preserved left ventricular volumes and ejection fraction, and significantly fewer adverse cardiac events compared with the control group after 1 year (13). The Cardiac CARE trial (ISRCTN24439460), a multicenter prospective randomized study, aims to investigate whether HF medications can reduce the risk of cardiotoxicity when given to breast cancer patients who develop elevated troponin levels during anthracycline treatment (14).

Genomics

Relying on cardiac biomarkers alone to predict the risk of cardiotoxicity is insufficient in light of the various caveats discussed earlier. There is growing research in the field of genomics with the aim of identifying genetic markers that can improve cardiotoxicity risk stratification and guide cancer and cardioprotective treatment strategies. Aminkeng et al. have singled out a coding variant in *RARG* (retinoic acid receptor γ) that increases the risk of anthracycline-induced cardiotoxicity in patients

treated for childhood cancer (15). A recent study by Hildebrandt et al. identified two hypertension susceptibility gene variants that may protect one from anthracycline cardiotoxicity (16). In addition to circulating biomarkers and imaging parameters, the ongoing SAPhIRE study aims to identify genetic mutations that predispose Asian patients to anthracycline cardiotoxicity (17).

Physicians should also consider sending cancer patients with suspected inheritable cardiac diseases for genetic testing. This is because a two-hit mechanism of cardiomyocyte injury may occur when patients with preexisting genetic cardiomyopathy predispositions receive cardiotoxic cancer therapies even in low doses. This is analogous to patients who develop alcohol-induced or peripartum cardiomyopathy, where for example titin-truncating variants have been implicated. Risk prediction models (18) that incorporate cardiac biomarkers, genomic factors, imaging indices, and patient demographics are necessary as we head toward the era of precision medicine.

IMAGING

Left ventricular ejection fraction (LVEF) is the imaging parameter that is most frequently used to guide the management of cardio-oncology patients. It is easily acquired from different imaging modalities and is reproducible. Expert consensus statements and clinical trials define cardiotoxicity based on LVEF measurement (19,20), but there are inconsistencies in the proposed values for the absolute and percentage reduction in LVEF. There are also no fixed recommendations on the most appropriate imaging modality to use. LVEF is an insensitive marker for the early detection of cardiotoxicity. The presence of appreciable LVEF reduction on cardiac imaging implies that significant myocardial damage has already occurred and the window of opportunity for the initiation of cardioprotective treatment and any chance of LVEF recovery may have already been missed (21).

At present, echocardiography is a key imaging tool in the field of cardio-oncology. It is widely available, relatively low-cost, and does not involve radiation exposure. However, the accuracy and consistency of LVEF measurement is dependent on the availability of good acoustic windows and the experience of the operator and/or reader. There are also geometric assumptions made in the biplane method of disks summation (modified Simpson's rule), which is the current recommended method for LVEF calculation (22). Thus, it is not wise to base important clinical decisions on a single LVEF parameter, further highlighting the need for novel imaging indices with greater sensitivity and specificity.

Echocardiography: Myocardial deformation parameters

GLOBAL LONGITUDINAL STRAIN

Studies have shown that global longitudinal strain (GLS) is a sensitive marker of subclinical cardiotoxicity. Sawaya et al. demonstrated that longitudinal strain by speckle-tracking echocardiogram was less than −19% in all breast cancer patients who developed HF after chemotherapy (23). A systemic review showed that a 10%–15% drop in GLS from baseline predicted the occurrence of subsequent left ventricular (LV) systolic dysfunction in patients during chemotherapy (24). The latest expert consensus paper for multimodality imaging in cancer patients by the American Society of Echocardiography and European Association of Cardiovascular Imaging has thus proposed a >15% reduction in GLS from baseline to be significantly abnormal (19).

Although GLS measurement is precise regardless of operator experience (25), reproducible, and has less interobserver variability compared with LVEF (26), the normal reference range for GLS is not clearly defined. Patient factors such as age, gender, and loading conditions can affect strain values (27). The issue of intervendor variability and different software versions also limits the comparability of strain measurements (26). In addition, the majority of existing evidence is derived from patients with breast cancer and hematological malignancies who were treated with anthracycline. Before the role of GLS as a marker of subclinical cardiotoxicity can be firmly established, more studies involving patients with other malignancies and receiving different forms of cancer therapies should be conducted. The BACCARAT (BreAst Cancer and Cardiotoxicity Induced by RAdioTherapy) Study (ClinicalTrials.gov identifier: NCT02605512) is an ongoing prospective study looking at the change in myocardial strain values in breast cancer patients at baseline and 2 years after adjuvant radiotherapy (28). We also eagerly await the results of the SUCCOUR (Strain sUrveillance of Chemotherapy for improving Cardiovascular OUtcomes) Study (ACTRN12614000341628), which will hopefully shed light as to whether early cardioprotective strategies initiated based on abnormal myocardial strain values observed during chemotherapy will reduce future HF events (29).

OTHER MYOCARDIAL DEFORMATION PARAMETERS

There are other upcoming myocardial deformation parameters that are being evaluated. Ventricular-arterial coupling, which displayed prognostic value in chronic HF (30), was strongly predictive of LV dysfunction in cancer patients receiving anthracycline and/or trastuzumab (31,32). A small study of 25 patients revealed significant reductions in LV torsion and twisting/untwisting velocities 1 month after chemotherapy (33). Mornos and Petrescu showed that deterioration in a novel index (GLS × LV twist) occurred early after the initiation of chemotherapy and was a strong predictor of subsequent cardiotoxicity (area under curve 0.93) (34). As evidence regarding the clinical utility of circumferential strain is conflicting (24,31), further studies are needed for more definitive results.

Cardiac magnetic resonance imaging

Cardiac magnetic resonance imaging (CMR) is the gold standard for the quantification of ventricular volumes and ejection fraction (35). In addition to the advantages of being radiation-free and not affected by limitations of poor acoustic windows, CMR can detect subtle alterations within the myocardium. It can also provide detailed assessment of other cardiac structures (e.g., heart valves and pericardium) and cardiac perfusion status. CMR appears to be an ideal "one stop for all" imaging tool, but its use is hindered by high cost and reduced availability, and it is not suitable for patients with claustrophobia or noncompatible implantable cardiac devices.

LATE GADOLINIUM ENHANCEMENT

At present, a well-recognized role of CMR in a cardio-oncology practice is the assessment of LV volumes and ejection fraction. This is especially important in the cardiac monitoring of patients on active cancer treatments as minor changes in these LV parameters can affect clinical management. Late gadolinium enhancement (LGE) on CMR reflects the presence of myocardial fibrosis, which is pertinent in the detection of cardiac injury. The presence of LGE has prognostic significance in patients with ischemic heart disease (36). Unfortunately, the clinical significance of LGE in the setting of chemotherapy-induced cardiomyopathy is unclear. Data from published studies show that the incidence of LGE in cancer patients with LV dysfunction varies from 6% (37) to 100% (38). Additional research is hence required to clarify the value of LGE.

EXTRACELLULAR VOLUME FRACTION

LGE can detect areas of focal myocardial fibrosis easily, but subtle diffuse myocardial fibrosis, which occurs in chemotherapy-induced cardiotoxicity, can be missed. Extracellular volume (ECV) fraction is calculated from pre- and post-contrast T1-mapping relaxation times and is a potential marker of diffuse myocardial fibrosis. Among adult cancer survivors, ECV fraction remained elevated even after adjusting for age and other cardiovascular risk factors, suggesting that prior anthracycline exposure was associated with the presence of diffuse myocardial fibrosis (39). Increased ECV fraction was shown to be associated with increased left atrial volumes and diastolic dysfunction (40). In a subgroup of patients from the PRADA trial, those with higher cumulative anthracycline doses had elevated ECV fraction and total ECV (41). Prophylactic candesartan treatment during active chemotherapy also led to a significant reduction in LV total cellular volume (41).

Cardiac positron emission tomography imaging

Some of the most frequent adverse cardiac complications associated with cancer therapies include LV dysfunction and ischemia/infarction. Cardiac positron emission tomography (PET) imaging is able to provide detailed information regarding cardiac perfusion and metabolism; hence it can possibly detect early cardiotoxicity, monitor disease progression, and guide clinical decisions with regard to future oncological and cardioprotective treatments.

However, the utility of PET imaging in cardio-oncology is still in its infancy stage. In a recent study looking at mice and rats being exposed to sunitinib, cardiac PET scans post-sunitinib showed increased glucose uptake and reduced myocardial perfusion in association with increased myocardial lipid deposition on electron microscopy (42). In another study, similar changes in glucose metabolism and perfusion indices, together with LVEF reduction and histological findings of HF, were present in mice treated with doxorubicin but absent in the control group (43). A pilot study by Nehmeh et al. suggests that myocardial flow reserve assessed using ^{13}N-ammonia PET imaging may be a predictor of early radiation-induced cardiotoxicity in breast cancer patients (44).

These preliminary studies demonstrate that cancer therapies have a direct toxic cardiac effect, and PET imaging can likely be a very effective non-invasive tool to diagnose subclinical cardiotoxicity. It may also lead to the discovery of previously unknown crucial cellular metabolic pathways and the development of more efficacious therapeutic options.

Imaging protocols

There are currently no fixed guidelines on the timing of cardiac imaging and preferred imaging modality for patients during cancer treatment and for the long-term surveillance of cancer survivors. An important consideration in the development of future protocols is the availability of imaging technology and expertise. Imaging modalities such as CMR and PET scans are often only available in tertiary specialist centers. There are, however, many patients being managed in local hospitals that lack such facilities; the echocardiography lab in local hospitals may not possess the necessary software to obtain myocardial strain readings. While we do not wish to deny patients of specialized cardiac scans whose results might have an impact on the clinical decisions, we should not refer patients for all scans as this may cause unnecessary treatment delays, increased patient anxiety, and higher healthcare costs. Guidelines to identify accurately high-risk patients who will gain the most benefit from these specialized imaging techniques are required.

EPIDEMIOLOGY AND HEALTHCARE DELIVERY

Survival rates of cancer patients have improved over the years with the introduction of more efficacious cancer treatments. Approximately half of cancer patients diagnosed in 2010–2011 in England and Wales are expected to live for at least 10 years

(45). As a result, there are increasingly more cancer survivors presenting with chronic health issues that arise as sequelae of their previous life-saving cancer therapies. Examples of these chronic medical conditions include cardiovascular complications, second malignancy, endocrinopathies, and mental health issues. Childhood cancer survivors are 9 to 15 times more likely to experience severe or life-threatening cardiotoxic events (namely congestive HF, coronary artery disease, and cerebrovascular accidents) when compared to their siblings, and the incidence progressively increases with time (46).

Registry data

Although there are registry studies looking at long-term cardiotoxic events following cancer treatment, direct comparisons are often not possible due to inconsistent definitions of cardiotoxicity and missing data elements. Current statistics on anthracycline cardiomyopathy and radiation heart disease are also most likely an underestimate as these conditions are often asymptomatic and are diagnosed incidentally when patients undergo investigations for another condition.

Therefore, large national and international registries dedicated to the field of cardio-oncology are imperative for physicians to understand better the incidence, severity, and progression of these cardiotoxic events. A universal consensus nomenclature agreed on by both oncologists and cardiologists will facilitate the uniform collection of data elements in retrospective and prospective clinical trials and registries. This will serve as a common platform for the monitoring of adverse events associated with established and upcoming cancer therapies, and may lead to the discovery of vital cellular signaling pathways.

Survivorship clinics

There are published papers proposing various clinical algorithms regarding cardiac surveillance of cancer survivors (47,48); however, these recommendations are largely based on expert opinion. Further validation is needed in the following areas: (1) how to risk-stratify patients; (2) which screening tests to order; (3) when should cardiac surveillance begin, at what frequency, and for how long; and (4) the overall cost-effectiveness.

At present, there is a paucity of strong evidence to guide clinical management after abnormalities in cancer survivors are detected. Current treatment strategies of chemotherapy-induced cardiomyopathy have been extrapolated from previous HF trials that have unfortunately excluded cancer patients. In addition, it is unclear if patients initiated on cardioprotective medications for new-onset HF during cancer therapy can be safely weaned off their cardiac medications upon completion of cancer treatment. Results from a pilot study consisting of cancer survivors who recovered their LVEF with HF treatment showed that the majority of patients remained asymptomatic with no significant change in LVEF and cardiac biomarkers at 6 months post-withdrawal of HF treatment (49). More evidence in the setting of well-designed trials is required to address these important clinical questions.

Apart from actively screening for cardiotoxic events and titration of pharmacological therapies, survivorship clinics should also focus on nonpharmacological measures. Both cancer and cardiovascular disease share many similar risk factors such as hypertension, diabetes, smoking, and obesity. Cancer patients should be educated on the importance of healthy lifestyle measures, and this should ideally begin at the time of cancer diagnosis, continue during cancer treatment and persist throughout survivorship. While exercise reduces mortality and HF hospitalizations in HF patients (50) and improves fitness level and quality of life in cancer patients (51), there is mixed evidence regarding the benefits of exercise in the prevention and treatment of anthracycline cardiomyopathy (52). Little is also known about the role of screening exercise tests and the appropriate levels of exercise intensity in cancer survivors with and without cardiac disease (52).

Having a dedicated survivorship clinic is also an avenue for research opportunities. Suitable patients can be easily approached for participation in research trials during routine clinic visits, collection of any blood specimens can be performed simultaneously, and information regarding long-term clinical outcomes can be readily obtained.

Healthcare networks

There is a need to educate both healthcare providers and cancer patients on the importance of long-term surveillance for cardiotoxic events. Cancer

Table 15.1 Summary of areas for future research in cardio-oncology

Biomarkers

- Well-powered prospective clinical trials with sufficiently long follow-up testing the diagnostic and prognostic roles of available cardiac biomarkers (high-sensitivity troponin and natriuretic peptides) and their use in predicting response to HF therapies.
- Identification of novel biomarkers with sensitivity and specificity profiles to allow detection of early myocardial injury before overt HF develops.
- Further genome-based studies that identify genotypes (including single-nucleotide polymorphisms and genes known to be involved in inherited cardiomyopathies) that predict the development of cardiotoxicity.

Imaging

- Understanding the diagnostic and prognostic roles of echocardiographic measurements other than left ventricular ejection fraction (e.g., global longitudinal strain and other myocardial deformation parameters).
- More imaging studies conducted in broader cancer populations receiving a range of chemotherapeutic agents.
- Additional research using cardiac MRI to confirm the role of late gadolinium enhancement and extracellular volume fraction in cardiac toxicity.

Treatment

- Dedicated prospective studies testing commonly used HF and novel therapies in participants with chemotherapy-induced cardiotoxicity.
- More research on whether HF treatments need to be continued long-term in cancer survivors who have recovered cardiac function, and if not, how therapies should be weaned and with what monitoring.

Epidemiology and healthcare delivery

- Universal consensus definitions agreed upon by cardiologists and oncologists will allow registry and cohort data to be collected and analyzed uniformly.
- Before patients start cancer treatment, there need to be consensus recommendations on how patients should be risk stratified and which screening tests should be used.
- In patients having cancer treatment and who have been risk stratified, there need to be consensus recommendations on the timing, frequency, and modality of cardiac monitoring.
- In patients who have completed cancer treatment, there need to be consensus recommendations on when cardiac surveillance should begin, its frequency and method, and for how long after completion of treatment.
- With an increasingly aging population and improved cancer outcomes, the cost-effectiveness and burden on healthcare systems need to be investigated. Guidelines should take into account available healthcare resources across different healthcare systems.
- Education for healthcare providers and cancer patients on the significance of cardiac toxicity and importance of long-term surveillance.
- Cancer survivorship clinics are one method which could ensure individuals are not lost to follow-up, though their clinical and cost-effectiveness need to be tested.

survivors are easily lost to follow-up once they are given the all-clear by their oncologists, with primary care doctors likely to remain their first and main point of medical contact. Doctors should consider whether symptoms reported by cancer patients are due to cardiac injury, especially young childhood cancer survivors of whom a large majority have been exposed to anthracycline and radiotherapy (53). In addition, as cardiotoxic events are often asymptomatic for many years, primary care doctors should make a conscious effort in screening cancer survivors so that timely intervention can be implemented to delay or prevent the onset of symptomatic disease.

Efforts are needed to set up local networks of healthcare providers comprised of primary care doctors, nurse practitioners, oncologists, and cardiologists. Depending on the needs of the local community and availability of resources, the most appropriate care delivery model can be adopted to coordinate the care of the patients. With the increase in medical tourism, the use of information technology facilitates the creation of a global healthcare network by bridging links between cancer patients and multiple healthcare professionals worldwide. The Survivorship Passport established by the European Society for Paediatric Oncology and its partners is an example of a survivorship initiative dedicated to the long-term care of European childhood cancer survivors (54).

In summary there are a range of future research strategies and avenues which are being explored in cardio-oncology, which hopefully will deliver improvements in clinical care and outcomes for cancer patients with cardiovascular disease (see Table 15.1).

REFERENCES

1. Cowie M. Clinical applications of B-type natriuretic peptide (BNP) testing. *Eur Heart J.* 2003;24(19):1710–8.
2. Galasko GI, Lahiri A, Barnes SC, Collinson P, Senior R. What is the normal range for N-terminal pro-brain natriuretic peptide? How well does this normal range screen for cardiovascular disease? *Eur Heart J.* November 2005;26(21):2269–76.
3. Takase H, Dohi Y. Kidney function crucially affects B-type natriuretic peptide (BNP),

   N-terminal proBNP and their relationship. *Eur J Clin Invest.* 2014;44(3):303–8.
4. Christenson ES, James T, Agrawal V, Park BH. Use of biomarkers for the assessment of chemotherapy-induced cardiac toxicity. *Clin Biochem.* March 2015;48(4–5):223–35.
5. Marini MG, Cardillo MT, Caroli A, Sonnino C, Biasucci LM. Increasing specificity of high-sensitivity troponin: New approaches and perspectives in the diagnosis of acute coronary syndromes. *J Cardiol.* October 2013;62(4):205–9.
6. Wang GK, Zhu JQ, Zhang JT, Li Q, Li Y, He J, Qin YW, Jing Q. Circulating microRNA: A novel potential biomarker for early diagnosis of acute myocardial infarction in humans. *Eur Heart J.* March 2010;31(6):659–66.
7. Vegter EL, van der Meer P, de Windt LJ, Pinto YM, Voors AA. MicroRNAs in heart failure: From biomarker to target for therapy. *Eur J Heart Fail.* May 2016;18(5):457–68.
8. Weber JA, Baxter DH, Zhang S, Huang DY, Huang KH, Lee MJ, Galas DJ, Wang K. The microRNA spectrum in 12 body fluids. *Clin Chem.* November 2010;56(11):1733–41.
9. Ruggeri C, Gioffre S, Achilli F, Colombo GI, D'Alessandra Y. Role of microRNAs in doxorubicin-induced cardiotoxicity: An overview of preclinical models and cancer patients. *Heart Fail Rev.* 2018 January;23(1):109–22.
10. Horie T et al. Acute doxorubicin cardiotoxicity is associated with miR-146a-induced inhibition of the neuregulin-ErbB pathway. *Cardiovasc Res.* September 01, 2010;87(4):656–64.
11. Rigaud VO et al. Circulating miR-1 as a potential biomarker of doxorubicin-induced cardiotoxicity in breast cancer patients. *Oncotarget.* 2017;8(4):6994–7002.
12. Delpy E, Hatem S, Andrieu-Abadie N, de Vaumas C, Henaff M, Rucker-Martin C, Jaffrezou J, Laurent G, Levade T, Mercadier J. Doxorubicin induces slow ceramide accumulation and late apoptosis in cultured adult rat ventricular myocytes. *Cardiovasc Res.* 1999;43:398–407.
13. Cardinale D, Colombo A, Sandri MT, Lamantia G, Colombo N, Civelli M, Martinelli G, Veglia F, Fiorentini C, Cipolla CM. Prevention of high-dose chemotherapy-induced cardiotoxicity in high-risk

patients by angiotensin-converting enzyme inhibition. *Circulation*. December 05, 2006;114(23):2474–81.

14. ISRCTN registry. The Cardiac CARE Trial - can heart muscle injury related to chemotherapy be prevented? 2017 [cited November 28, 2017]; Available from: https://www.isrctn.com/ISRCTN24439460?q=&filters=conditionCategory:Cancer&sort=&offset=2&totalResults=1958&page=1&pageSize=10&searchType=basic-search.

15. Aminkeng F et al. Consortium. TCPNfDS. A coding variant in *RARG* confers susceptibility to anthracycline-induced cardiotoxicity in childhood cancer. *Nat Genet*. 2015;47(9): 1079–84.

16. Hildebrandt MAT, Reyes M, Wu X, Pu X, Thompson KA, Ma J, Landstrom AP, Morrison AC, Ater JL. Hypertension susceptibility loci are associated with anthracycline-related cardiotoxicity in long-term childhood cancer survivors. *Sci Rep*. August 29, 2017;7(1):9698.

17. SAPhIRE (Surveillance And Pharmacogenomics of Adverse Drug Reactions). Research Focus: Clinical Studies (Ongoing Trials): Doxorubicin/Herceptin. 2014 [cited December 12, 2017]; Available from: http://www.saphire.sg/doxorubicinherceptin/.

18. Skitch A, Mital S, Mertens L, Liu P, Kantor P, Grosse-Wortmann L, Manlhiot C, Greenberg M, Nathan PC. Novel approaches to the prediction, diagnosis and treatment of cardiac late effects in survivors of childhood cancer: A multi-centre observational study. *BMC Cancer*. August 03, 2017;17(1):519.

19. Plana JC et al. Expert consensus for multimodality imaging evaluation of adult patients during and after cancer therapy: A report from the American Society of Echocardiography and the European Association of Cardiovascular Imaging. *J Am Soc Echocardiogr*. September 2014;27(9):911–939.

20. Seidman A, Hudis C, Pierri MK, Shak S, Paton V, Ashby M, Murphy M, Stewart SJ, Keefe D. Cardiac Dysfunction in the Trastuzumab Clinical Trials Experience. *J Clin Oncol*. 2002;20(5):1215–1221.

21. Cardinale D, Colombo A, Lamantia G, Colombo N, Civelli M, De Giacomi G, Rubino M, Veglia F, Fiorentini C, Cipolla CM. Anthracycline-induced cardiomyopathy: Clinical relevance and response to pharmacologic therapy. *J Am Coll Cardiol*. January 19, 2010;55(3):213–20.

22. Lang RM et al. Recommendations for cardiac chamber quantification by echocardiography in adults: An update from the American Society of Echocardiography and the European Association of Cardiovascular Imaging. *J Am Soc Echocardiogr*. January 2015;28(1):1–39, e14.

23. Sawaya H et al. Assessment of echocardiography and biomarkers for the extended prediction of cardiotoxicity in patients treated with anthracyclines, taxanes, and trastuzumab. *Circ Cardiovasc Imaging*. September 01, 2012;5(5):596–603.

24. Thavendiranathan P, Poulin F, Lim KD, Plana JC, Woo A, Marwick TH. Use of myocardial strain imaging by echocardiography for the early detection of cardiotoxicity in patients during and after cancer chemotherapy: A systematic review. *J Am Coll Cardiol*. July 1, 2014;63(25 Pt A):2751–68.

25. Negishi T, Negishi K, Thavendiranathan P, Cho GY, Popescu BA, Vinereanu D, Kurosawa K, Penicka M, Marwick TH, SUCOUR Investigators. Effect of experience and training on the concordance and precision of strain measurements. *JACC Cardiovasc Imaging*. May 2017;10(5):518–22.

26. Farsalinos KE, Daraban AM, Unlu S, Thomas JD, Badano LP, Voigt JU. Head-to-head comparison of global longitudinal strain measurements among nine different vendors: The EACVI/ASE inter-vendor comparison study. *J Am Soc Echocardiogr*. October 2015;28(10):1171–81, e1172.

27. Collier P, Phelan D, Klein A. A test in context: Myocardial strain measured by speckle-tracking echocardiography. *J Am Coll Cardiol*. February 28, 2017;69(8):1043–56.

28. ClinicalTrials.gov. BreAst Cancer and Cardiotoxicity Induced by RAdioTherapy: The BACCARAT Study (BACCARAT). 2017 [January 2018]; Available from: https://clinicaltrials.gov/ct2/show/NCT02605512?cond=strain+and+cardiotoxicity&rank=6.

29. Australian New Zealand Clinical Trials Registry (ANZCTR). SUCOUR Study. 2016. [January 2018]; Available from: https://www.anzctr.org.au/Trial/Registration/TrialReview.aspx?id=366020.

30. Ky B et al. Ventricular-arterial coupling, remodeling, and prognosis in chronic heart failure. *J Am Coll Cardiol.* September 24, 2013;62(13):1165–72.

31. Narayan HK et al. Noninvasive measures of ventricular-arterial coupling and circumferential strain predict cancer therapeutics-related cardiac dysfunction. *JACC Cardiovasc Imaging.* October 2016;9(10):1131–41.

32. Narayan HK, Wei W, Feng Z, Lenihan D, Plappert T, Englefield V, Fisch M, Ky B. Cardiac mechanics and dysfunction with anthracyclines in the community: Results from the PREDICT study. *Open Heart.* 2017;4(1):e000524.

33. Motoki H, Koyama J, Nakazawa H, Aizawa K, Kasai H, Izawa A, Tomita T, Miyashita Y, Kumazaki S, Takahashi M, Ikeda U. Torsion analysis in the early detection of anthracycline-mediated cardiomyopathy. *Eur Heart J Cardiovasc Imaging.* January 2012; 13(1):95–103.

34. Mornos C, Petrescu L. Early detection of anthracycline-mediated cardiotoxicity: The value of considering both global longitudinal left ventricular strain and twist. *Can J Physiol Pharmacol.* August 2013;91(8):601–7.

35. Pennell DJ, Sechtem UP, Higgins CB, Manning WJ, Pohost GM, Rademakers FE, van Rossum AC, Shaw LJ, Yucel EK, Society for Cardiovascular Magnetic Resonance, Working Group on Cardiovascular Magnetic Resonance of the European Society of Cardiology. Clinical indications for cardiovascular magnetic resonance (CMR): Consensus Panel report. *Eur Heart J.* November 2004;25(21):1940–65.

36. Kwong RY, Chan AK, Brown KA, Chan CW, Reynolds HG, Tsang S, Davis RB. Impact of unrecognized myocardial scar detected by cardiac magnetic resonance imaging on event-free survival in patients presenting with signs or symptoms of coronary artery disease. *Circulation.* June 13, 2006;113(23):2733–43.

37. Neilan TG, Coelho-Filho OR, Pena-Herrera D, Shah RV, Jerosch-Herold M, Francis SA, Moslehi J, Kwong RY. Left ventricular mass in patients with a cardiomyopathy after treatment with anthracyclines. *Am J Cardiol.* 2012;110(11):1679–86.

38. Fallah-Rad N, Lytwyn M, Fang T, Kirkpatrick I, Jassal DS. Delayed contrast enhancement cardiac magnetic resonance imaging in trastuzumab induced cardiomyopathy. *J Cardiovasc Magn Reson.* January 22, 2008;10:5.

39. Jordan JH et al. Anthracycline-associated T1 mapping characteristics are elevated independent of the presence of cardiovascular comorbidities in cancer survivors. *Circ Cardiovasc Imaging.* August 2016;9(8).

40. Neilan TG et al. Myocardial extracellular volume by cardiac magnetic resonance imaging in patients treated with anthracycline-based chemotherapy. *Am J Cardiol.* March 1, 2013;111(5):717–22.

41. Heck SL et al. Effect of candesartan and metoprolol on myocardial tissue composition during anthracycline treatment: The PRADA trial. *Eur Heart J Cardiovasc Imaging.* May 1, 2018;19(5):544–52.

42. O'Farrell AC et al. A novel positron emission tomography (PET) approach to monitor cardiac metabolic pathway remodeling in response to sunitinib malate. *PLOS ONE.* 2017;12(1):e0169964.

43. Gascon S, Croteau E, Sarrhini O, Tremblay S, Benoit-Biancamano M, Turcotte E, Lecomte R. Cardiac PET imaging of perfusion, metabolism and function in a mouse model of cardiotoxicity induced by doxorubicin chemotherapy. *J Nucl Med.* 2015;56(supplement 3):1475.

44. Nehmeh S, Fox J, Schwartz J, Ballangrud A, Schoder H, Strauss H, Yu A, Gupta D, Powell S, Humm J, Ho A. Value of cardiac 13N-Ammonia PET in assessing early radiation-induced cardiotoxicity in breast cancer patients undergoing radiotherapy: A feasibility study. *J Nucl Med.* 2017;58(supplement 1):517.

45. Cancer Research UK. Cancer Survival. 2014 [cited December 2017]; Available from: http://www.cancerresearchuk.org/sites/default/files/cstream-node/surv_1_5_10yr_all.pdf.

46. Oeffinger K et al. Chronic health conditions in adult survivors of childhood cancer. *N Engl J Med.* 2006;355:1572–82.

47. Armenian SH et al. Prevention and monitoring of cardiac dysfunction in survivors of adult cancers: American Society of Clinical Oncology clinical practice guideline. *J Clin Oncol.* March 10, 2017;35(8):893–911.

48. Groarke JD, Nguyen PL, Nohria A, Ferrari R, Cheng S, Moslehi J. Cardiovascular complications of radiation therapy for thoracic malignancies: The role for non-invasive imaging for detection of cardiovascular disease. *Eur Heart J*. March 2014;35(10):612–23.

49. Fadol AP, Banchs J, Hassan SA, Yeh ET, Fellman B. Withdrawal of heart failure medications in cancer survivors with chemotherapy-induced left ventricular dysfunction: A pilot study. *J Card Fail*. June 2016;22(6):481–2.

50. Piepoli MF, Davos C, Francis DP, Coats AJ, ExTraMATCH Collaborative. Exercise training meta-analysis of trials in patients with chronic heart failure (ExTraMATCH). *BMJ*. January 24, 2004;328(7433):189.

51. Mustian KM, Sprod LK, Palesh OG, Peppone LJ, Janelsins MC, Mohile SG, Carroll J. Exercise for the management of side effects and quality of life among cancer survivors. *Cur Sports Med Rep*. 2009;8:325–30.

52. Smith SM, Carver JR. Exercise intensity in cancer survivors: A matter of the heart. *Cardio-Oncology*. 2017;3(1).

53. Armenian SH et al. Recommendations for cardiomyopathy surveillance for survivors of childhood cancer: A report from the International Late Effects of Childhood Cancer Guideline Harmonization Group. *Lancet Oncol*. 2015;16(3):e123–36.

54. European Society for Paediatric Oncology. The Survivorship Passport. 2017 [cited December 2017]; Available from: https://www.siope.eu/activities/joint-projects/survivorship-passport/.

16

Cardio-oncology: Future directions in clinical care and education

SUSAN F. DENT, GRETCHEN KIMMICK, AND JOE CARVER

INTRODUCTION

Cancer and cardiovascular disease are the top two causes of mortality in North America, accounting for over 45% of deaths in the USA (1). The population is aging—by 2050 more than 20% of the U.S. population will be over 65 years of age (2). Given the overlap of risk factors for both cancer and heart disease, patients may have established cardiovascular disease prior to the detection of their cancer, placing them at greater risk of cardiovascular complications (3).

Our improved understanding of cancer biology has led to an exponential increase in the number of cancer therapeutics available to individuals facing a cancer diagnosis (4). Novel targeted agents, such as monoclonal antibodies and tyrosine kinase inhibitors, have achieved better clinical outcomes, but are associated with unique toxicities, including cardiovascular toxicity (5). The establishment of cardio-oncology as a discipline has led to the emergence of cardio-oncology clinics across North America and globally (see Figure 16.1); yet, there is a paucity of information in the literature on the benefits of this multidisciplinary approach. Cardio-oncology guidelines and position statements have helped to define current best practices; however, these documents are based largely on expert opinion rather than rigorous science (6–9). Education

of healthcare providers, in this field, has been limited to lectures, conferences, and continuing medical education events sponsored by larger academic institutions. Training programs in cardio-oncology are still being developed and refined. The field of cardio-oncology will continue to grow. The establishment of quality indicators for cardio-oncology programs, and education of healthcare providers and patients, will ensure the continued success of this novel treatment approach to patient care.

CLINICAL CARE

Cardio-oncology clinics have emerged as a result of a multidisciplinary effort between oncology and cardiology, mainly in larger academic institutions (10). While general principles on the establishment of a cardio-oncology clinic have been previously described (11–13) (see Figure 16.2), little information is available on the success of these models. Are cardio-oncology clinics really improving the care of cancer patients? Are patients satisfied with their care? How do we define a "successful" cardio-oncology clinic/program? Quality indicators are needed to determine the short- (e.g., completion of cancer therapy) and long-term benefits (e.g., prevention of heart failure) of these programs. Given the heterogeneity of cancers, and the different mechanisms of cardiotoxicity of cancer treatments,

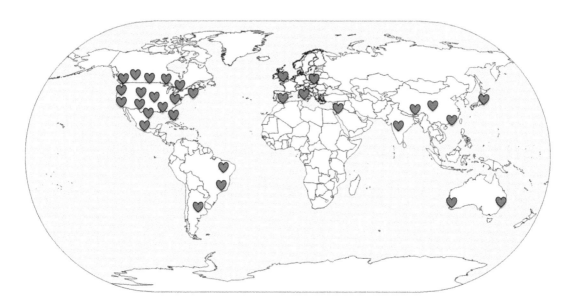

Figure 16.1 Growth of cardio-oncology clinics.

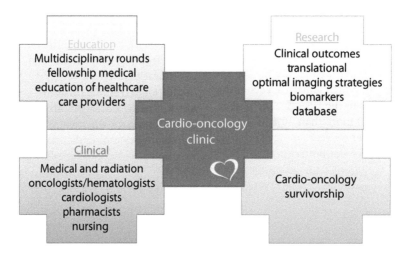

Figure 16.2 Components of a cardio-oncology program.

common quality indicators may be difficult to define. Importantly, the sustainability of cardio-oncology clinics/programs depends on the support of respective institutions and healthcare administrators who need to measure the success of a novel program and financial return on investment. Further research is needed to define appropriate quality indicators or measures for cardio-oncology clinics, which can be used to inform the success of clinics/program within and across institutions. Standardized measures, if reported by institutions who operate cardio-oncology clinics, could provide

more "robust" data to facilitate the development of "best practices" in this population and provide the basis for quantification of quality metrics.

Few cardio-oncology clinics/programs have been established in community cancer centers, where the majority of cancer care is delivered in the USA. Clinicians have reported barriers to the formation of cardio-oncology clinics, including lack of institutional support and resources (14). For certain healthcare facilities, it may not be possible to establish cardio-oncology clinics due to lack of medical expertise and/or low patient volumes. Novel strategies are needed for those cancer patients who do not have readily available access to cardio-oncology services.

Telemedicine provides medical care for patients with limited access to major healthcare facilities in many cities across North America. The American Academy of Family Physicians (AAFP) supports expanded use of telemedicine as an appropriate and efficient means of improving health, when conducted in a manner supportive of longitudinal care and within the context of appropriate standards of care (15). Telehealth refers to the broad collection of electronic and telecommunications technologies that support healthcare delivery and services from distant locations. Telemedicine can be divided into three basic platforms: asynchronous telemedicine, remote patient monitoring, and real-time medicine (16,17). Asynchronous telemedicine permits healthcare providers to share patient medical information such as lab reports, imaging studies, videos, and other records with a physician, radiologist, or specialist at another location. It is similar to email, but is done using a system that has built-in, sophisticated security measures to ensure patient confidentiality. A similar approach could be used to provide cardio-oncology services for cancer patients in centers where this expertise is not available. Patient services could range from comprehensive consults to specific cancer therapy–related questions such as: should I hold trastuzumab if a patient has a left ventricular ejection fraction of 49%?; or how should I manage hypertension in a cancer patient on a tyrosine kinase inhibitor? The use of telemedicine in cardio-oncology is an area where further research is clearly needed.

The majority of patients who have completed their cancer therapy are eventually discharged from the cancer center to their primary care provider. The Institute of Medicine suggests that once a person has completed cancer therapy, they should be provided with a summary of the treatments received and a follow-up "survivorship plan" (18). These plans usually summarize the details of an individual's cancer diagnosis, treatment plan, and recommended surveillance. Including information on possible late- and long-term effects of cancer treatment and symptoms of such effects is recommended. But is this enough? Patients who receive potentially cardiotoxic cancer therapy and those patients with preexisting cardiovascular disease are at risk of long-term cardiovascular morbidity and mortality (19). How can these patients be monitored for cardiovascular health? Should primary or secondary prevention strategies be considered? Should cancer patients at high risk of long-term cancer therapy–related dysfunction be followed in a "cardio-oncology survivorship clinic" (see Chapter 8)? These are important questions that need to be addressed in the field of cardio-oncology.

EDUCATION

Cardio-oncology remains, for the majority of healthcare providers and patients, an unknown entity. There is a clear need to educate health care providers and cancer patients on the potential impact of cancer therapy on cardiovascular health. Several societies, including the International Cardio-Oncology Society (ICOS), the Canadian Cardiac Oncology Network (CCON), and the British Cardio-Oncology Society (BCOS), have been established with the goal of educating healthcare providers and cancer patients. The Global Cardio-Oncology Summit (GCOS), an annual scientific meeting established in 2015, gives clinicians, researchers, basic scientists, and trainees from around the world the opportunity to share their knowledge and best practices. ICOS sponsors monthly webinars in cardio-oncology, and academic institutions in the USA, including Memorial Sloan Kettering in New York and the Mayo Clinic in Rochester, Minnesota, host annual continuing medical education (CME) events.

Cardio-oncology is now recognized by professional cardiology and oncology organizations around the world, including the American College of Cardiology (ACC), European Society for Medical Oncology (ESMO), European Society of Cardiology (ESC), and the American Society of Clinical Oncology (ASCO) (see Figure 16.3). Cardio-oncology has become an established entity within these organizations, which often support special workshops and mini-symposiums in cardio-oncology within their annual meetings. The ACC has established a special chapter in cardio-oncology as well as an annual workshop for individuals with an interest in this field.

Clinical practice guidelines and position statements in cardio-oncology have been published by a number of societies (ESC, ASCO, ESMO, Canadian Cardiology Society) (6–9) to help guide clinicians in the assessment and management of cancer patients who are at risk of, or who have developed,

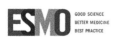
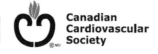
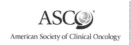

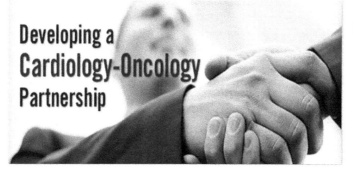

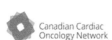
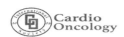
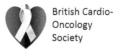

Figure 16.3 Endorsement of cardio-oncology as a discipline.

cancer therapy–related cardiac dysfunction. The American Society of Echocardiography (ASE) expert consensus specifically addresses cardiac imaging strategies in this patient population (20). Several of these guidelines/position statements address current recommendations on cardiovascular surveillance after completion of cancer therapy. The majority of these recommendations, however, are based on either consensus from experts in the field, or low to moderate levels of evidence. While, these guidelines/position statements clearly outline best practices today, research is needed to generate the high-quality data necessary to develop more rigorous evidence-based guidelines.

Despite efforts by academic institutions and professional organizations, the penetration of cardio-oncology into community hospitals and institutions remains low. CME events in cardio-oncology have been limited mainly to large academic institutions, and conferences often take place in major cities that are out of reach for many community healthcare providers. Exploration of strategies to improve engagement of community healthcare providers (e.g., videoconferencing or webinars) is needed in order to meet their educational needs in cardio-oncology.

Allied healthcare providers (e.g., pharmacists, nurses, exercise physiologists) are integral members of the cardio-oncology team. Participation in cardio-oncology CME events should be encouraged by supervisors and hospital administration. Ideally, professional societies of these allied healthcare disciplines should be encouraged to include cardio-oncology within their educational framework. The MacMillan Cancer Support group in the UK has published a guide which provides basic recommendations on the management of heart health during and after cancer treatment for both primary care professionals and patients. This guide has been endorsed by the British Cardio-Oncology Society, the British Heart Foundation, and the UK Oncology Nursing Society (21).

As the field of cardio-oncology expands, so will the need for more individuals with expertise in this area. There are currently no "board-certified" training programs in cardio-oncology; however, several major centers (e.g., Vanderbilt, Dana-Farber, University of Pennsylvania) in North America have developed 1–2 year fellowship training programs in cardio-oncology. ICOS and CCON developed a consensus document that outlines the ongoing efforts for training the next generation of cardio-oncologists. The necessary elements of cardio-oncology training are outlined, including the expectations for exposure necessary to develop adequate skills in this new field. Further refinements of these recommendations will be needed as this discipline evolves (22).

There is a paucity of information in the literature on the education of cancer patients (on active cancer therapy or cancer survivors) in cardio-oncology. Most cancer patients are introduced to this field at the time they are referred to a cardio-oncology clinic. There is currently no evidence to suggest that oncologists are discussing cardiovascular risk factors with cancer patients beyond the cardiac risk associated with the specific cancer therapy prescribed. Currently, there are no standardized recommendations to include information in cancer survivorship plans, on cardiac surveillance strategies, or cardiovascular risk optimization for patients treated with cancer therapy and/or radiation therapy. This is in contrast to pediatric cancer survivors who, based on the Children's Oncology Group (COG) long-term follow-up guidelines (www.survivorshipguidelines.org), are given survivorship plans in which there are evidence-based guidelines on recommended cardiac surveillance and cardiac risk modification strategies (23). The Canadian Cardiac Oncology Network provides information for patients on its website (www.cardiaconcology.ca); however, this is limited to frequently asked questions such as—what is an echocardiogram? The cardio-oncology section of the ACC provides patient-level information on cancer treatment and heart disease on a web-based platform (www.cardiosmart.org).

Patient advocacy organizations serve the purpose of educating patients and the community. They also advocate for funding of treatment and research by lobbying government officials and advising medical organizations and researchers. Therefore, it is of paramount importance that patient advocacy groups are included in educational efforts in cardio-oncology because of the potential impact of cancer treatments on cardiovascular health. Only recently have organizers of CME events in cardio-oncology reached out to patients and patient advocates to share their experiences. There is a clear need for cardio-oncologists and patient advocates to partner in moving the field forward.

The evolution of targeted cancer therapies provides increasing optimism for those individuals facing a cancer diagnosis. More individuals are surviving a cancer diagnosis and those with advanced cancer are living longer. Cardio-oncology has emerged as a clinically-based discipline focused on the cardiovascular health of cancer patients and cancer survivors. The institution of cardio-oncology clinics/programs provides the framework for optimizing clinical care delivery, education, and research. The goals of this new subspecialty should include improved patient access to effective multidisciplinary care, education of healthcare providers and the public, application of guideline-based diagnosis and treatment, and commitment to collective research in this field. The future of cardio-oncology will depend on the cohesive efforts of all healthcare providers to achieve these goals.

REFERENCES

1. DeSantis CE et al. Cancer treatment and survivorship statistics. *CA Cancer J Clin.* 2014;64:252–71.
2. Heron M et al. Changes in the leading causes of death: Recent patterns in heart disease and cancer mortality. 2016. cdc.gov/nchs/products/databriefs/db254.htm.
3. Cubbon RM, Lyon AR. Cardio-oncology: Concepts and practice. *Indian Heart J.* 2016;68.
4. Sparreboom A, Verweij J. Advances in cancer therapeutics. *Clin Pharmacol Ther.* 2009;85(2):113–17.
5. Curigliano G, Cardinale D, Dent S, Criscitiello C, Aseyev O, Lenihan D, Cipolla CM. Cardiotoxicity of anticancer treatments: Epidemiology, detection, and management. *CA Can J Clin.* July 2016;(66):309–25.
6. Zamorano JL et al. ESC Position Paper on cancer treatments and cardiovascular toxicity developed under the auspices of the ESC Committee for Practice Guidelines: The Task Force for cancer treatments and cardiovascular toxicity of the European Society of Cardiology (ESC). *Eur J Heart Fail.* 2016;37(36):2768–801.
7. Virani S, Dent S, Brezden-Masley C. Canadian Cardiovascular Society Guidelines for evaluation and management of patients at risk for cardiovascular complications of cancer therapy. *Can J Cardiol.* July 2016;32(7).

8. Armenian S et al. Prevention and monitoring of cardiac dysfunction in survivors of adult cancers: American Society of Clinical Oncology Clinical Practice Guidelines. *J Clin Oncol.* 2017;35(8):893–911.

9. Curigliano G et al. Cardiovascular toxicity induced by chemotherapy, targeted agents and radiotherapy: ESMO Clinical Practice Guidelines. *Ann Oncol.* 2012;23(supplement 7).

10. Barac A, Mayer E. Future clinical and professional directions in cardio-oncology. In Chapter 13. (*Cardio-Oncology: The Clinical Overlap of Cancer and Heart Disease*). Springer; 2016; 303–10.

11. Okwuosa TM, Barac A. Challenges and opportunities for early career cardiologists/faculty directors. *JACC.* 2016;66(10).

12. Barros-Gomes S, Hermann J, Mulvagh S, Lerman A, Lin G, Villarraga H. Rationale for setting up a cardio-oncology unit: Our experience at Mayo Clinic. *Cardio-oncology.* April 2016;2:5.

13. Dent S, Law A, Aseyev O, Ghosh N, Johnson C. Coordinating cardio-oncology care. In Chapter 15. *Cardio-Oncology: Principles, Prevention and Management.* Elsevier; 2017; 221–36.

14. Barac A et al. Cardiovascular health of patients with cancer and cancer survivors. *J Am Coll Cardiol.* June 2015;65(25).

15. American Association of Family Physicians. What's the difference between telemedicine and telehealth? 2019. https://www.aafp.org/media-center/kits/telemedicine-and-telehealth.html.

16. Van Dyk L. A review of telehealth service implementation frameworks. *J Environ Res Public Health.* 2014;11(2):1279–98.

17. Broens THF et al. Determinants of successful telemedicine implementations: A literature study. *J Telemed Telecare.* 2007;13(6):303–9.

18. *From Cancer Patient to Cancer Survivor: Lost in Transition.* Institute of Medicine of the National Academies; November 3, 2005.

19. Patnaik JL et al. Cardiovascular disease competes with breast cancer as the leading cause of death for older females diagnosed with breast cancer: A retrospective cohort study. *Breast Cancer Res.* 2011;12(3):R64.

20. Plana JC et al. Expert Consensus for Multimodality Imaging Evaluation of adult cancer patients during and after cancer therapy: A report from the American Society of Echocardiography and the European Association of Cardiovascular Imaging. *J Am Soc Echocardiogr.* 2014;27:911–39.

21. MacMillan Cancer Support. Cancer Treatment and your heart. 2019. https://www.macmillan.org.uk/information-and-support/coping/side-effects-and-symptoms/cancer-treatment-and-your-heart#.

22. Lenihan D et al. Cardio-oncology training: A proposal from the International Cardio-Oncology Society and Canadian Cardiac Oncology Network for a new multidisciplinary specialty. *J Card Fail.* March 2016;22(6).

23. Children's Oncology Group. Long-term follow-up guidelines for survivors of childhood, adolescent, and young adult cancers. Version 5.0. October 2018. www.survivorshipguidelines.org

Index